Biological Additive Manufacturing of Bone Implants

生物增材制造骨植入物

帅词俊　杨友文　彭淑平　杨文静　著

中南大学出版社
www.csupress.com.cn
·长沙·

图书在版编目(CIP)数据

生物增材制造骨植入物／帅词俊等著. —长沙：
中南大学出版社，2020.8
ISBN 978 - 7 - 5487 - 4023 - 0

Ⅰ.①生… Ⅱ.①帅… Ⅲ.①生物材料－应用－骨骼
－移植术(医学)－研究 Ⅳ.①R687.3

中国版本图书馆 CIP 数据核字(2020)第 053189 号

生物增材制造骨植入物
SHENGWU ZENGCAI ZHIZAO GUZHIRUWU

帅词俊　杨友文　彭淑平　杨文静　著

□责任编辑　　刘　辉
□责任印制　　易红卫
□出版发行　　中南大学出版社
　　　　　　　社址：长沙市麓山南路　　　　邮编：410083
　　　　　　　发行科电话：0731 - 88876770　　传真：0731 - 88710482
□印　　装　　长沙雅鑫印务有限公司

□开　　本　　787 mm×1092 mm　1/16　□印张 14.25　□字数 434 千字
□版　　次　　2020 年 8 月第 1 版　□2020 年 8 月第 1 次印刷
□书　　号　　ISBN 978 - 7 - 5487 - 4023 - 0
□定　　价　　68.00 元

内容简介

本书系统介绍了生物增材制造骨植入物的研究现状，针对临床骨修复的要求，从增强力学性能、调控降解速率、赋予抗菌性能和促进成骨性能四个方面详细阐述激光增材制造技术在骨修复方面的研究进展，以期对骨组织的再生修复与功能重建提供理论支撑和科学依据。本书可为增材制造、生物制造、组织工程、再生医学等领域的研究人员提供一定借鉴作用。

Preface

Tissue repair and regencration after tissue damage has been a worldwide problem that human beings have been endlessly pursuing and exploring. With the aging of population, the development of publie service, the demand for artificial bone grafts continues to grow. For this reason, the 13th Five-Year Plan for Biotechnology Innovation emphasizes the acceleration of innovative breakthroughs in advamced technologies such as regenerative medicine and additive manufacturing. The Outline of the National Mid-and Long-term Plan for Science and Technology Development puts emphasis on the development of new biomedical materials such as human tissue and organ substitution. "Made in China 2025" plan emphasizes the development of medical devices such as orthopaedic implants and medical additive manufacturing. "Healthy China 2030" proposes to strengthen the innovation capacity of high-performance medical devices and international competitiveness.

At present, the bone grafts used in clinical includes autogenous bone, allogenic bone and artificial bone. Among them, artificial bonresearch has become an important direction in the development of bone transplantation, because it can avoid the pain and complications of harvesting autogenous bone as well as the immune rejection of allogenic bone. Its basic principle is to firstly make three-dimensional porous scaffolds firstly formed by biodegradable materials. Stem cells are then implanted in the scaffolds to reproduce, grow and induce osteogenesis. As the scaffolds gradually degraded and fully absorbed, the defects of bone repair and functional reconstruction are also realized. In general, the ideal artificial bone should have appropriate degradation rate consistent with the growth of new bone, sufficient mechanical strength providing structural support for the defect site, three-dimensional porous structure for the growth of new bone, and individualized shape to match the artificial bone in the defect site.

Laser additively manufacturing is a new technology based on discrete/stack forming, with new technologies being integrated such as computer, numerical control, laser and new materials. Its basic process is to discretize the three-dimensional model into a series of ordered two-dimensional layers along a certain direction. The forming machine then builds a series of layers through laser cladding, sintering, deposition and so on, and automatically which connected to obtain three-dimensional physical entities. As it applied to fabricate bone implants, laser additively manufacturing is can accurately control the overall outline and internal fine structure, for meeting the individual customization needs of different patients. At the same time, it can easily realize the control of material components during laser forming, so as to obtain bone implants with excellent comprehensive performance.

In the past decades, our team has been devoting to the research of biological additive manufacturing of bone implants. Our thirteen papers were selected from the journal papers published, which described biological additive manufacturing of bone implants on the following four aspects:

1) Improvement of mechanical properties;

2) Regulation of degradation rate;

3) Addition of anti-bacterial function;

4) Promotion of osteogenic ability.

It should be stated that our research is funded by the following funds: (1) The Natural Science Foundation of China (51575537, 81572577, 51705540); (2) Hunan Provincial Natural Science Foundation of China (2016JJ1027); (3) The Project of Innovation-driven Plan of Central South University (2016CX023); (4) National Postdoctoral Program for Innovative Talents (BX201700291); (5) The Project of State Key Laboratory of High Performance Complex Manufacturing, Central South University; (6) The Project of Hunan Provincial Science and Technology Plan (2017RS3008); (7) The China Postdoctoral Science Foundation (2018M632983).

We are also very grateful to every teammate in our research team, because of their great efforts to the research work and the subsequent publication of this book. Finally, it is expected that this book will benefit the teachers, students and medical staff who work in the field of bio-manufacturing.

Contents

Chapter 1

Improvement of Mechanical Properties

Bone implants should have appropriate strength, stiffness and modulus to provide structural support during healing, and maintain a certain time until the new tissue produces its own biomechanical properties. In order to improve the mechanical properties, a series of methods including nanoparticle strengthening, composites design and interface optimization, has been proposed in this chapter.

1.1 Biodegradable Metallic Bone Implants

1.1.1 Introduction

Bone fracture and defect are becoming more and more common with the rapid increase of aging population, traffic accidents, sport injuries, and illness. Although autologous bone and allogeneic bone are considered to be ideal candidates for bone repair, they are restricted by either limited source or immunologic rejection. In view of this, numerous research efforts have been done to develop implants as bone substitutes. A desired bone implant is supposed to uniformly degrade in the human body and be progressively replaced by the growing tissue until the bone repair process is completed. The mechanical properties, such as strength, elastic modulus, or hardness, should be comparable or slightly better than those of natural bone for sufficient load-bearing capacity without looseness or displacement. Moreover, it should be no toxicity or inflammation in the human body, and meanwhile, bone regeneration could be promoted by osteoinduction and osteogenesis.

To date, various kinds of bone implant materials have been developed, including biopolymers, bioceramics, and biomedical metals. Biopolymers are a type of materials with good plasticity and biocompatibility. Nevertheless, low strength, poor hydrophilicity, and aseptic inflammation risk, restrict their applications in bone repair. Bioceramics that combine the excellent activity and biocompatibility, are usually limited by their disadvantage of brittleness. Compared with biopolymers and bioceramics, biomedical metals have integrated mechanical properties, being more suitable for load-bearing applications. Metals used commonly in clinical applications include titanium alloys, stainless steels, and cobalt-chromium alloys, etc. Although these metals can serve as partial functional substitutes for natural bone, they could not degrade and remain as permanent implants. As a result, a second surgery is always needed to remove the implants after bone healing. Repeated surgery inevitably incurs additional costs and pains to patients. So people are looking for biomedical metals that can degrade progressively in the human body and dissolve completely without residue after bone repair.

In this condition, biodegradable metals are proposed for use as bone implants, including Mg and Mg alloys (Mg-based alloys), Fe and Fe alloys (Fe-based alloys), and Zn and Zn alloys (Zn-based alloys). Mg is one of the most abundant cations in the human body and exists primarily in bone, positively affecting the metabolism of enzymes and the structures of RNA and DNA. As one of the group IIA elements, Mg has high chemical activity and easily corrodes to form porous oxidation film on its surface. Afterwards, the oxidation film tends to fall off, especially in solutions containing chlorine ions, accelerating the degradation process. Fe is one of essential trace elements in the human body and plays a major role in oxygen transport and many enzymatic reactions. Moreover, Fe is sensitive to oxidation in humid condition, which is regarded as a degradable property. As another essential element, Zn plays a key role in physiological functions such as bone metabolism, gene expression, and synthesis of various transcriptional factors. In recent years, it is also recognized to be biodegradable and exhibits potential application for bone repair. Considering of a combination of biosafety and biodegradability, the three types of metals are becoming a research focus in the field of bone repair.

This chapter systemically introduces the characteristics of biodegradable metals. And their potentials for bone implants are evaluated in terms of biodegradability, mechanical properties, and biocompatibility. Moreover, attempts are summarized and discussed to regulate the biodegradability and mechanical properties. The future development trends are also prospected for biodegradable metallic bone implants.

1.1.2　Types of Biodegradable Metals

A series of biodegradable metals have been investigated based on Mg, Fe, and Zn. Mg-based alloys, known as revolutionary metals in biomedical applications, are prime targets for studies on biodegradable metallic implants in the past decade. As bone implants, they have inherent advantages owing to the density and elastic modulus similar to those of natural bone, but meanwhile, their applications are severely restricted by high degradation rates and inadequate mechanical properties. Till now, a series of Mg-based alloys have been developed to solve the above deficiencies, including Mg-Al, Mg-Ca, Mg-Zn, Mg-Sr, Mg-RE (rare earth), Mg-Mn, Mg-Cu, Mg-Ag, Mg-Si, etc., Fe is usually mixed with other elements to form alloys for accelerating the biodegradation process, and the alloying elements should be carefully selected for biosafety consideration. So far, Fe-based alloys for bone repair can be classified into binary alloys and ternary alloys including Fe-Mn, Fe-W, Fe-Al, Fe-C, Fe-Ag, Fe-Mn-C, Fe-Mn-Pd, Fe-Mn-Si, etc. Zn, as a new kind of biodegradable metal reporte lately, receives more and more attentions. Commonly used Zn-based alloys in industry usually contain a large quantity of toxic elements, for example, ZA typed Zn alloys contain toxic Al element up to 40% (mass fraction) of inevitability reducing biosafety issues. On account of biosafety of Zn-based alloys for bone repair, current studies mainly concentrate on a few number of newly developed alloys, Zn-Mg, Zn-Ca, Zn-Cu, Zn-Sr, which have shown acceptable biosafety as well as appropriate mechanical properties for use as bone implants.

1.1.3 Biodegradability

It is expected that once biodegradable metals are implanted in the human body, they would gradually degrade at a suitable rate meitehing the recovery rate of bone tissue. Therefore, it is necessary to investigate the degradation mechanisms, degradation behavior, and corresponding regulation methods of biodegradable metals.

1.1.3.1   Degradable Mechanisms

Many degradation phenomena of metals are driven by electrochemical reactions. Therefore, electrochemical principles are used commonly to describe the degradation mechanisms of metallic implants.

1.1.3.1.1   Mg-based Alloys

Mg-based alloys degradation are susceptible to acidic or neutral aqueous solutions via electrochemical reaction. The main degradation products of Mg-based alloys are H_2 and $Mg(OH)_2$. The degradation process principally involves the following reactions:

Anodic reaction $\qquad\qquad\qquad Mg \longrightarrow Mg^{2+} + 2e^-$ $\qquad\qquad\qquad$ (1-1)

Cathodic reaction $\qquad\quad 2H_2O + 2e^- \longrightarrow H_2\uparrow + 2OH^-$ $\qquad\qquad$ (1-2)

Overall reaction $\qquad\quad Mg + 2H_2O \longrightarrow Mg(OH)_2\downarrow + H_2\uparrow$ $\qquad$ (1-3)

At the same time, porous $Mg(OH)_2$ on the surface of Mg-based alloys is easily eroded by solution containing chlorine ions owing to the following reaction:

$$Mg(OH)_2 + 2Cl^- \longrightarrow MgCl_2 + 2OH^- \qquad\qquad (1-4)$$

Thus, the $Mg(OH)_2$ layers can't protect Mg matrix against further corrosion, which greatly accelerates the degradation process. The degradation types of Mg-based alloys strongly depend on the composition and structural states of the alloys. And pitting corrosion is usually undesirable due to the possible stress concentration and significant reduction in the mechanical properties of Mg-based alloys.

1.1.3.1.2   Fe-based Alloys

In comparison with the hydrogen evolution reaction of Mg-based alloys, the degradation of Fe-based alloys are characterized by oxidation absorption corrosion in an aqueous environment. When Fe-based alloys are exposed to solution, Fe will be oxidized to Fe^{2+} based on the following reactions:

Anodic reaction $\qquad\qquad\qquad Fe \longrightarrow Fe^{2+} + 2e^-$ $\qquad\qquad\qquad$ (1-5)

Cathodic reaction $\qquad\quad O_2 + 2H_2O + 2e^- \longrightarrow 4OH^-$ $\qquad\qquad$ (1-6)

Overall reaction $\qquad\quad 2Fe + 2H_2O + O_2 \longrightarrow 2Fe(OH)_2\downarrow$ $\qquad$ (1-7)

Fe^{2+} may be transformed to Fe^{3+} under alkaline and oxygen environment, and new products form as follows:

$$Fe^{2+} \longrightarrow Fe^{3+} + e^- \tag{1-8}$$

$$Fe^{3+} + 3OH^- \longrightarrow Fe(OH)_3 \downarrow \tag{1-9}$$

$$Fe(OH)_2 + 2FeO(OH) \longrightarrow Fe_3O_4 \downarrow + 2H_2O \tag{1-10}$$

At the early stage, Fe-based alloys degrade gradually according to the reactions (1-5) – (1-10), and the degradation products mainly consist of $Fe(OH)_2$, $Fe(OH)_3$, and Fe_3O_4, etc. These degradation products are compact and have a good protective effect on Fe matrix. As a result, further degradation is retarded, leading to a slow degradation rate for bone repair. Compared with Mg-based alloys, no gas is produced during the degradation process of Fe-based alloys. Meanwhile, Fe always undergoes a uniform degradation process so that Fe-based alloys might show local corrosion owing to inhomogeneous chemical composition, non-uniform stress distribution etc.

1.1.3.1.3　Zn-based Alloys

Similarly, Zn-based alloys undergo a chemical anode reaction when exposed in solution, and the cathodic reaction occurs with reduction of oxygen:

Anodic reaction $\qquad Zn \longrightarrow Zn^{2+} + 2e^- \tag{1-11}$

Cathodic reaction $\qquad 2H_2O + O_2 + 4e^- \longrightarrow 4OH^- \tag{1-12}$

Overall reaction $\qquad 2Zn + 2H_2O + O_2 \longrightarrow 2Zn(OH)_2 \downarrow \tag{1-13}$

As a result, insoluble $Zn(OH)_2$ is formed on the surface as a intermediate layer. However, the $Zn(OH)_2$ will be converted into soluble salt due to the presence of chlorine ions, according to the following reaction:

$$6Zn(OH)_2 \downarrow + Zn^{2+} + 2Cl^- \longrightarrow 6Zn(OH)_2 \cdot ZnCl_2 \tag{1-14}$$

This reaction reduces the area protected by $Zn(OH)_2$ layer and fresh Zn matrix is exposed to solution again, causing a new cycle of electrochemical reactions. Similar to Mg-based alloys, the degradation types of Zn-based alloys also depend on their composition and structure.

To conclude, these three kinds of alloys generally degrade in terms of electrochemical corrosion, as shown in Fig. 1-1. In the solution, biodegradable metals release electrons and are oxidized to metal ions (M^{n+}) according to the anodic reactions. The electrons participate subsequently in the cathodic reactions (i. e., water reduction of Mg-based alloys, oxygen reductions of both Fe-based and Zn-based alloys), resulting in local alkalization. The organic molecules in the solution may be absorbed on the metal surface, affecting the anodic reactions, as illustrated in Fig. 1-1(a). Subsequently, degradation layers of $M(OH)_n$ form on the metal surface, accompanying with the continuous invasion of media and M^{n+} release, as illustrated in Fig. 1-1(b). It is worth noting that the degradation layers of $M(OH)_n$ could be eroded by chloride ions [Fig. 1-1(c)], especially for Mg-based alloys. At the same time, the Ca^{2+} and PO_4^{3-} in the solution can induce apatite formation on the degradation layers because of the local alkalization, which is beneficial for cell adhesion. With the prolongation of time, the cells gradually proliferate and new tissues will be formed at the metal surface. As the degradation proceeds, more degradation products form on the surface and the metal matrix continues to dissolve, which may lead to the partial fall-off of matrix, as illustrated in Fig. 1-1(d). As a result, fresh matrix is exposed to the media and undergoes a new

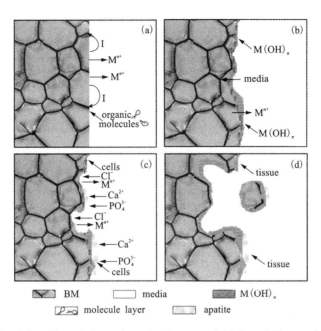

Fig. 1-1　Degradation schematic diagram of biodegradable metals.
Reproduced with permission from ref. [2]7. Copyright 2014 Elsevier.

round of degradation.

1.1.3.2　Degradation Behavior

1.1.3.2.1　In Vitro Degradation

In vitro degradation tests including electrochemical tests and immersion tests, are usually carried out as effective evaluation methods for the degradation behavior of metallic implants on the strength of convenience and short term consuming. And a suitable medium should be selected to precisely simulate the degradation behavior in human physiological environment. So far, the degradation tests of metallic implants are generally done in 0.9% NaCl solution, Hank's solution, simulated body fluid (SBF) solution, or phosphate buffered saline (PBS) solution.

In electrochemical tests, transient current response is collected digitally, and inherent corrosion properties, can be obtained including corrosion potential, corrosion current density, impedance, etc. ,. Afterwards, the corrosion potential and current density are used to calculate the degradation rates according to the following equation:

$$R = K \frac{J_{corr}}{\rho} m_e \qquad (1\text{-}15)$$

In which, R, K, J_{corr}, ρ and m_e represent the corrosion rate (mm/a), a constant, the corrosion current density ($\mu A/cm^2$), the density (g/cm^3), and the equivalent weight (g), respectively.

In comparison, immersion tests can simulate relatively long-lasting degradation behavior of metallic implants. In this method, the degradation rates of biodegradable metals are determined by mass loss based on the following equation:

$$R = K\frac{W}{AT} \tag{1-16}$$

Where, R, A, T, K, and W represent the degradation rate $[g/(m \cdot h)^{-1}]$, surface area (cm^2), immersion time (h), a constant, and mass loss (g), respectively.

The mass loss can be determined by means of H_2 formation, direct weighing, or ion concentration. For Mg-based alloys, released H_2 during immersion is collected to estimate the mass loss according to equation (1-3). Specifically, one mol H_2 is generated by the degradation of one mol of Mg, which corresponds to 24 loss of Mg. This method can easily acquire numerous and detailed degradation data by real-time observing the volume of H_2 formation. Another method to determine mass loss is weighing the mass change before and after immersion directly. To obtain the accurate mass data after immersion, the degradation products need to be removed primarily with chromic acid and distilled water. This method has been extensively applied to Mg-based alloys, Fe-based alloys, and Zn-based alloys. The mass loss can also be obtained by ion concentration. Specifically, the samples are removed from the immersion solution, and the degradation products are separated. Afterwards, the degradation products and an appropriate amount of acid (nitric acid) are added together into the immersion solution. The concentrations of ions, such as Zn^{2+}, Mg^{2+}, Fe^{2+}, and Fe^{3+}, etc., are analyzed by using inductively coupled plasma atomic emission spectrometer, and then used to determine mass loss based on the following equation:

$$W = CV \tag{1-17}$$

Where, W, C, and V represent the mass loss (g), ion concentration (g/L), and volume of solution (L), respectively. It should be noted that the mass loss and consequent degradation rates obtained by directly weighing and ion concentration are closely related to the disposal of degradation products, which is susceptible to the cleaning, washing, and weighing process.

The degradation rates of metallic implants should be maintained within a reasonable range in order to ensure their functions during the service period. Too slow degradation will hinder the growth of new bone while too fast degradation cannot provide structural support in the defect site. The size and shape of the implant depend on that of the defect bone, resulting in different repair period. For bone repair, it has been reported that the degradation rates of bone implants should be lower than 0.5 mm/a and higher than 0.2 mm/a to match the bone healing. The degradation rates of typical metallic implants are summarized in Fig. 1-2. It can be seen that Mg-based alloys exhibit the highest degradation rates, approximately ranging from 0.8 to 2.7 mm/a, which is above the tolerable degradation rates of bone implants. The degradation rates of Zn-based alloys are mainly between 0.1 and 0.3 mm/a, appearing as prospective alternates. In contrast, the slowest degradation rates, less than 0.1 mm/a, are observed for Fe-based alloys. Hence, the degradation rates of these alloys, especially Mg-based alloys and Fe-based alloys, need to be regulated to meet the clinical requirements of bone implants.

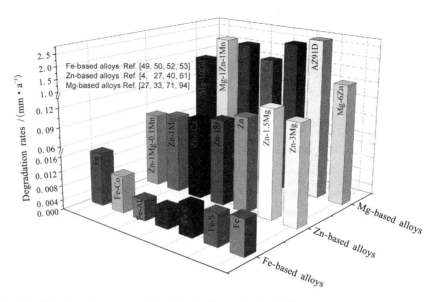

Fig. 1-2   The degradation rates of Mg-based alloys, Fe-based alloys, and Zn-based alloys.

1.1.3.2.2   In Vivo Degradation

In vivo animal studies are imperative to assess the degradability, safety, and feasibility of metallic bone implants prior to clinical applications. At present, most in vivo animal studies focused on Mg-based alloys while only a few studies on Fe-based alloys and Zn-based alloys.

Biodegradable Mg was first employed as internal fixation plate to fix bone fracture in 1907. This attempt failed because the Mg plate degraded too fast and generated a lot of hydrogen in vivo. Subsequently, Troitskii and Znamenski used Mg alloys as bone repair materials to treat bone fracture, which did not achieve satisfactory results because of subcutaneous bubbles and severe loss of mechanical strength caused by rapid degradation. These studies have shown that Mg-based alloys degraded too fast to reach an effective repair of damaged bones, which restricted their applications in bone repair.

In recent years, the corrosion resistance of Mg-based alloys has been significantly improved by smelting and surface treatment technology. Accordingly, Mg-based alloys have again aroused worldwide attentions. The in vivo degradation behaviors of WE43 Mg alloy implants were also studied by Torroni et al. in sheep cranial bones. They found that Lymph-node Mg accumulation showed no differences between studied sheep and the control (no implants) groups after implantation for 6 weeks, indicating good biocompatibility. Moreover, there was no hydrogen bubble in the degradation process and new bones surrounding the implants were found, suggesting osteogenesis promoting properties. They further investigated their histo-morphologic characteristics of artificially aged WE43 Mg alloys on the calvarial bone of sheep. Histomorphological analysis of the bone-implant after 6 weeks showed greater interface stability between the bone and WE43 Mg alloy implants, indicating that WE43 Mg alloy seemed to be suitable for use as biodegradable bone implants. Witte et al. studied the degradation behaviors of LAE442 Mg alloy in the medial femur condyle of rabbits. They did not find subcutaneous gas cavities at 2, 4, 6 and 12 weeks postoperatively. Meanwhile, the LAE442 Mg alloy implants were observed in direct bone contact and there was no a fibrous capsule, which had an acceptable host response. Duygulu et al. studied the in vivo degradation of AZ31 Mg alloy as bone implants. They implanted AZ31 Mg alloy into sheep hip bone. Three months later, it was found that the degradation of AZ31 Mg alloy could guide osteoblast growth at the implant site. Mg alloy rods (AZ31, AZ91, WE43, and LAE442) were implanted into the femora of guinea pigs with a size of 1.5 mm in diameter and 20.0 mm in length to investigate the mechanical properties of bone-implant interaction after degradation, and degradable self-reinforced poly-96L/4D-lactide rods were also implanted as a control. Fluoroscopic images of the bone-implant [Fig. 1-3(a1)] indicated that the Mg alloy rods degraded non-uniformly compared to the polymer rods. What's more, the mineral apposition rate around the Mg alloy rods, especially for WE43 Mg alloy, was higher than that around the polymer rods [Fig. 1-3 (a2)]. In vivo mechanical properties and implant-bone interface strength of AZ31 Mg alloy after degradation were also studied by Tan et al. They implanted AZ31 Mg alloy with Si-containing coating, AZ31 Mg alloy, and poly-L-lactide (PLLA) respectively into rabbit femurs, and then assessed the interfacial strength after degradation by extraction torque [Fig. 1-3 (b1)]. It could be observed that the extraction torque of as-coated AZ31 Mg alloy at 21st week was much higher than those of AZ31 Mg alloy and PLLA [Fig. 1-3(b2)], indicating a stronger osteosynthesis activity during the degradation process. This was attributed to the moderate degradation rate of coated AZ31 Mg alloy. Moreover, one-point bending test [Fig. 1-3(c1)] showed that the PLLA implant broke down at 4th week owing to bulk degradation and the AZ31 implants lost 26.4% of their original bending strength at 4th week, 35.8% at 12th week, and 42.4% at 21st week [Fig. 1-3(c2)], respectively, due to fast degradation. In contrast, the coated AZ31 implants showed significantly higher mechanical stability with a loss of 13.4% at 4th week, 17.1% at 12th week, and 29.9% at 21st week, respectively, due to the improved degradation resistance, which facilitated the osteosynthesis process as evidenced by a higher Ca/P atomic ratio than other implants [Fig. 1-3(d1) and Fig. 1-3(d2)].

Fe-based implants have also attracted close attention for bone repair. Fe, Fe-5% TCP (Fe-TCP), Fe-5% hydroxyapatite (Fe-HA), Fe-5% (40% TCP : 60% HA) (Fe-BCP)implants were prepared respectively by powder metallurgy and implanted into sheep femurs [Fig. 1-4(a)]. It was observed that black degradation products were formed on the Fe-based implants, as denoted by white arrows. Surface appearance and roughness of these implants at day 70 in Fig. 1-4(b) showed that Fe-HA, Fe-TCP, Fe-BCP had rougher surfaces than those of Fe, indicating higher degradation rates after the incorporation of bioceramics. Meanwhile, the degradation layers of Fe-HA, Fe-TCP, and Fe-BCP were thicker than that of Fe [Fig. 1-4(c)], also indicating that faster degradation rates occurred on the former, especially for Fe-BCP. A Fe-Mn-Si alloy with 25.3 mm in length, 2.45 mm in width, and 0.45 mm in thickness, was implanted in a rabbit bone for 30 days. It was found that the implant weight reduced from the initial 0.2284 g to 0.2277 g due to degradation. The SEM images of the implant in Fig. 1-5(a) and Fig. 1-5(b) presented a corroded surface with types of

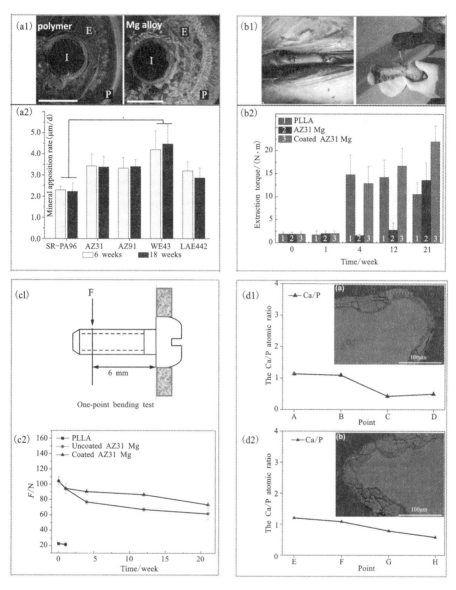

Fig. 1-3　Implantation trails of Mg-based alloys. （a1）Fluoroscopic images of Mg alloy rods at week 18 （I, E, and P representing implant residual, endosteal bone formation, and periosteal bone formation, respectively. ）, and （a2）mineralized area of AZ31, AZ91, WE43, and LAE442 Mg alloy rods at week 6 and week 18 post-implantation in guinea pig, and a polymer rod served as control. （b1）Representative digital images of AZ31 Mg alloy and coated AZ31 Mg alloy implanted in rabbit femurs, and subsequent extraction torque test, （b2）extraction torque of AZ31 Mg and coated AZ31 Mg alloy implants at week 0, 1, 4, 12, and 21, respectively, and PLLA implants served as control; （c1）Schematic diagram of one-point bending test, and （c2）bending strength of AZ31 Mg, coated AZ31 Mg at week 0, 1, 4, 12, and 21 post-implantation in rabbit femurs, respectively, and PLLA served as control; Cross-section morphology and element composition of the implant-bone interface after implantation of （d1）AZ31 Mg alloy and （d2）coated AZ31 Mg alloy in rabbit femurs at week 21. Reproduced with permission from ref. ［34, 117］. Copyright 2005 2014 Elsevier.

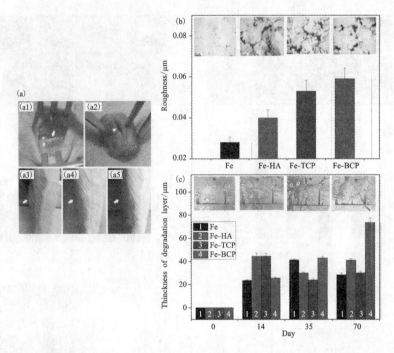

Fig. 1-4　Implantation trails of Fe-based alloys. (a) Implantation in sheep leg bones： (a1) implantation insertion showing bone (＊), periosteum (#), and implant (arrow), (a2) implant extraction (arrow head); (a3), (a4), and (a5) swelling observation (arrow) after 9, 14, and 35 days, respectively; (b) Surface morphology and corresponding roughness of Fe, Fe-HA, Fe-TCP, and Fe-BCP implants after 70 days; (c) Surface morphology, element composition, and degradation layer thickness after 0, 14, 35, and 70 days, respectively. Reproduced with permission from ref. [118]. Copyright 2014 John wiley and Sons.

compounds. On the implant surfaces before and after sonication cleaning, the element distributions of Fe, Mn, and Si elements, etc. , were shown in Fig. 1-5 (c) and Fig. 1-5 (d), where a large number of oxides were observed after degradation. Moreover, the element content of Mn was lower than that of Si, indicating that degradation of Mn compounds were more than Si compounds in the Fe-based alloy.

　　Zn-based alloys have been considered as promising biodegradable bone implants in recent years. In 2011, Zn-based alloys were first proposed by Vojtech et al. for potential bone repair owing to the satisfactory biodegradability. Afterwards, Zn-1Sr, Zn-1Ca, Zn-1Mg alloys were implanted into mouse femurs by Li et al. Cross-section histology at 8th week showed that the periosteum and cortical bone around Zn-1Sr, Zn-1Ca, Zn-1Mg implants, especially Zn-1Sr implant, were more than that of sham control group [Fig. 1-6(a), green fluorescence represented new bone]. In addition, micro-CT images of Zn-1Sr, Zn-1Ca, Zn-1Mg implants at 8th week showed higher bone volume [Fig. 1-6(b)]. Moreover, the degradation in vivo rates of Zn-1Sr, Zn-1Ca, and Zn-1Mg implants were 0. 22, 0. 19, and 0. 17 mm/a, respectively, similar to bone healing rate. Another study implanted Zn and Zn-0. 05Mg (mass fraction) alloys into rabbit femurs to investigate their

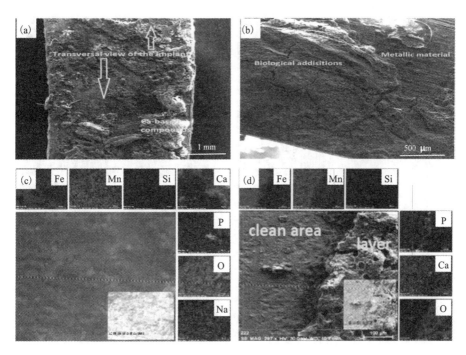

Fig. 1-5   SEM images and EDS analysis showing themicrographs and distributions of Fe, Mn, and Si elements, etc., on the surface of Fe-Mn-Si alloy after implantation in rabbit for 30 days: (a) the implant surface at macro scale, (b) the implant surface at micro scale, (c) before sonication cleaning, and (d) after sonication cleaning. Reproduced with permission from ref. [119]. Copyright 2017 IOP org.

degradability. The histology of implant-bone interface at 12th week and 24th weeks was shown in Fig. 1-6(c), (implant with white arrow, cortical bone with blue arrow). At 12th week, new bone formed (red arrow) around the implants and at week 24 bone trabecula (with green arrow) formed as a junction between the new bone and cortical bone. It was also found that a lot of Ca element (red area) enriched near the bone-implant interface, indicating that both the degradation of Zn and Zn-0.05Mg alloys could induce new bone formation.

Taking into account the influence of oxygen, cells, proteins, phosphates, amino acids, and other molecules, the degradation in vivo behavior of biodegradable metallic bone implants are complex and thus still need subsequent interest.

1.1.3.3   Regulation of Degradation Behavior

Ideal bone implants ought to have appropriate degradation rates to match the restoration process of new bone after implantation. Thus, many studies have been carried out in recent years to regulate the degradation rates of biodegradable metals.

1.1.3.3.1   Mg-based Alloys

The degradation of Mg-based alloys can be slowed down by various methods, including alloying, heat treatment, and surface treatment, etc. Alloying (RE, Al, Zn, Mn, Ca, Si, Sr, Zr, etc.) can control the phase distribution, grain size and microstructure of Mg-based alloys,

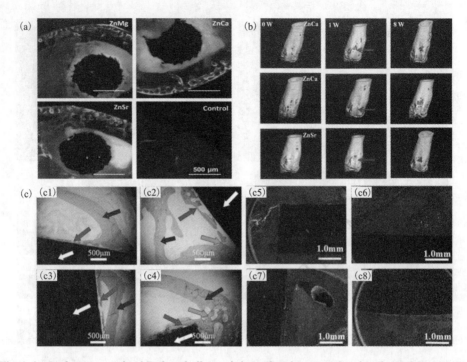

Fig. 1-6 Implantation trails of Zn-based alloys. (a) Implant-bone interface histology of Zn-Mg, Zn-Ca, Zn-Sr alloys at week 8, and the sham served as control; (b) Micro-CT 3D images of Zn-Mg, Zn-Ca, and Zn-Sr implants at week 0, 1, and 8. (c) Implant-bone interface histology of (c1) Zn at week 12, (c2) Zn at week 24, (c3) Zn-0.05Mg alloy at week 12, and (c4) Zn-0.05Mg alloy at week 24 (implant with white arrow, cortical bone with blue arrow, new bone with red arrow, and bone trabecula with green arrow), respectively; Element distributions at implant-bone interface of (c5) Zn at week 12, (c6) Zn at week 24, (c7) Zn-0.05Mg alloy at week 12, and (c8) Zn-0.05Mg alloy at week 24 (Ca element with red area, C element with green area, and Zn element with blue area), respectively. Reproduced with permission from ref. 63. Copyright 2015 Nature publishing group; Reproduced with permission from ref. [120]. Copyright 2018 Elsevier.

fundamentally improving the corrosion resistance. When 1% RE was added into AZ91 Mg alloy, the second phase $Mg_{17}Al_{12}$ along grain boundaries evolved from discontinuous reticulation to diffuse skeletal distribution, thereby increasing the corrosion resistance of AZ91 Mg alloy. Wang et al. reported that the degradation rate of AZ91 Mg alloy with RE elements was obviously decreased. The reason was that the addition of RE reduced the amount of second phase in the Mg alloy by forming new phase, thereby decreasing the amount of cathode of galvanic corrosion. Moreover, RE can reduce the negative effect of cathodic impurities and increase the protective function of the surface layer of corrosion products, further enhancing the corrosion resistance of Mg alloys. As for heat treatment, the second phase can be dissolved or uniformly distributed in matrix, which not only reduces the adverse impact of galvanic corrosion between second phase and Mg matrix, but also contributes to uniform corrosion by mitigating pitting corrosion. Liu et al. observed that $Mg_{17}A_{12}$ phase distributed uniformly in as-cast AZ63 alloy after solution treatment and aging. As a result, relative uniform corrosion with a half reduced corrosion rate was achieved compared with the untreated alloy. Kuwahara et al. studied the effect of heat treatment on the corrosion resistance of Mg. Mg with a purity of 99.9% was annealed at 803 K for 9 – 25 h and then immersed in Hank's solution. Whereafter, it was found that corrosion resistance of Mg increased because of the homogenized microstructure after annealing.

Surface treatment mainly refers to the use of physical or chemical methods to generate a surface film or a passivation layer on Mg matrix, which improves the corrosion resistance of Mg-based alloys at the initial stage of implantation. The wide methods include micro-arc oxidation, alkali heat treatment, electrochemical treatment, phosphate layers, and fluoridation treatment, etc. Zhang et al. coated a ceramic layer on AZ91 Mg alloy through microarc oxidation. And the corrosion potential of AZ91 Mg alloy rose from -1.5786 V to -0.43019 V after the treatment. Immersion tests in Hank's solution showed that the average weight loss rate of treated AZ91 Mg alloy was 15 times lower than that of the untreated, which indicated the significant effect of microarc oxidation in improving corrosion resistance. To investigate the effect of alkaline heat treatment on corrosion resistance, Mg-Ca alloys were immersed in three different alkaline solutions ($NaHCO_3$, Na_2CO_3, and Na_2HPO_4) for 24 h, and then treated at 773 K for 12 h. It was found that MgO layers with thickness of approximately 26, 9, and 13 μm, respectively, were formed on the surface of alloys after the treatment. In vitro degradation tests verified that the corrosion resistance of Mg-Ca alloys was effectively improved as a result of these MgO layers, with the sequence: Na_2CO_3 heated > Na_2HPO_4 heated > $NaHCO_3$ heated. Wang et al. investigated Mg-Zn-Ca alloy coated with HA by pulse electrodeposition. They discovered that the current density of the alloy decreased from 110 to 25 μA/cm^2 and the potential increased from -1645 to -1414 mV, indicating corrosion resistance of the Mg alloy improved by HA coating. Hiromoto et al. investigated Mg alloy coated with octacalcium phosphate by chemical solution deposition. They found that the degradation rate was restricted by approximately one-half with suppressed Mg-ion release. And a nearly uniform corrosion occurred. Xu et al. coated Mg alloy with a calcium phosphate (Ca-P) layer through a phosphating process. The Ca-P layer on the alloy surface was composed of netlike $CaHPO_4 \cdot 2H_2O$, which reduced the corrosion of Mg alloy. Fluoridation coating, mainly composed of MgF_2 and MgO, was prepared on Mg alloy by Yan et al. using hydrofluoric acid. And electrochemical impedance spectroscopy tests demonstrated significantly increased corrosion resistance of Mg alloy. Corrosion inhibition of Mg alloys by fluoride treatments were also confirmed by Pereda et al. They found that the protective characteristics of MgF_2 layer ensured the gradual degradation process of Mg alloys. Moreover, the influences of MgF_2 layer on the corrosion rate of LAE442 Mg alloy were studied in vivo. The results showed that the MgF_2 layer could effectively reduce the degradation rate during the first 6 weeks of implantation without subcutaneous bubbles and elevated fluoride content in the adjacent bone. Besides, purification to reduce galvanic corrosion between Mg matrix and impurity, and deformation treatment to induce microstructure evolution, etc., are also effective ways to decelerate the degradation process of Mg-based alloys. To conclude, the strategies, techniques, and corresponding mechanisms for regulating the degradation rates of Mg-based alloys are summarized in Fig. 1-7.

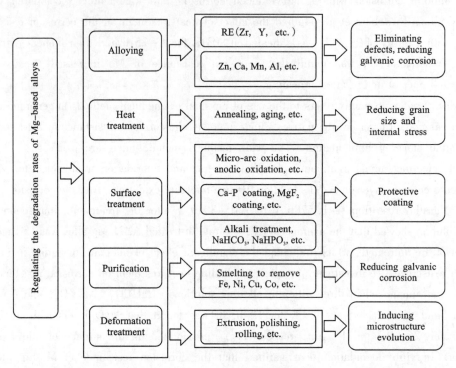

Fig. 1-7　Strategies, techniques, and corresponding mechanisms for regulating the degradation rates of Mg-based alloys.

1.1.3.3.2　Fe-based Alloys

So far, many methods have been proposed to accelerate degradation of Fe-based alloys: 1) alloying active elements to Fe matrix to reduce the standard electrode potential of Fe matrix, making the matrix easier to corrode; 2) adding noble metal elements into Fe matrix to form dispersed intermetallic phases as cathodes for galvanic corrosion. The first method has been tried by Liu et al. through alloying Mn, Co, W, B, C, and S elements. It was found that W, C, and S could accelerate the degradation rate of Fe while Mn, Al, and B slightly decreased. However, another study by Capek et al. reported an enhanced degradation rate of Fe after alloying Mn. Therefore, more studies are needed to reveal the effect of alloying Mn on the degradation of Fe-based alloys. Cheng et al. fabricated Fe-W alloy, in which W acted as cathodes and Fe matrix acted as anodes to generate galvanic corrosion. Results indicated that the current density increased after alloying W, thereby improving the degradation rate of Fe. Fe-Zn powders containing 15% (mass fraction) Zn were prepared by Wang et al. and then sintered into alloys by spark plasma sintering. Tests showed that Fe-15Zn alloy [at a rate of 0.73 mg/(cm^2 · d)] degraded much faster than Fe [at a rate of 0.35 mg/(cm^2 · d)] in SBF. Schinhammer et al. fabricated Fe-Mn-Pd alloys by casting. The results showed that Fe-Pd and Mn-Pd intermetallic compounds were formed and dispersed in the alloys, which were responsible for the fast degradation of Fe-Mn-Pd alloys. Ag was chosen by Huang et al. as the second phase isolated to Fe matrix. It was found that Fe-Ag alloy corroded much faster than Fe, attributing to the galvanic corrosion with Ag as cathodes and Fe as anodes. This galvanic corrosion mechanism was also reported in Fe-Au alloys. Apart from the aforementioned methods, many preparation methods, such as spark sintering, electroforming etc., were also proposed to promote galvanic corrosion via grain refinement, thereby improving the degradation rates of Fe-based alloys.

1.1.3.3.3   Zn-based Alloys

Compared to Mg-based and Fe-based alloys, Zn-based alloys degrade at more moderate rates, close to that of bone healing. Therefore, only a few studies have been reported on the regulation of the degradation behavior of Zn-based alloys. Mg, Ca and Sr were chosen as the alloying elements to accelerate the degradation of Zn by Li et al. They found that the corrosion potentials of Zn-Mg, Zn-Ca and Zn-Sr alloys were -0.999, -1.019, and -1.131 V, respectively, lower than that of Zn (-0.988 V). Mass loss by immersion tests showed that Zn-Mg, Zn-Ca and Zn-Sr alloys degraded significantly faster than Zn. Gong et al. found that as-cast Zn-1Mg alloy was less corrosion-resistant compared with extruded Zn-1Mg in SBF, leading to a much higher degradation rate of as-cast Zn-1Mg alloy (0.28 mm/a) than that of extruded Zn-1Mg (0.12 mm/a) owing to non-uniform microstructure. Vojtech et al. pointed out that the degradation rate of Zn-Mg alloys was tens of microns per year at different pH values, significantly lower than those of Mg and AZ91 Mg alloy because Zn was much inerter in nature than Mg. In general, Zn-based alloys have shown proper degradation rate for bone repair in comparison with Mg-based alloys and Fe-based alloys, but more studies are still needed to precisely regulate their degradation behavior for different requirements.

1.1.4   Mechanical Properties

As bone implants, mechanical support are required for efficient load-bearing. It is proposed that yield strength (YS), ultimate tensile strength (UTS), and elongation rate (E), etc. are the major indicators for mechanical properties. To satisfy these requirements, a lot of studies have been carried out on the mechanical properties of Mg-based, Fe-based, and Zn-based alloys.

1.1.4.1   Mg-based Alloys

"Young" modulus of Mg-based alloys (35 – 45 GPa) is close to that of natural bone (3 – 20 GPa), which prevents stress shielding effect. Additionally, Mg-based alloys are also known for high specific strength and high specific stiffness. However, Mg-based alloys generally possess hexagonal close packed (HCP) structure with only a small amount of slip planes, which results in relatively low ductility for bone implant applications. For example, the E of Mg is less than 6%. Besides, the UTS of Mg is poor, about 50 MPa. Thus, various methods, such as grain refinement, deformation, and heat treatment, etc., have been proposed to improve the mechanical properties.

Grain refinement can enhance the mechanical properties of Mg-based alloys mainly through the blockage of dislocation motion and the dispersion of internal stress. Grain refinement are commonly achieved by adding refiner such as RE (Ce, Y, etc.), Ca, Zr, Sr, and Zn, etc. It was found that the second phase in AZ91D Mg alloy transformed from a thick mesh into a fine granular shape after adding 0.6% Ce and 0.3% Y (mass fraction), which improved the UTS of the alloy from 124 MPa to 213 MPa. Brar et al. also confirmed that the grain size of matrix became small with the addition of Sr, improving the mechanical properties of Mg. Besides, deformation (extrusion, forging, rolling, etc.) and heat treatment (solid solution, annealing, and aging, etc.) are important ways to regulate the microstructure and reduce the internal stress within Mg-based alloys. The mechanical properties of extruded EW75M Mg alloy were studied under different extrusion conditions. At an extrusion temperature of 400℃, a extrusion speed of 12 m/min, and an extrusion ratio of 20, the UTS, YS, and E of the alloy reached up to 335 MPa, 240 MPa, and 16.5%, respectively, owing to the refined microstructure. Zhang et al. investigated the effects of hot extrusion and aging on the mechanical properties of Mg-3Nd-0.2Zn-0.4Zr alloy. The alloy was first extruded with a extrusion ratio of 25 to induce grain recrystallization, and then aged at 200℃ for 10 h to reduce the residual stress generated in extrusion process, during which grain refinement and second phase precipitation occurred. As a result, the YS, UTS, and E of the alloy were improved to 137 MPa, 236 MPa, and 17%, respectively.

1.1.4.2 Fe-based Alloys

Fe-based alloys have better mechanical properties, such as strength and plasticity, than Mg-based and Zn-based alloys, basically meeting the requirements for use as bone implants. Studies on the mechanical properties are inferior to the degradation rates of Fe-based alloys. Several methods, including new preparation technologies, heat treatment, and alloying, etc., have been exerted on Fe-based alloys for the purpose objective of mechanical properties. Moravej et al. reported that a grain size of 4 μm in electroformed Fe resulted in high YS (360 MPa) and UTS (423 MPa). After annealing at 550℃, its ductility was improved by 18% because of recrystallization and stress relief. Fe and Mn powders were sintered and rolled to fabricate Fe-Mn alloys by Capek et al. Results showed that the YS (235 MPa) of the fabricated alloys was higher than that of as-casted Fe-Mn alloys, and the UTS was comparable to that of SS316L. Meanwhile, the maximum E reached to 31%, about 60% of that of as-casted Fe-Mn alloys (50%). Fe-Mn alloys (0, 0.5%, 2.7%, 6.9% Mn, mass fraction) with 250 mm in height and 60 mm in diameter were prepared by sand casting, and then forged at 1050℃. All of the alloys exhibited good mechanical properties compared to Mg-based alloys, for example, Fe-2.5Mn alloy had UTS of 495 MPa, YS of 295 MPa, and E of 28%, respectively. Besides, the mechanical properties of Fe-Mn alloys with other Mn contents, including Fe20Mn, Fe25Mn, Fe35Mn, etc., are also systematically evaluated, which further confirmed the positive effect of alloying Mn on the mechanical properties of Fe-based alloys.

1.1.4.3 Zn-based Alloys

As for Zn-based alloys, the low strength and poor plasticity significantly restrict their applications as bone implants. It is known that Zn has a HCP crystal structure, which brings about brittleness. Zn is also soft with low mechanical strength, for instance, the tensile strength of as-cast Zn is only about 30 MPa. Furthermore, Zn-based alloys would undergo a recrystallization process under stress, resulting in low resistance to creep. Therefore, the mechanical properties of Zn-based alloys have been a focus in the study for use as bone implants.

Similar to Mg-based alloys, alloying, deformation, and heat treatment, are also the common methods to improve the mechanical properties of Zn-based alloys. Given to the high solubility of Mg in Zn, Kubasek et al. prepared Zn-Mg alloys with various Mg contents (0. 5% ~ 3% , mass fraction) through hot extrusion. It was found that the Zn-Mg alloys consisted of fine grains of 12 μm. The strength and hardness were improved with increasing Mg content, from 120 MPa and 44 HV for Zn to 380 MPa and 97 HV for Zn-1.6Mg alloy, however, Zn-1.6Mg alloy showed no plasticity owing to excess brittle Mg_2Zn_{11} phase. In comparison, Zn-0. 8Mg alloy exhibited a good combination of strength and plasticity (YS of 203 MPa, UTS of 301 MPa, and E of 15% , respectively) due to the absence of brittle Mg_2Zn_{11} phase. Effects of alloying and deformation on the mechanical properties of as-cast Zn-Mg alloys were studied by Liu et al. Compared to Zn, the YS and UTS were improved to 114 MPa and 131 MPa, respectively, owing to the increased volume fraction of eutectic mixture. Moreover, the coarse dendrites primary grains were mostly transformed into strip grains after hot rolling. Consequently, the YS, UTS, and E of Zn-Mg alloy were further enhanced to 195 MPa, 299 MPa, and 26% , respectively. Alloying Ag was also found to obviously reduce the grain size of Zn matrix and the relationship between the grain size and Ag content shown in Fig. 1-8(a). It is well established that grain refinement can enhance the mechanical properties of Zn-based alloys. Jasinska et al. prepared Zn-xAg (x from 2. 5% to 7. 0% , mass fraction) alloys to investigate the relationship between mechanical properties and Ag contents [Fig. 1-8(b)]. The YS and UTS showed an upward trend with the increase of Ag contents. Due to the grain refinement of Zn matrix and the increased volume fraction of $AgZn_3$ second phase, a maximum YS (236 MPa) and UTS (367 MPa) for Zn-7Ag alloy were achieved. Nevertheless, the addition of Ag to Zn also brought about a reduction in elongation, from 60% for Zn down to 32% ~ 36% for Zn-xAg alloys. In spite of the above efforts, it remains a challenge to improve the mechanical properties of Zn-based alloys for application in bone implants.

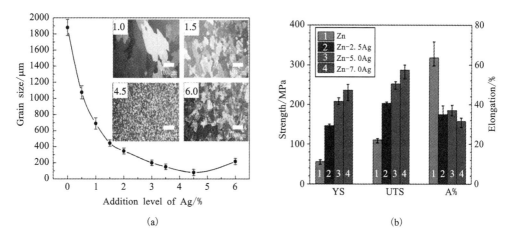

(a)   (b)

Fig. 1-8   Effect of alloying Ag on the microstructure and mechanical properties of Zn-based alloys. (a) Microstructural involution and grain size of Zn matrix with Ag content increasing. (b) Mechanical properties of Zn-Ag alloys with different Ag contents. Reproduced with permission from ref. [169]. Copyright 2014 Elsevier.

In general, the mechanical properties of biodegradable alloys have been improved by novel preparation methods (rapidly solidified, electroforming etc., alloying, processing deformation (extrusion, rolling, and forging, etc.), and heat treatment (solution treated, annealing, and aging, etc.), etc.), to meet the requirements of bone implants. The representative enhancing strategies and resulting mechanical properties of biodegradable metals are summarized in Tab. 1-1.

Tab. 1-1 Representative enhancing strategies and resulting mechanical properties of biodegradable metals

Compositions /%	Preparation methods	Post treatments	YS /MPa	UTS /MPa	E /%	References
Mg-3Al	Casting	Solid solution treatment	150	255	3	54
Mg-2Ca	Rapid solidification	—	—	380	7.3	35
Mg-Zn-0.8Sr	Zone solidification	Heat treatment	117	210	12	37
LAE442	Casting	—	148	247	18	173
AZ31	Casting	—	—	260	15	35
Mg-2Sr	Casting	Hot rolling	147	213.3	—	41
Mg-6Zn	Casting	Heat treatment & extrusion	280	170	19	39
Mg-Y-RE-Zr	Powder metallurgy	—	250	275	10	44
Mg-5.0Y-7.0Gd-1.3Nd-0.5Zr	Casting	Extrusion	162	234	26	164
Mg-Y	Casting	—	156	257	14	41
Mg-5.0Y-7.0Gd-1.3Nd-0.5Zr	Casting	Extrusion & aging	189	243	21	164
Mg-3Sn-0.5Mn	Casting	Extrusion	150	240	13	29
ZW21	Casting	Squeezing	200	270	17	161
WE43	Casting	Heat treatment	170	220	44	64
WE43	Casting	Extrusion & heat treatment	195	280	10	20
Mg-1Zn	Casting	—	89	187	11	37
Mg-Zn-Mn	Zone solidification	Extrusion	246	280	22	29
Mg-Y-Zn	Casting	Extrusion	—	250~270	17~20	174
Mg-Zn-1Sr	Zone solidification	Heat treatment	130	249	13	37
AZ31	Casting	—	110~180	255~290	15~21	4
WE43A	Casting	Heat treatment	162	250	—	173

Continued to Tab. 1-1

Compositions /%	Preparation methods	Post treatments	YS /MPa	UTS /MPa	E /%	References
Fe-30Mn-C	Casting	Hot rolling	373	1010	88	175
Fe-30Mn-C	Casting	Forging	—	205	16	176
Fe-30Mn-6Si	Casting	Solution treatment	180	450	16	62
Fe-30Mn	Casting	Forging	299	372	94	82
Fe-30Mn	Casting	Rolling	—	530	15	14
Fe-C	Casting	Rolling	440	600	7	52
Fe-35Mn	Casting	Annealing	230	430	30	54
Fe-10Mn-Pd	Casting	Heat treatment	850 ~ 950	1450 ~ 1550	2 ~ 8	55
Fe	Casting	Rolling	—	310	15	14
Fe	Electroforming	Annealing	270	290	18	149
Zn-3Cu-0.5Fe	Casting	—	232	284	33	68
Zn-0.8Mg	Casting	Extrusion	203	301	15	68
Zn-4Cu	Casting	Extrusion	250	270	51	67
Zn-Mg-Mn	Casting	Rolling	195	300	26	29
Zn-1Ca	Casting	Rolling	7	253	13	63
Zn-1Mg	Casting	Rolling	—	300	16	177
Zn-1Mg	Casting	Rolling	190	237	12	63
Zn-0.05Mg	Casting	Extrusion	160	225	26	120
Zn-1Sr	Casting	Rolling	188	229	20	63
Zn-1Mg-1Ca	Casting	Extrusion	138	198	9	177
Zn-5Mg-1Fe	Casting	Extruded-draw tube	150 ~ 187	180 ~ 230	5 ~ 26	65
Zn-1Mg-1Sr	Casting	Extrusion	140	201	10	177

1.1.5 Biocompatibility

Biocompatibility is a vital property of metallic implants for bone repair. It is generally known that Mg, Fe, Zn are essential elements for human body. Although this can be regarded as the evidence of good biocompatibility, metallic implants directly release ions into human body, affecting the surrounding cells, tissues, and blood. Therefore, cytocompatibility, histocompatibility, and hemocompatibility have been the primary evaluation indicators of the biocompatibility of biodegradable metallic implants.

1.1.5.1　Cytocompatibility

As metallic implants degrade in the human body, metal ions will be released and impact on cells. Cytocompatibility can be evaluated in terms of cytotoxicity by the extracts of biodegradable metals. It was reported that the extracts of Mg-1Sn, Mg-1Zn, and Mg-1Al alloys reduced the viability of fibroblasts and osteoblasts, but the extracts of Mg-1Zn and Mg-1Al alloys did not show negative effects on the viability of the cells. Marrow cells in touch with alkali-treated and heat-treated Mg gave the evidence of common morphology, and cellular lysis and inhibitory effect on cell growth was not detected. It is known that Mg-based alloys may exhibit certain cytotoxicity because of the influences of ion concentrations and pH values of the extracts. Even so, Mg-2Sr alloy showed a cytotoxicity of Grade I, which was acceptable for bone implants. Li et al. revealed that murine fibroblast viability decreased with the increase of extract concentration of Mg-Zn-Sr alloy at the first day while became basically equivalent in all the extracts at the third day, indicating the normal proliferation of murine fibroblasts in the extracts of Mg-Zn-Sr alloy. As for Mg-Zn alloy, the extracts showed little impact on the morphology and proliferation of murine fibroblasts with cytotoxicity of Grade 0 – 1, which indicated the favorable cytocompatibility of Mg-Zn alloy. Chen et al. incubated preosteoblasts in the extracts of Mg and Mg-Cu alloys for 12 h. The cell cytoskeleton in Fig. 1-9(a) showed that the cells had normal morphology in all the extracts, implying little cytotoxicity of Mg and Mg-Cu alloys. Thus, it can be concluded that most Mg-based alloys have acceptable cytotoxicity as bone implants.

As for Fe-based alloys, although they exhibit a slow release of ions during degradation, Liu et al. found that the viability of smooth muscle cells was reduced in Fe extracts after alloying S, Co, Sn, C, B, or Al. Moreover, Fe-W extracts also showed mildly cytotoxicity to smooth muscle cells in terms of cell viability. Another research also showed that the proliferation of smooth muscle cells decreased owing to the degradation of Fe. In vitro cytotoxicity of Fe-30Mn alloys to murine fibroblasts was studied by Hermawan et al. Owing to the presence of Mn, the extracts of the alloys were slightly more toxic than that of Fe; however, metabolic activity of the cells was still above the tolerable 70% limit. Huang et al. found that after culture in the extracts of Fe-Au or Fe-Ag alloys, the viability of smooth muscle cells was evidently suppressed while the viability of murine fibroblasts always maintained around 100% during incubation. Hermawan et al. assessed the viability of mouse fibroblasts in terms of metabolic activities by incubation in the medium with different Fe concentrations. The assay showed the cell viability remained up to 95% along the tested concentrations, which resembled the control. Metabolic activity assay of smooth muscle cells was also performed for 24, 48, and 72 h, respectively, to study the cytotoxicity of electroformed Fe. Results showed that the electroformed Fe induced no obvious inhibition effect on metabolic activity compared to 316 L SS owing to its inert property. The cytocompatibility of Fe, Fe-20CS (mass fraction, calcium silicate), and Fe-40CS was evaluated by Wang et al. , and the results were presented in Fig. 1-9(b). It can be seen that the cytoskeleton of human bone mesenchymal stem cells was well-defined and did not exhibit significant difference in distribution or morphology. It seems that the endurance capacity of cells for cytotoxicity differs with the types of Fe-based alloys.

The contents of alloyed elements need to be carefully considered according to biomedical science (for instance, the daily intake of elements and ion concentrations in the human body) and material science (for instance, the Fe phase diagram to obtain suitable mechanical properties for bone implants).

The cytotoxicity of Zn-based alloys as bone implants has also draw close attention. Kubasek et al. verified that the maximum concentration of Zn^{2+} was 80 μmol/L and 120 μmol/L for human osteosarcoma cells and formurine fibroblasts, respectively. Gong et al. reported that fibroblast viability was not obviously effected after incubation in the Zn-1 Mg extracts for 24 h and 48 h, compared with that of the control group, which indicated Zn-Mg had nontoxicity to the cells. Li et al. investigated the effects of alloying Mg, Ca, or Sr elements into Zn on human umbilical endothelial cells, smooth muscle cells, and human osteoblast cells. It was found that the viability of human umbilical endothelial cells and human osteoblasts increased significantly, whereas the viability of smooth muscle cells did not show prominent promotion. The cytotoxicity of Zn alloy was also evaluated by culturing murine fibroblasts in the extracts for 1, 3, and 5 days, respectively. It was found that the proliferation rate of murine fibroblasts showed little statistical significance compared with the control. Murni et al. incubated human osteoblasts in the extracts of Zn, Mg, and Zn-3 Mg alloy for 7 days, respectively, and the cytoskeleton morphology revealed that Zn-3 Mg alloy

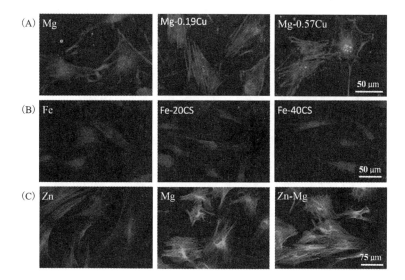

Fig. 1-9   Cytoskeletal morphology showing the cytocompatibility of biodegradable metals. (a) Preosteoblasts cultured with Mg and Mg-Cu alloy extracts for 12 h (nuclei with blue and actin with red). (b) Human bone mesenchymal stem cells exposed to Fe, Fe-20CS, and Fe-40CS alloys for 24 h (nuclei with blue and actin with red). (c) Human osteoblasts exposed to Zn, Mg, and Zn-3 Mg alloy for 7 days (nuclei with blue, actin with red, and microtubule with green). Reproduced with permission from ref. 48. Copyright 2016 Nature publishing group; Reproduced with permission from ref. [192]. Copyright 2017 Elsevier; Reproduced with permission from ref. [194]. Copyright 2015 Elsevier.

had lower toxicity compared to Zn and Mg, as illustrated in Fig. 1-9(c). In general, different cell types are different in response to metal ions, and the activity of cells decreases with the increase of metal ion concentration. Here, the physiology, total amount in the human body, ion concentration limit, and daily allowance of metals are summarized in Tab. 1-2.

Tab. 1-2　The physiology, total amount in the human body, ion concentration limit, and daily allowance of metals

Elements	Physiology	Total amount	Ion concentration limits or blood serum level	Daily allowance	References
Mg	Maintaining nucleic acid structure stability, regular cell proliferation stabilizer of RNA, DNA	25 g	$0.73 \sim 1.06$ mmol/L	400 mg	[27,173, 176]
Fe	Transfer of oxygen by blood, essential 000for metabolism	5 g	$5.0 \sim 17.6$ g·L^{-1}	10 mg	[173,176]
Zn	Co-factor for enzyme reaction, bone, and muscle, essential for immune system	2 g	$12.4 \sim 17.4$ μmol·L^{-1}	6.5 – 40 mg	[54,144, 196]
Al	Factor of Alzheeimer's disease, excess causing neurotoxicity	300 mg	$2.1 \sim 4.8$ μg·L^{-1}	60 mg	[173,197]
Mn	Activation of enzyme systems, involving in metabolism, influencing immune system, blood clotting, bone growth	12 mg	0.8 μg·L^{-1}	5 mg	[27,82, 173]
Si	promoting growth of bone and connective tissue	—	—	20 – 50 mg	[82,175]
Sr	osteogenesis effect	0.3 g	—	4 mg	[33,173]
Ca	Main Skeletal element abundant mineral in bone	1 ~ 1.1 kg	$2.1 \sim 4.8$ μg·L^{-1}	1000 ~ 1500 g	[173,198]
RE(Y, Gd, Ce, etc.)	Y, Nd, Gd, etc., trace nontoxic element, anticancerogenic properties	247 μg	—	—	[17,173, 197]
Zr	High concentrationin liver and gallbladder	250 mg	—	3.5 mg	[198]
Li	Overdose reducing kidney function and nervous system disorders, possible teratogenic effects	—	$2 \sim 4$ (μg·g^{-1})	0.2 ~ 0.6 mg	[175,198]
Ni	Genotoxicity, carcinogenicity	—	$0.05 \sim 0.23$ μg·L^{-1}	—	[173]
Be	Carcinogenicity	—	2 μg·m^{-3}	—	[173]
Cu	Involving in synthesis of enzymes, antiseptic effects	—	$74 \sim 131$ μmol·L^{-1}	—	[198]

1.1.5.2　Histocompatibility and Hemocompatibility

Histocompatibility and hemocompatibility are also considered as sensitive indicators of the biocompatibility of bone implants. Ideal bone implants should neither cause an inflammatory response in tissue, nor cause clotting, hemolysis, and destruction of platelets, etc. , in blood. Histocompatibility and hemocompatibility of biodegradable metals are usually evaluated in terms of biomarkers, hemolysis rate, and platelet adhesion, etc.

Porous AZ91D Mg alloys were implanted into rabbit femur by Med et al. and the results showed that the porous AZ91D Mg alloy implant promoted bone remodeling with no harmful effects on the surrounding tissues. WE43 Mg alloys were implanted randomly into femur of seventy-two rats for 4, 12, and 24 weeks by Castellani et al. And no relevant inflammatory in consequence of WE43 Mg alloy implantation was detected in the blood samples of the rats. Similar method was followed by Peng et al. , who implanted Mg-Y-Nd-RE alloy in rats for the same periods and did not observe any inflammatory either, indicating good hemocompatibility. For Fe-based alloys, hemocompatibility studies were carried out on Fe-W, Fe-CNT, Fe-Pd, Fe-Pt, Fe-Au, Fe-Ag, and $Fe-Fe_2O_3$, etc. It was found that the hemolysis rate was all lower than 5%, and the platelets adhering on the alloy surfaces showed no significant differences in both shape and number, compared to that of the control. Ulum et al. measured the swelling thickness caused by tissue response in sheep femur. It was found that Fe had the lowest degree of tissue response, compared to that of Fe-TCP and SS316. Meanwhile, the numbers of hemoglobin, white blood cells, and red blood cells were within the normal levels during the entire experimental period, indicating good histocompatibility. In a word, the majority of biodegradable Fe-based alloys have satisfactory histocompatibility and hemocompatibility with hemolysis rate less than 5%, appropriate clotting time, and no signs of thrombogenicity or obvious inflammatory response. As to Zn-based alloys, no inflammation was observed by radiographs analysis after the implantation of Zn-Mg, Zn-Ca, and Zn-Sr alloys into mouse femur for 8 weeks. Similar results were verified by Xiao et al. , who implanted Zn-0.05Mg alloy into in a rabbit bone and did not find any inflammatory at 4th, 12th and 24th week, respectively, demonstrating good histocompatibility. Jin et al. reported that fibrous tissue was detected at the interface of Zn-Ag alloy and bone tissue, proving the capability of bone formation. Liu et al. studied the hemolysis rates of Zn-Mg-Mn alloy. Results showed that the hot rolled Zn-Mg-Mn alloy had a hemolysis rate of 1.10%, much lower than that of Zn (4.10%). In vitro degradation test showed no harmful effect of the alloy on erythrocyte, and platelets on the alloy surface kept a round shape with no signs of thrombogenicity. Generally, Zn-based alloys do not induce obvious adverse reactions when they contact with tissue and blood, having a good combination of histocompatibility and hemocompatibility.

1.1.6　Conclusive Remarks

Biodegradable metals are emerging as promising candidates for bone implants. At present, the researches of biomedical Mg-based alloys and Fe-based alloys have a certain accumulation. In the light of these studies, Mg-based alloys are considered to possess proper elastic modulus and good biocompatibility. However, they degrade too fast compared to the growth of new bone. Fe-based alloys have a good combination of mechanical properties and biocompatibility while the main drawback is too slow degradation rate. As for Zn-based alloys, they are characterized by homogeneous corrosion process and moderate degradation rate, but limited by the insufficient strength and ductility.

In recent years, considerable efforts have been devoted to developing metallic implants with a combination of matched biodegradability, sufficient mechanical properties, and favorable biocompatibility for bone repair. For example, a series of commercial biodegradable Mg-based alloys, such as WE43, ZEK100 and LAE442 Mg alloys, etc., have been attempted and showed better corrosion resistance. Moreover, many in vivo studies also demonstrated the favorable degradation behavior and osteogenesis capacity for bone repair applications. Nevertheless, more studies are still needed with focus on the following aspects: 1) The impact of microstructure on degradation behavior deserving a prominent place in due to the complex human environment; 2) Evolution mechanisms of the mechanical properties after alloying; 3) Fatigue performance in human physiological environment to avoid early failure of implants; 4) The influence of alloying elements on biocompatibility of metallic implants serving for a long term; 5) Composition analysis and safety evaluation of degradation products; 6) The establishment of a more comprehensive in vitro evaluation criteria to provide accurate results.

To conclude, biodegradable metals, as a new generation of metallic biomaterials, have shown great potential in implants for bone repair and are getting more and more attention around the world. Due to the complexity of human physiological environment, the research of biodegradable metallic bone implants is a long-term process. With further development, they are expected to partially replace the traditional metallic bone implants used in clinic.

1.2　Refined Lamellar Eutectic in Biomedical Zn-Al-Zr Alloys for Mechanical Reinforcement

1.2.1　Introduction

Zinc is considered as an appropriate biodegradable metallic material for bone implants owing to its natural biodegradability and good biocompatibility. It is also an essential nutrient element in the human body with a daily intake of 15 mg and plays an important role in cell proliferation and bone formation, as well as the nervous and immune systems. Following this, Zn and its alloys such as Zn-Mg and Zn-Al-Mg have been under investigation for potential biomedical applications. Besides, it has been reported that the degradation rate of Zn was compatible with the bone healing process, and the degradation products were considered to be harmless to adjacent tissues. Bowen et al. found that the degradation rate of Zn in the first $2 \sim 3$ months was close to ideal degradation rate for medical implants (0.02 mm/a) and a uniform corrosion was detected. Nevertheless, its poor mechanical strength can't offer sufficient support for the defects when it was used as bone implants.

Many studies have reported that the eutectic in metals can effectively enhance their strength by hindering dislocation motion and forming dislocation pile-up at phase interfaces. Typical eutectic structures include rod-like, irregular and lamellar eutectic. Among them, lamellar eutectic shows the best reinforcing effect since it is composed of two alternating phases, which can provide more phase interfaces than rod-like and irregular eutectic. Schlieteret al. reported a lamellar eutectic Ti-Fe alloy composing of β-Ti(Fe) solid solution and TiFe, which showed 95% ~ 139% higher compressive strength than that of Ti. This motivates the researchers to explore the feasibility of introducing lamellar eutectic in Zn to improve its mechanical properties.

According to the Zn-Al binary phase diagram, Zn-Al lamellar eutectic forms between Zn and Al at appropriate ratios. The amount and corresponding reinforcing effect of the eutectic increase with the increase of Al content. On one hand, both the lamellar eutectic and primary Zn-enriched phase are coarse at a relatively low Al content, which is insufficient in the mechanical requirement for bone repair. On the other hand, as we all known, excess of Al concentration is harmful to nervous system. However, small amount of Al is tolerable because it can be excreted through the kidneys and these would not be accumulated to produce toxic effects. Wang has found that the commercial Zn-Al alloys exhibited good biocompatibility to human umbilical vein endothelial cells. Thus, there is an urgent need to take full advantage of the Zn-Al lamellar eutectic while to minimize the adverse effect of Al. A study by S. H. Seyed Ebrahimi et al. has been reported that Zr was beneficial for the refinement of Al grains in Al-based alloys. Because Al-enriched phase is the primary phase in Zn-Al lamellar eutectic, we thus assume that the introduction of Zr may also has the same refining effect on the Zn-Al lamellar eutectic.

In this chapter, a series of Zn-Al-Zr alloys were fabricated by selective laser melting (SLM). Their microstructures, mechanical strength, degradation performance, and cytocompatibility were investigated. What's more, the underlying evolvement mechanisms of the eutectic structure and resulting effects on the properties of the Zn-Al-Zr alloys were also discussed in detail.

1.2.2　Experimental Details

1.2.2.1　Powder Materials

The Zn-7Al alloy (7% Al) powder (average particle size of 70 μm) and Zr powder (particle size of 8 ~ 15 μm) were supplied from Naiou Nano technology Co., Ltd,. (Shanghai, China), shown in Fig. 1-10 (a-b). All the powders were produced by gas atomization. Herein, the Zr and Zn-7Al powders were mixed in four fixed weight ratios and then spun at a rate of 300 r/min for half an hour using a ball grinder. Subsequently, the mixed powders (denoted as Zn-7Al-xZr, where x = 0.1%, 0.2%, 0.3%, 0.4%, respectively) were used for alloy preparation. In addition, the Zn powder (average particle size 40 μm) was used as control.

1.2.2.2　Alloy Preparation

The preparation of all samples (size 10 mm × 10 mm × 5 mm) was performed on a homemade SLM machine. The SLM machine was mainly equipped with a computer-control system, a fiber laser (YLR-500 – WC-Y14, IPG, America) with maximum power 500 W, a scanning galvanometer (SSIIE-20, raylase, Germany) and an Argon protection system. The preparation process was carried out in argon with scanning speed of 15 mm/s, scanning line interval of 80 μm and laser power of 75 W. The schematical view of the machine was shown in Fig. 1-10(c).

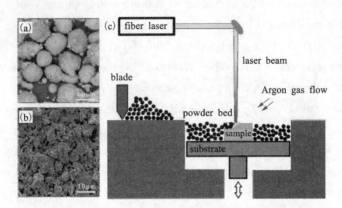

Fig. 1-10 （a-b）The morphology of Zn-7Al and Zr powders. （c）The schematical view of the machine.

1.2.2.3 Microstructure Characterization

According to the standard metallographic procedure, all alloys were grinded with 800, 1000 and 1500 SiC grit papers and then polished into a mirrorlike surface by diamond suspensions of 9, 3 and 1 μm sizes. Subsequently, the microstructures of the alloys were observed using an optical microscope (DM2500, Germany) and a scanning electron microscope (SEM, Phenom pure, Netherlands) equipped with an energy dispersive spectrometer (EDS). Before optical microscopy analysis, the alloys were etched with 4% HNO_3/alcohol solution for 5 ~ 10 s. The average grain sizes were analyzed in metallographic images by Image J software. The constituent phases were further analyzed via an X-ray diffractometer (XRD, Germany) by using Cu Kα radiation with scanning range from 30° to 80° at a scanning rate of 8°/min. The melting temperature of Zn and Zn-Al-Zr alloys was measured by differential scanning calorimetry (DSC) using a synchronous thermal analyzer (STA-200, China) with temperature range of 30℃ ~ 700℃ at a heatly rate of 20℃/min.

1.2.2.4 Mechanical Test

The compressive strength of Zn and Zn-7Al-Zr alloys was obtained on an electronic universal testing machine (ZLC-50M, China) with a 0.5 mm/min loading speed. The loading force of the compression test was applied to the upper surface (along the building direction) of each sample. The compressive strength after immersion test was also measured. And five tests were performed for each group.

1.2.2.5 Electrochemical Measurement

Electrochemical measurement was performed in a simulated body fluid (SBF) solution at 37℃ with an electrochemical workstation (gamry interface 1000, Germany). The chemical composition of SBF are 8.036 g/L of NaCl, 0.354 g/L NaHCO$_3$, 0.311 g/L MgCl$_2$ · 6H$_2$O, 0.292 g/L CaCl$_2$, 0.231 g/L K$_2$HPO$_4$ · 3H$_2$O and 0.225 g/L KCl. A traditional three-electrode cell system was used for the electrochemical measurement with a platinum foil and a saturated calomel electrode as counter electrode and reference electrode. The alloys in this book were used as working electrode. The open circuit potentials were monitored for 4800 s. Afterwards, the test was performed at a scanning rate of 3.33 mV/s. The corrosion current density (I_{corr}) and corrosion potential (E_{corr}) were obtained from the polarization curves by means of Tafel analysis. The corrosion rate was obtained using Equations (1-18):

$$CR = 3.27 \times 10^{-3} \frac{i_{corr}}{\rho} W_E \qquad (1\text{-}18)$$

where CR was the corrosion rate (mm/a), I_{corr} was the corrosion current density ($\mu A/cm^2$), ρ was the density (g/cm^3), W_E was the equivalent weight with the value of 32.6.

1.2.2.6   Immersion Test

To investigate the degradation behavior of Zn and Zn-7Al-Zr alloys, the immersion test with 3 duplicates was carried out in SBF with a ratio of the alloy surface area to the solution volume (S/V) at 1 cm^2 : 20 mL according to ASTM G31 – 72. At 7th d and 21st d, the alloys were taken out of the SBF and washed with deionized water. The pH values of the SBF after immersion for 7 d and 21 d were determined. Afterwards, the degradation products were removed by chemical reagents with 200 g/L of chromiumoxide according to ISO 8407: 2009. The degradation rate was then calculated according to ASTMG31 – 72. The surface morphologies of Zn and Zn-7Al-Zr alloys were analyzed with SEM and EDS, before and after removing degradation products.

1.2.2.7   Cytocompatibility Evaluation

Human osteosarcoma cells named as MG-63 cells were used in this book to investigate the cell response of Zn and Zn-7Al-Zr alloys. MG-63 cells were incubated in Dulbecco's modified Eagle's medium (DMEM) which was obtained from USA and supplemented with 100 U/mL penicillin, 10% fetal bovine serum (FBS), and 100 mg/mL streptomycin at 37℃ in humidified atmosphere with 5% CO_2. Zn and Zn-7Al-Zr alloys were separately soaked in DMEM for 72 h with an ratio of extraction volume to surface area of 1mL/1.25 cm^2 and then the extracts were collected. The extracts were diluted at concentrations of 10%, 50%, and 100%, respectively. For Cell Counting Kit-8 (CCK-8) test, the cells were digested and seeded in 96 well plates with 1000 cells per well at 37℃ in 5% CO_2 incubator. After 6 h cultured, the MG-63 cells were then cultured in the above diluted extracts. After incubation for 1, 3, and 5 days, the cells were incubated with CCK-8 for 2 h at 37℃, and then the absorbance was measured at 450 nm by Paradigm Detection Platform (Beckman Coulter, USA). For cell viability test, the MG-63 cells were cultured in the 100% extracts for 1, 3, and 5 days, and then the cells were digested and seeded upon glass slide in 6 well plates (5×10^3 cells per 100 mL). Afterwards, the cells upon glass slide were stained with Calcein-AM and Ethidium homodimer at room temperature for 30 min and then visualized by a fluorescence microscope (BX5O, Olympus, Japan). For morphological analysis, the Zn and Zn-7Al-Zr alloys were settled in 6 well plates and 1 mL MG-63 cells suspensions were added in each well. After being cultured for 6 h, the samples were fixed with 2.5% glutaraldehyde for 1 h at 25℃, followed by washing twice in PBS solution and dehydrating in a graded series of ethanol (75%, 80%, 95%, and 100%). The samples were then dried with CO_2 and observed by SEM.

1.2.2.8   Statistical Analysis

The experimental data were averaged from independent experiments and analyzed by using SPSS 19.0 software. And Student's t-tests were carried out between different groups to calculate the values of p, which were significant when $p < 0.05$.

1.2.3 Results and Discussions

1.2.3.1 Microstructures

The optical images and average grain size of the alloys were shown in Fig. 1-11(a)(b). The equiaxed grains replaced columnar grains after alloying with Al and Zr. Moreover, the grain size was reduced from (250 ±35) μm for Zn to (8 ±1) μm for 7% Al and 0.2% Zr. The reason was that the solute Al and Zr atoms enriched in the solid-liquid interface during solidification, which resulted in constitutional supercooling. This promoted the formation of crystal nuclei and subsequent refinement for primary Zn phase. However, the grain size of primary Zn became coarse to (12 ±4) μm for 0.3% Zr and increased to (19 ±6) μm for 0.4% Zr, respectively. To investigate the melting temperatures, the liquidus and solidus temperatures of Zn and Zn-7Al-Zr alloys were studied by DSC and the thermograms were presented in Fig. 1-11(c). It was observed that Zn started to melt at 420℃ without addition of Al and Zr, which corresponded to the melting point of Zn. And there was no other endothermic peak could be observed. After alloying Al and Zr, the endothermic peak shifted from 420℃ to 381℃. Corresponding to the eutectic phases of Zn-7Al-Zr alloy started melting at temperature 381℃. Moreover, the other endothermic peak at 277℃ appeared, corresponding to eutectoid transformation began at temperature 277℃. These results were consistent with Zn-Al binary diagram and conform with the formation of eutectic after alloying with Al and Zr.

The XRD patterns of Zn and Zn-7Al-Zr alloys were presented in Fig. 1-11(d). It was observed that Zn pattern merely presented peaks corresponding to the primary Zn phase, confirming that the Zn was pure. After alloying with Al and Zr, there were other diffraction peaks appeared, which represented the face centered cubic(FCC) Al-enriched phase and hexagonal close-packed (HCP) Zn-enriched phase. It must be pointed out that the appearance of Al-enriched phase might have the cytotoxicity. Moreover, peaks represented the Al_2ZnZr phase emerged in the Zn-7Al-0.3Zr alloy, and when the Zr content further increased, the diffraction intensity of the Al_2ZnZr phase increased. The Al_2ZnZr phase did not appear in the patterns with Zr contents of 0.1% and 0.2%, which might be the amount of the Al_2ZnZr phase was small and couldn't attained the minimum detectable limit of the XRD technique.

The microstructures of Zn and Zn-7Al-Zr alloys were characterized by SEM, as presented in Fig. 1-12. It was observed that Zn showed smooth surface with primary Zn phases. After alloying with Al and Zr, lamellar eutectic could be observed in the inter regions of primary Zn phases. As the Zr content increased, the size as well as the amount of the primary Zn phase decreased while the lamellar eutectic increased. When Zr content increased up to 0.2%, the microstructures of the Zn-7Al-Zr alloys mainly comprised lamellar eutectic. To quantitatively reveal the changes in eutectic structure with the Zr content, the lamellar spacing was calculated. The lamellar spacing was (0.51 ±0.05) μm for Zn-7Al-0.1Zr alloy, and decreased to (0.34 ±0.03) μm for Zn-7Al-0.2Zr alloy. With further increases of Zr content to 0.3% and 0.4%, the lamellar spacing increased to (0.37 ±0.02) μm and (0.93 ±0.07) μm, respectively.

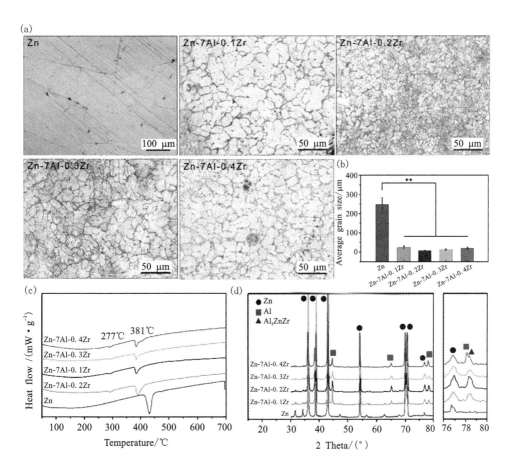

Fig. 1-11　(a) The optical images of Zn and Zn-7Al-Zr alloys showing the transformation of the columnar grains to equiaxed grains. (b) Average grain size. (c) DSC thermograms indicating the formation of eutectic after alloying with Al and Zr. (d) XRD patterns showing the formation of FCC Al-enriched phased and Al_2ZnZr phase.

To reveal the effect mechanisms of Zr and Al on the lamellar eutectic, the high magnifications SEM analysis was carried out in Fig. 1-13. And Fig. 1-13(a) detailed the element composition of the primary Zn. It could be seen that the primary Zn and white lamellae were Zn-enriched phase. The black lamellae were Al-enriched phase. It could be confirmed that the lamellar eutectic was composed of alternating layer Zn-enriched (white) and Al-enriched (black) phase. And addition of Zr could result in the precipitation of Al_2ZnZr phases from the melt. It was known that the structure of Al_2ZnZr phase and the Al-enriched phase were both face centered cubic. According to the disregistry model of two-dimensional lattices, the disregistry between the Al-enriched and Al_2ZnZr phase could be calculated and the smallest disregistry was 0.47%. So the Al_2ZnZr phase could act as the effective heterogeneity nucleation substratum and promote the formation of Al-enriched phase. This would certainly lead to the increase in the amount and the decrease in the lamellar spacing of lamellar eutectic, because Al-enriched phase mostly existed in the lamellar eutectic. Moreover, the increase of the lamellar eutectic consumed primary Zn phase, and the lamellar eutectic distributing

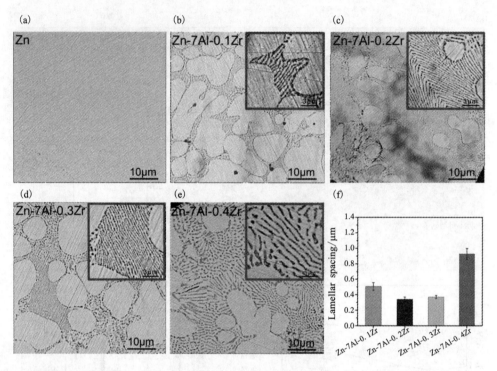

Fig. 1-12 The SEM micrographs and calculated lamellar spacing of Zn and Zn-7Al-Zr alloys.

in the inter-dendritic regions inhibited continued dendritic growth of primary Zn phase. These two aspects make the grain refinement after alloying with Al and Zr. Besides, Al_2ZnZr phase was observed in eutectic structure in Fig. 1-13(b). The Al_2ZnZr phase was spherical and coarse which could cause the decrease of nuclei sites for Al-enriched phases, thus the grain size and the lamellar spacing increased. What's more, the Al_2ZnZr phase was difficult to degrade in the body fluid. Therefore, with the gradual degradation of the matrix, the Al_2ZnZr phase would disintegrate from the matrix and fall into surrounding media. The macrophages would play an important role in removing the Al_2ZnZr phase. It has been reported that another difficult-dissolved $Mg_{17}Al_{12}$ phase leaching into the physiological environment accompanied with the degradation of the matrix could be phagocytized by the macrophages and digested by the lysosomes further. As for the Al_2ZnZr phase, it might also be digested in the same way.

1.2.3.2　Compressive Strength

To investigate the effect of the lamellar eutectic on the mechanical strength, compressive test was carried out (Fig. 1-14). It was obvious that the addition of Al and Zr could improve the compressive strength of Zn. Moreover, the compressive strength of Zn-7Al-Zr alloys increased gradually with Zr content increasing, and the compressive strength peaked at (250 ± 30) MPa with 0.2% of Zr. However, a decrease of compressive strength was noticed with the Zr content further increased to 0.3% and 0.4%. It should be pointed out that the lamellar eutectic played an important role in improving the compressive strength. On one hand, the strength value of Al-

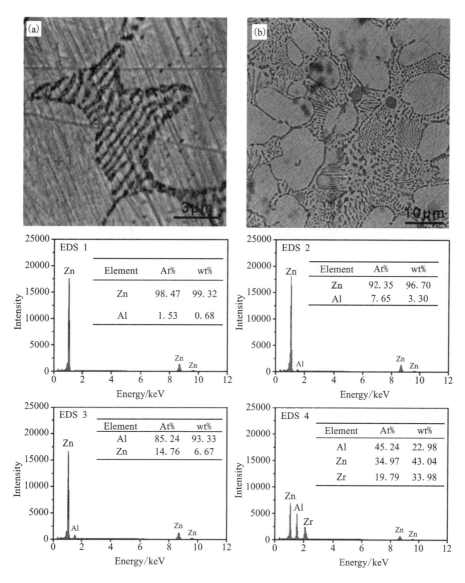

Fig. 1-13　The SEM and EDS analysis results of the lamellar eutectic and secondary phase: (a) lamellar eutectic and (b) black and circular shape particle.

enriched phase was higher than that of Zn-enriched phase. As mentioned above, Al-enriched phase was the main component in the lamellar eutectic, and thus the increase in the amount of the lamellar eutectic would lead to the improvement of compressive strength. On the other hand, the phase interface could effectively hinder the dislocation motion through the interface and have a pinning effect on the dislocation motion. Because the fine lamellar eutectic provided more phase interfaces, the fine lamellar spacing yielded better compressive strength than a coarse lamellar eutectic. Fig. 1-12 shows that the lamellar spacing of 0.2% Zr content was the minimum, and accordingly the compressive strength was the highest. What's more, the coarse Al_2ZnZr phases [Fig. 1-13(b)] might detrimentally affect the compressive strength of the alloy as the interface between the coarse Al_2ZnZr phases and the primary Zn phases was prone to crack.

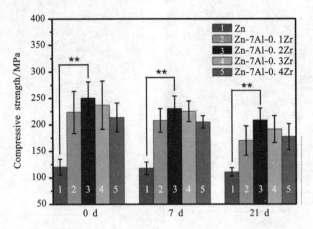

Fig. 1-14   The compressive strengths of Zn and Zn-7Al-Zr
alloys before and after immersion in SBF solution.

For all bone implants, it was important to maintain their strength until the damaged bone healed. To investigate the change of compressive strength during the degradation process, compression tests were also performed on Zn and Zn-Al-Zr alloys after immersion for 7 d and 21 d (Fig. 1-14). For all the alloys, compressive strength decreased after immersion, in spite of the different Zr content. It could be seen that Zr content increasing from 0.1% to 0.4% gave large reductions of compressive strength after immersion 21 d. For Zn-7Al-0.2Zr alloy, the compressive strength decreased from (250 ± 30) MPa to (204 ± 22) MPa, compared to the strength criteria for bone implants.

For a more intuitive understanding of the alloy strengths we learned in this book, we summarized the compressive strength of some alloys and composites of Zn of Fig. 1-15. Previously studies have shown the compressive strength of 120 ~ 160 MPa in Zn-Al alloys, 132 ~ 290 MPa in Zn-Mn alloy, 70 ~ 158 MPa in Zn-HA composites, 90 – 123 MPa in Zn-Mg alloys, and 59 ~ 74 MPa in Zn-ND composites. For instance, Yu added ND into Zn and found that the compressive strength of Zn decreased. That is because the porosity of the composites increased with increasing the ND content, which reduced the compressive strength of Zn. Compared to the study in this book, Zn-7Al-Zr alloys showed higher compressive strength. From the perspective of compressive strength, the Zn-7Al-0.2Zr alloy [(250 ± 30) MPa of compressive strength] was superior to the other previously studied alloys and composites. Besides, there are other researches indicated that alloying with Mg, Ca and Sr into Zn could improve the strength because of the grain boundary strengthening and precipitation strengthening. But with the increase of alloying elements, more intermetallic acts as which cracks presented along the grain boundaries and region of stress concentration, leaded the alloys more brittle.

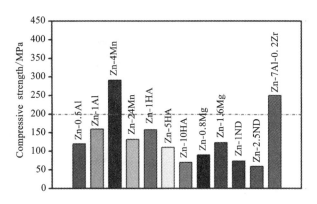

Fig. 1-15   Comparison of the compressive strength among various biodegradable Zn-based alloys and Zn-based metal matrix composites.

1.2.3.3   Potentiodynamic Degradation Characterization

The Tafel potentiodynamic polarization curves of Zn and Zn-7Al-Zr alloys were shown in Fig.1-16(a). The electrochemical parameters were obtained from the curves (Tab. 1-3). The corrosion potentials of Zn-7Al-Zr alloys were lower than Zn, which indicated a higher corroding tendency after the addition of Al and Zr. In addition, higher I_{corr} values were thought to be higher corrosion rate. It could be seen from Tab. 1-3 and Fig. 1-16(b) that the I_{corr} and corrosion rate of Zn-7Al-0.2Zr alloy (0.065 ± 0.002) mm/a) and (5.01 ± 0.25) $\mu A/cm^2$ were higher than those of Zn (1.26 ± 0.09) $\mu A/cm^2$ and (0.016 ± 0.001) mm/a.

Tab. 1-3   Electrochemical parameter values of Zn-7Al-Zr alloys in SBF solution

Alloy	E_{corr}/V	$I_{corr}/(\mu A \cdot cm^{-2})$
Zn	-1.09 ± 0.21	1.26 ± 0.09
Zn-7Al-0.1Zr	-1.25 ± 0.56	3.98 ± 0.41
Zn-7Al-0.2Zr	-1.36 ± 0.49	5.01 ± 0.25
Zn-7Al-0.3Zr	-1.35 ± 0.74	4.47 ± 0.11
Zn-7Al-0.4Zr	-1.30 ± 0.15	1.58 ± 0.22

The results of pH values and degradation rates after immersion tests were presented in Fig. 1-16(c)-(d). It was obvious that the degradation rate of Zn-7Al-Zr alloys was higher than that of Zn. The degradation rate of Zn was the lowest [(0.08 ±0.01) mm/a] and the addition of Al and Zr increased the degradation rate. The Zn-7Al-0.2Zr alloy showed the highest degradation rate [(0.15 ±0.03) mm/a]. The accelerated degradation rate could be explained by the formation of micro-galvanic corrosion among Al-enriched phases and Zn-enriched phases. As for 0.2% of Zr, the lamellar spacing was minimal, and the maximum volume fraction of lamellar eutectic was in Zn-7Al-0.2Zr compared with the other Zr content, which mean more micro-galvanic couples formed in it

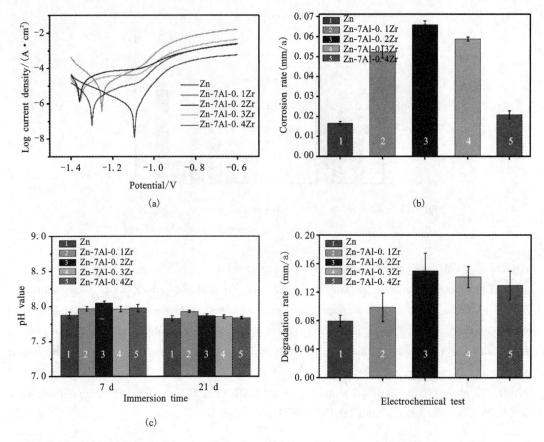

Fig. 1-16 （a）Tafel potentio dynamic polarization，（b）Degradation rate calculated by I_{corr}，（c）Changes of the pH value after immersion in SBF solution for 7 d and 21 d（d）Degradation rate after immersion for 21 d.

and accelerated the degradation rate. The higher degradation rate formed the more amount of the OH^- ion. Thus, the pH value of SBF solutions for Zn was lower than Zn-7Al-Zr alloys. However, with the immersion time increasing, the pH values for 21st d were lower than those for 7th d, due to the formation of calcium-phosphorus phosphates and Zn-oxide/hydrated oxides which consumed the OH^- and blocked the release of OH^- ions.

The degradation morphologies after immersion for 7 d and 21 d were presented in Fig. 1-17, before and after removing degradation products of Zn and Zn-7Al-Zr alloys. After immersion for 7 d, the surface of Zn presented the scratches formed by being polished and visible substrates with few degradation products. With Zr content increasing, massive degradation products were accumulated on the surface and the scratches were almost invisible. When the Zr was added up to 0.2%, the degradation products were almost covered the surface of the alloy. With the Zr content further increasing to 0.4%, the degradation products decreased. After 21 d immersion, more products formed and the degradation products layer became thick. A representative EDS analysis of degradation product indicated the presence of the elements C, O, Zn, P and Ca. Therefore, we assumed that the degradation products were composed of ZnO, $Zn(OH)_2$, $ZnCO_3$ and $Zn_3(PO_4)_2$, which was consistent with the previous reports.

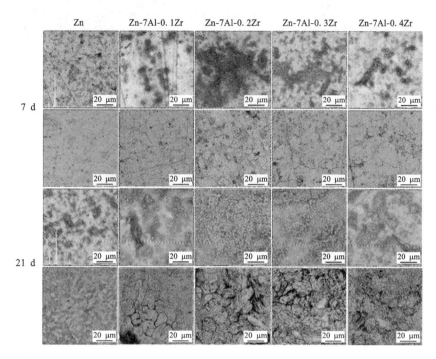

Fig. 1-17　The surface morphologies before and after removing degradation products of Zn and Zn-7Al-Zr alloys after immersion in SBF solution for 7 d and 21 d.

The effect of Al and Zr addition on degradation behavior of the investigated alloys, was further assessed by SEM after removing degradation products. Zn showed small pits after 7 d immersion and the pits continued to expand and connected together with the increasing immersion time. As for Zn-7Al-Zr alloys, the surfaces severely corroded with the anode were the main corrosion parts. The reason was that the standard potentials of Al and Zn were -1.662 V and -0.762 V, respectively. Therefore, the Al-enriched phase was tending to be more negative potential than that of Zn-enriched phase. The active Al-enriched phase was prone to corrode when immersed in solution. The Al-enriched phases were corroded by micro-galvanic coupling between Al and Zn-enriched phases.

1.2.3.4　Cytocompatibility

To observe the effect of Al and Zr on the cell activity, the cytocompatibility evaluation was carried out. The fluorescence images of the MG-63 cells were presented in Fig. 1-18(a), after being cultured in the 100% extracts of Zn and Zn-7Al-Zr alloys for 1 d. The live cells were stained in green and the dead cells were stained in red. The MG-63 cells exhibited classical fusiform shape, suggesting good cells spreading and only a small number of cells were dead. Moreover, with Zr content increasing, the live cells increased. These results indicated that the Zn-7Al-Zr alloys could improve the cell proliferation.

After being cultured in the 10%, 50% and 100% extracts of Zn and Zn-7Al-Zr alloys for 1 d,

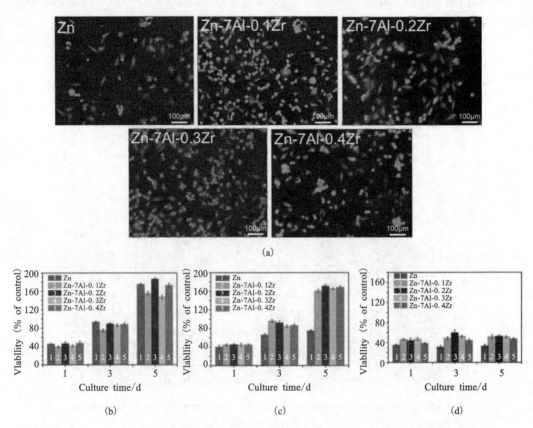

(a)

(b)   (c)   (d)

Fig. 1-18   Fluorescence images of MG-63 cells after cultured in 100% extracts of Zn and Zn-7Al-Zr for 1 d. Quantitative viability results of MG-63 cells culture in 10%, 50% and 100% extracts of Zn and Zn-7Al-Zr alloys for different period.

3 d and 5 d, the cell viability results are presented in Fig. 1-18 (b)-(d). According to ISO standards, the alloys could be considered as cytocompatibility when the cell viability was higher than 75%. The 100% extracts of Zn and Zn-7Al-Zr alloys reduced the viability of MG-63 cells to below 60% for all period. While the extracts were diluted to 50% and 10%, the cell viability increased with prolonged culture days. It could be seen that the cell viability of these extracts was higher than 75% after cultured for the 3 d and 5 d. It was reported that Zn alloying with nutrient elements such as Mn, Mg, Ca and Sr revealed good biocompatibility. Similarly, the results in the present study also showed that Zn alloying with Al and Zr presented good biocompatibility to MG-63 cells and had a positive effect on cell growth.

In order to investigate the adhere ability, MG63 cells were cultured on the surfaces of Zn and Zn-7Al-0.2Zr alloy for 24 h and the cell morphology was shown in Fig. 1-19. It could be seen that cell generated pseudopods in order to adhere to the Zn surface, whereas cell was rounded up shape in Zn-7Al-0.2Zr. It was reported that Zn^{2+} could enhance cell viability, proliferation but decreased cell adhesion strength. As mentioned earlier the degradation rate of Zn-7Al-0.2Zr was higher than

Zn which made it release more Zn^{2+}, so the accumulation of these ions near the surface of Zn-Al-0.2Zr alloy could be disadvantageous and cell became spherical shape. But this result could be acceptable.

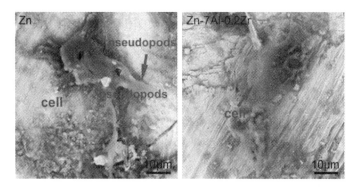

Fig. 1-19   Cell adhesion of Zn and Zn-7Al-0.2 Zr alloy.

1.2.4   Conclusions

In the present study, Al and Zr were introduced into Zn to form refined lamellar eutectic to improve its mechanical properties. The results showed that the addition of Al and Zr could form lamellar eutectic and the amount of lamellar eutectic increased with Zr content increasing. Besides, the lamellar spacing decreased to (0.34 ± 0.03) μm with the 0.2% of Zr. As a result, the compressive strength of Zn-7Al-Zr alloys was significantly improved. Particularly, the compressive strength of the Zn-7Al-0.2Zr reached to (250 ± 30) MPa, which meet the strength standards of orthopedic implants. The compressive strength still maintained higher than 200 MPa after immersion for 21 d. The degradation rate of Zn-7Al-0.2Zr alloy immersion in SBF solution increased to (0.15 ± 0.025) mm/a. Cytocompatibility evaluation showed that Zn-7Al-0.2Zr alloy presented good biocompatibility to MG-63 cells. As far as the high mechanical strength, proper degradation rate and acceptable cytocompatibility, the Zn-7Al-0.2Zr alloy could be a promising material for biodegradable bone implant.

1.3 nMgO-incorporated PLLA Bone Scaffolds: Enhanced Crystallinity and Neutralized Acidic Products

1.3.1   Introduction

Poly-l-lactic acid (PLLA) has received extensive attention in the field of bone repair application, because of its good biocompatibility and natural degradability. Up to now, it has already been used in a series of Food and Drug Administration-approved implants. Nevertheless, two critical shortcomings: relatively poor mechanical properties and excessive acidic products, restrict its further application. The relatively poor mechanical properties malice it hard to provide effective mechanical support in long term bone repair. On the other hand, the excessive acidic degradation products of PLLA usually cause local inflammatory response, which is harmful to the growth of new bone tissue.

The insufficient mechanical properties of PLLA are believed to be closely related with its poor crystallinity. From this point of view, a workable strategy is to introduce inorganic nano-nucleating agents to enhance the crystallinity. For instance, Shieh et al. reported the incorporated carbon nanotube promoted the orderly arrangement of PLLA molecular chains, which reduced the amorphous layer thicknesses. Pei et al. prepared PLLA/cellulose nanocrystal composites by solution casting method. Results indicated that the crystallinity of PLLA was effectively increased from 14.3% to 20.7%. The tensile strength and tensile modulus were increased by 21% and 27%, respectively. Gay et al. prepared PLLA/hydroxyapatite (HA) composites by hot pressing method. Results confirmed that HA effectively increased the mechanical properties, with the Young's modulus and compressive strength reaching to 6 GPa and 100 MPa, respectively. Nevertheless, the inorganic nano-nucleating agents mentioned above exhibited rather poor ability to solve the other problem, namely, excessive acidic products during degradation.

Magnesium oxide nanoparticle (nMgO), as another typical inorganic nano-nucleating agent, is able to release alkaline products in body fluid, which can effectively consume acidic production form the degradation of biopolymer materials. Lin et al. prepared a poly (lactic-co-glycolic acid) (PLGA)/MgO-alginate core-shell microsphere system. The results confirmed that MgO effectively neutralized the acidic degradation products of PLGA. Shuai et al. introduced MgO into poly (3-hydroxybutyrate-co-3-hydroxyvalerate) to fabricate composite scaffold. Immersion tests were found that the pH value maintained at -7.5 during the 4 weeks' soaking period. Moreover, nMgO shows no toxic to human body. In the body fluid environment, the released Mg ions could participate in the synthesis of various proteases, thereby favoring of bone healing.

In this study, nMgO was incorporated into PLLA, with an aim to enhance the mechanical properties and simultaneously reduce excessive acidic products. PLLA/nMgO scaffolds were manufactured using selective laser sintering (SLS), which was known as a typical additive manufacturing technique. It was able to prepare parts with complex porous structure as well as customized shape. It was well accepted that the porous structure could create a microenvironment which was conducive to cell activity and reproduction, while a customized external shape could avoid the excess removal of bone tissue during implantation. Moreover, SLS was suitable for processing a wide range of materials, including metals, polymers, ceramics. The crystallization behavior, mechanical properties and degradation behavior were comprehensively studied. The mechanisms of crystallization behavior on mechanical properties and degradation behavior were elaborated.

1.3.2 Materials and Methods

1.3.2.1 Materials

PLLA powder ($M_w = 150000$ Da, $T_m = 175 \sim 185^{\circ}\text{C}$) was obtained from Polymtek Biomaterial

Co. Ltd. (Shenzhen, China). nMgO powder with a mean size of 60 nm and density of 3.58 g/cm^3 was obtained from Shanghai Macklin Biochemical Co. Ltd. (Ningbo, China).

1.3.2.2 Scaffold Fabrication

The fabrication process of scaffolds was illustrated in Fig. 1-20(a). The PLLA/nMgO mixed powders were obtained after the process of magnetically stirring, ultrasonic dispersing and ball milling. Then scaffolds were fabricated by a homemade SLS system. The processing parameters were as follows: laser power of 3.6 W, scanning speed of 800 mm/s, spot size of 300 μm and layer thickness of 100 μm. Finally, the PLLA and PLLA/nMgO scaffolds were obtained. The prepared scaffolds had nominal nMgO contents of 1%, 3%, and 5%, which were designated as PLLA/1nMgO, PLLA/3nMgO and PLLA/5nMgO, respectively.

1.3.2.3 Microstructural Characterization

PLLA and PLLA/nMgO scaffolds were analyzed using FTIR (Tianjin Gang Dong Technology Co. Ltd., China). The surface morphologies were analyzed using a scanning electron microscopy (SEM, EVO 18, ZEISS, Germany) combined with an energy dispersive spectroscopy(EDS, X-Max 20, Oxford Instruments, UK). Meanwhile, the phase structure of the scaffolds was characterized using an X-ray Diffraction (XRD, Karlsruhe, Germany) at a scanning rate of 8°/min from 10° to 80°. The surface hydrophilicity was measured by utilizing an Attension Theta Lite optical tensiometer (Bio lin Scientific Co. Ltd., Stockholm, Sweden).

1.3.2.4 Thermal Property Analysis

The thermal behaviors of PLLA and PLLA/nMgO powders were investigated using a differential scanning calorimeter (DSC, Q20, TA, USA). For non-isothermal behavior analysis, a small amount of powders (5~8 mg) placed in a sealed aluminum pot, were firstly heated to 200 ℃ at a rate of 10 ℃/min for 5 min to remove the thermal history. Then, the samples were cooled to 25 ℃ at a rate of 5 ℃/min. Subsequently, the samples were heated to 200 ℃ at a rate of 10 ℃/min. The DSC curves were recorded during heating and cooling process.

For isothermal behavior analysis, the samples were firstly heated to 200℃ at a rate of 10℃/min for 5 min to remove the thermal history. Then the samples were quickly cooled to 110℃ at a cooling rate of 30℃/min for 10 min. Finally, the samples were heated to 200℃ at a heating rate of 10 ℃/min. Finally, the DSC curves were recorded. Moreover, the crystal morphologies of the samples at 110℃ were observed using a polarized optical microscopy (DM2500P, Leica, Germany) equipped with a hot stage (THMS600, Linkam Scientific Instruments Ltd., UK).

1.3.2.5 Mechanical Tests

Tensile tests were carried out on a universal testing machine (Metes industrial systems Co. Ltd., China) with a loading rate of 1 mm/min. The stress-strain curves were recorded. The hardness was tested on a micro-hardness tester (Beijing TIME High Technology Co. Ltd., China). All the samples were measured for three times.

1.3.2.6 Degradation Behavior

The immersion tests were performed in simulated body fluid (SBF, 37℃, pH 7.4) at a mass to volume ratio of 0.1 g/mm^3 without changing the SBF. The pH of immersion solution was detected

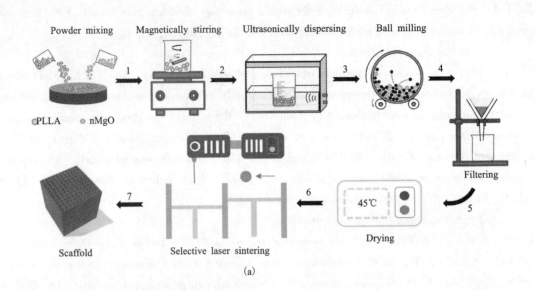

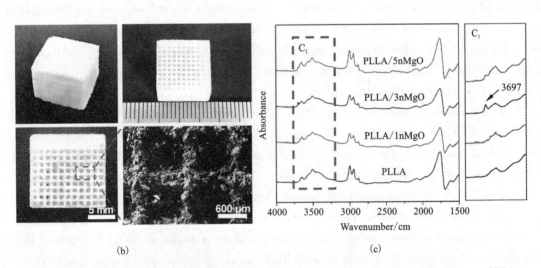

Fig. 1-20 (a) The fabrication process of scaffolds, (b) the digital photographs of representative PLLA/ nMgO scaffold, and (c) Fourier transform infrared spectrometer (FTIR) analysis results of the scaffolds.

using a pH meter at 1st, 2ed, 3th, 4th weeks, respectively. Weight loss method was utilized to quantitatively study the degradation rate of the scaffolds. The scaffolds (8 mm × 8 mm × 3 mm) were weighed before immersion, as recorded W_0. Then, the scaffolds were placed in a sealed tank contained 10 mL of SBF (37℃, pH 7.4), with SBF replaced twice a week. After soaked for 1st, 2ed, 3th, 4th weeks, the scaffolds were taken out and weighed, as recorded W_t. Finally, the weight loss (W_L) was calculated by the following equation:

$$W_L = (W_0 - W_t)/W_0 \times 1 \tag{1-19}$$

1.3.2.7 Cytocompatibility

Human osteoblastic MG-63 cells (ATCC, Rockville, MD, USA) and Dulbecco's modified

Eagle's medium (DMEM), supplemented with 10% fetal bovine serum, 100 U/mL penicillin and 100 mg/mL streptomycin, were used as tested cells and culture medium, respectively. The MG-63 cells were incubated in DMEM in a 12 – well plate. Meanwhile, the DMEM was used as control. Before seeding, the scaffolds were sterilized at high temperature and placed in the 12 – well plate. Then the cells were cultured for 1, 4 and 7 days (5% CO_2, $37\,^{\circ}\!C$), with culture medium updated every other day.

LIVE/DEAD viability assay: After culture for 1, 4 and 7 days, the scaffolds were removed out and rinsed twice with phosphate buffer solution (PBS). Then the cells were rinsed and stained using 4 μmol/L of calcein acetoxymethyl for 25 min at $37\,^{\circ}\!C$. Ultimately, a fluorescence microscope (BX60, Olympus, Japan) was used to observe the cells.

Cell activity assay: After culture for 1, 4 and 7 days, the scaffolds were removed out and rinsed with PBS twice. Afterwards, the cell counting kit-8 (CCK-8) reagent was incorporated into culture plates, and then cultured for 2 h. Finally, a microplate reader (Beckman, USA) was used to measure the absorbance at 450 nm.

Alkaline phosphatase (ALP) activity tests: After culture for 1, 4 and 7 days, the scaffolds were washed twice, and then fixed using paraformaldehyde. The ALP staining was performed using staining reagents. Then the stained cells were observed using a microscope (TE2000U, Nikon, Japan).

1.3.2.8   Statistical Analysis

All data were expressed as the mean ± errors. Student's t-test was used to study the statistical significance. And it was considered to be statistically significant with p-value less than 0.05.

1.3.3   Results and Discussion

1.3.3.1   Microstructure Characteristics

The PLLA/nMgO scaffold (13 mm × 13 mm × 10 mm) prepared by SLS was shown in Fig. 1-20 (b), which presented a three-dimensional porous structure with a mean pore size of -600 μm. As known to all, the porous structure could provide a vital microenvironment favoring to cellular adhesion, proliferation and exchange nutrients after implantation.

The infrared spectrum of PLLA and PLLA/nMgO scaffolds were depicted in Fig. 1-20(c). The obtained spectra of all PLLA/nMgO scaffolds were basically consistent with that of PLLA. It was worth noting that a new peak at 3697 cm^{-1} was observed as nMgO increasing up to 3%. The appearance of this new peak revealed that there were some interactions occurred between nMgO and PLLA, which facilitated to their interfacial bond strength. However, this peak strength became weakened with nMgO further increasing to 5%.

The surface and cryo-fractured morphologies of PLLA and PLLA/nMgO scaffolds were presented in Fig. 1-21 (a). Smooth surface morphology with no other substance was observed for PLLA scaffold. With nMgO increasing to 3%, some nano-scale particles were observed to homogeneously distributein the PLLA matrix with relative rough surfaces. The corresponding EDS analysis revealed these particles mainly contained O and Mg elements, which confirmed that they were MgO.

Nevertheless, as the content of nMgO reached to 5%, they tended to aggregate in PLLA matrix, as marked in Fig. 1-21(a) by red arrows. The large specific surface and high surface energy should be responsible for the agglomeration of nanoparticles.

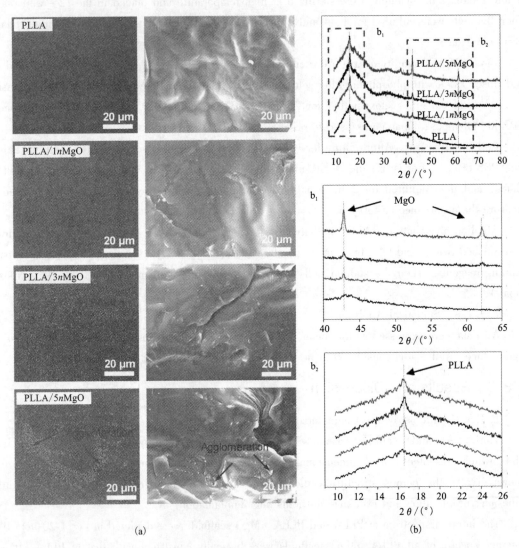

(a)　　　　　　　　　　(b)

Fig. 1-21 (a) Surface (left) and cryo-fractured (right) morphologies of PLLA/nMgO scaffolds; (b) XRD spectrums of PLLA/nMgO scaffolds.

The XRD spectra of PLLA and PLLA/nMgO scaffolds were depicted in Fig. 1-21(b). Clearly, strong peak corresponding to PLLA was detected for all the scaffolds. And some characteristic peaks at $-42.7°$ and $-62.1°$ corresponding to MgO were detected in PLLA/nMgO scaffolds. A more detailed view of the characteristic peaks corresponding to MgO and PLLA were presented in the Figs. 1-21(a) and 1-21(b), respectively. It could be seen that the peak intensities corresponding to MgO were gradually increased with the increase of MgO. Interestingly, as shown in Fig. 1-21(b), the peak intensities corresponding to PLLA (located at $2\theta = 16.2°$) were firstly increased and then decreased with the increase of MgO. This phenomenon was considere to be closely related with the heterogeneous nucleation of the MgO, which would be comprehensively discussed in the subsequent chapter.

1.3.3.2　Thermal Behavior

The non-isothermal crystallization behaviors of PLLA and PLLA/nMgO were investigated by DSC, with cooling curves presented in Fig. 1-22(a) and heating curves presented in Fig. 1-22(b). During cooling from 160℃ to 50℃, an exothermic peak located at −104.2℃ was detected from PLLA. As a comparison, the exothermic peak gradually shifted to high temperature with the content of nMgO gradually increasing to 3%, with an −106.9℃ for PLLA/1nMgO and −107.7℃ for PLLA/3nMgO. The appearance of exothermic peaks indicated the occurrence of crystallization behavior. The location of exothermic peak corresponded to its maximum crystallization temperature. Thus, it was reasonable to deduce that nMgO increased the maximum crystallization temperature of PLLA. It was well known that an enhanced maximum crystallization temperature indicated an accelerated crystallization rate. Nevertheless, the exothermic peak shifted to lower temperature with nMgO further increasing to 5%. The appearance of endothermic peak revealed the melting behavior of polymer. Usually, the initial melting of polymers began from the amorphous region. And an improved crystallinity resulted in an enhanced melting point (T_{m}). As shown in Fig. 1-22(b), the endothermic peak of PLLA/nMgO gradually shifted to higher temperature with nMgO gradually increasing to 3%. The PLLA matrix exhibited a low T_{m} of 178.95℃, whereas PLLA/3nMgO exhibited a relative high T_{m} of 179.16℃. As for PLLA/5nMgO, the T_{m} was 178.65℃. These results revealed the enhanced crystallinity of PLLA/3nMgO.

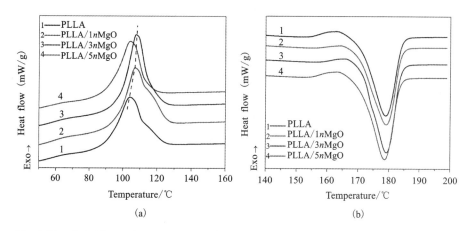

Fig. 1-22　(a) The cooling curves and (b) the heating curves of PLLA and PLLA/nMgO during non-isothermal crystallization.

The isothermal crystallization behaviors of PLLA and PLLA/nMgO were also investigated, with DSC curves depicted in Fig. 1-23(a). At determined temperature of 110℃, the stronger exothermic peaks were obtained in heat flow curves for all samples, where exothermic peak location corresponded to the necessary temperature for maximum crystallization. It was clearly to observe that the necessary temperature for maximum crystallization decreased significantly with nMgO increasing. The relative crystallinity (X_t) as a function of crystallization time deduced from the isothermal crystallization curves were depicted in Fig. 1-23(c). And $t_{1/2}$, which represented the time required for semi-crystallization, was listed in Tab. 1-4. Particularly, PLLA had a $t_{1/2}$ of 3.30 min, whereas PLLA/$3n$MgO exhibited a reduced $t_{1/2}$ of 1.81 min.

Avrami plots were also deduced from isothermal crystallization DSC curves, as presented in Fig. 1-23(d). The curves for all samples were linear at initial stage of crystallization, suggesting that the isothermal crystallization kinetics could be well described by Avarmi equation. Moreover, Avrami exponent (n) was calculated, with results shown in Tab. 1-4. For all samples, n ranged from 1.29 to 1.84, indicating that PLLA grew into two dimensions during isothermal crystallization testing. It revealed that nMgO exerted had no effect on the crystallization mechanism of PLLA.

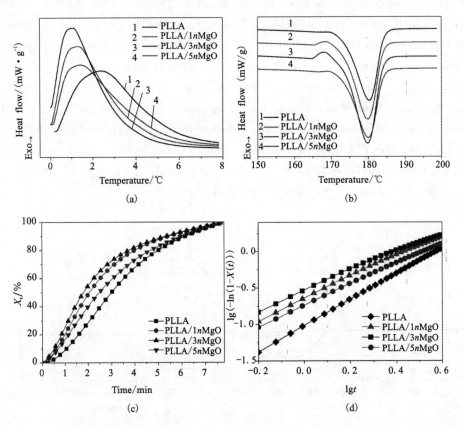

Fig. 1-23 (a) DSC isothermal crystallization curves and (b) subsequent heat curves. (c) Relative crystallinity versus the crystallization time and (d) Avrami plots.

The subsequent heat curves after isothermal crystallization were depicted in Fig. 1-23(b). From the heat flow curves, the melting peak intensity of PLLA evidently increased after the addition of nMgO. Meanwhile, the crystallinity (X_c) was calculated, with results summarized in Tab. 1-4. The obtained crystallinity of PLLA was 47.41%. The crystallinity gradually increased to 50.21% for

PLLA/3nMgO, and subsequently reduced to 47.91% for PLLA/5nMgO. These results were consistent with previous non-isothermal crystallization behavior analysis.

Tab. 1-4　Crystallization kinetic parameters of PLLA and PLLA/nMgO

Samples	X_c(100%)	K/min	N	$t_{1/2}$/min
PLLA	47.41	7.54×10^{-2}	1.84	3.30
PLLA/1nMgO	49.78	2.54×10^{-1}	1.39	2.06
PLLA/3nMgO	50.21	3.22×10^{-1}	1.29	1.81
PLLA/5nMgO	47.91	1.94×10^{-1}	1.40	2.48

The crystal morphologies of PLLA and PLLA/nMgO after isothermal crystallization at 110℃ were shown in Fig. 1-24. For PLLA, a small amount of spherulites with maltese-cross appearance distributed in the matrix. After incorporating 1% and 3% of nMgO, more spherulites with refined grain were observed in the matrix. Nevertheless, coarsened spherulites were presented in the matrix of PLLA/5nMgO, suggesting the nucleation density of PLLA decreased.

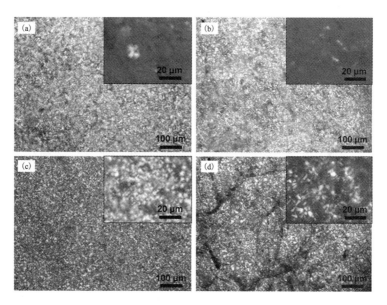

Fig. 1-24　Polarized optical microscopy images of (a) PLLA, (b) PLLA/1nMgO, (c) PLLA/3nMgO and (d) PLLA/5nMgO at 110℃.

In this study, the non-isothermal behavior and isothermal crystallization behavior were investigated to study the effect of nMgO on the crystallinity of PLLA. Results definitely revealed that nMgO effectively enhanced the crystallinity, with the evidence of increased melting point, maximum crystallization temperature and reduced crystallization time. In general, the crystallization behaviors of polymers involved two kinds of nucleation process: homogeneous nucleation and heterogeneous nucleation. In present study, PLLA exhibited a homogeneous nucleation process, in which its own molecular chains orderly arranged in the melt and subsequently formed crystal nucleus. Nevertheless, after incorporating nMgO, the nucleation process changed to heterogeneous nucleation, which referred to a fast and stable ordered arrangement by produced some chemical bonds between other substances and matrix. In detail, the incorporated nMgO provided more nucleation sites, which induced PLLA macromolecule chain to easier nucleate on it, thus enhancing the crystallization efficiency. It should be stated that further increasing nMgO to 5% led to a reduced crystallinity. A fact was that the crystallization of polymers was a process of orderly stacking of molecular chains. The excessive nMgO resulted in aggregation in PLLA matrix, which might hinder the movement of molecular chains and deteriorate crystallization behavior.

1.3.3.3 Hydrophilicity and Degradation

The water contact angles measured by surface water droplet deposition were presented in Fig. 1-25(a). The water contact angle of PLLA scaffold was $86.60° \pm 1.23°$, which was consistent with the results reported in other literatures. The water contact angles were gradually reduced to $44.23° \pm 2.20°$ for PLLA/$3n$MgO scaffold and $27.20° \pm 1.44°$ for PLLA/$5n$MgO scaffold, respectively, which revealed that nMgO enhanced the surface hydrophilicity of PLLA/nMgO scaffolds. It was known that the surface hydrophilicity was closely related to surface micro texture and chemical composition. For PLLA/nMgO scaffolds, the incorporated nMgO particles orderly exposed to the surface, which definitely changed the surface micro texture and chemical composition. Particularly, the exposed nMgO particles could attract water molecules by hydrogen bonding, which promoted the penetration of water into PLLA matrix. For bone scaffolds, the enhanced surface hydrophilicity was considered to be favorable to absorb nutrient substance and bioactive factors, thus accelerating bone healing as implanted in vivo.

Immersion tests were performed to study the degradation behavior of PLLA and PLLA/nMgO scaffolds. The pH value in immersion solution was presented in Fig. 1-25(b). For PLLA scaffold, the pH of SBF solution gradually decreased from 7.40 to 6.82, with soaking period extending to 4 weeks. It was well known that the degradation of PLLA resulted in the formation of acidic products, thus reducing the pH value of SBF solution. As a comparison, a significant increase in pH was observed for PLLA/nMgO scaffolds after immersion for 1 week. The pH values were upped to 7.78 for PLLA/$1n$MgO, 8.29 for PLLA/$3n$MgO, and 8.33 for PLLA/$5n$MgO. The increased pH value might be derived from the OH$^-$ produced by the hydration of nMgO. It was considered that Mg (OH)$_2$ was formed by the degradation of MgO, which effectively neutralized the acidic substances produced by the degradation of PLLA, and enhanced the pH value of SBF solution. Subsequently, the pH value gradually decreased with soaking period extending, which was due to the continuous release of acidic products. Interestingly, the pH value of PLLA/$5n$MgO was considerably lower than that of PLLA/$3n$MgO after immersion for 3 weeks, which might be due to the fact that PLLA/$5n$MgO had more amorphous regions compared with PLLA/$3n$MgO, resultly in a rapid consumption of nMgO during soaking period. In addition, the pH value obtained from PLLA/$3n$MgO stabilized at -8.02 after 4 weeks' immersion, which was a statistically significant high pH value ($^*p < 0.05$) compared

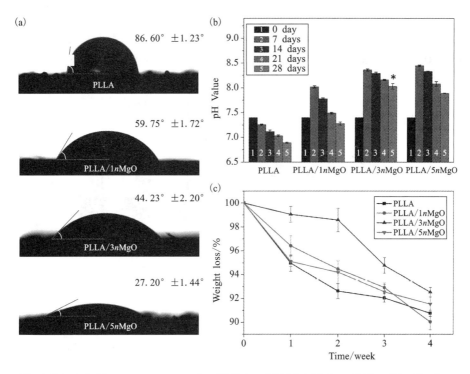

Fig. 1-25　(a) The water contact angle of PLLA and PLLA/nMgO scaffolds; (b) pH value and (c) weight loss of scaffolds during immersion. The values were expressed as mean ± errors, $n = 3$, $^{*}p < 0.05$.

with that from PLLA.

　　Weight loss was also evaluated during the immersion to further study the degradation behavior. All the scaffolds presented evident weight loss with soaking period extending. As compared with PLLA scaffold, the PLLA/nMgO scaffolds exhibited a lower weight loss at initial degradation stage, indicating that the incorporated nMgO slowed down the degradation. It was easy to understand that the reduced amorphous region, caused by the incorporating of nMgO, improved the stability of PLLA/nMgO scaffolds. After 2 weeks' immersion, the degradation rate of PLLA/$3n$MgO began to accelerate. It was possibly because the alkaline environment promoted the degradation of PLLA. And the co-degradation of MgO and PLLA played a positive role in the degradation reaction.

　　1.3.3.4　Mechanical Properties

　　The tensile stress-strain curves of PLLA and PLLA/nMgO were presented in Fig. 1-26(a). There was no obvious yield deformation zone, indicating their brittle fracture characteristics. And the peak stress obtained from PLLA/nMgO was clearly higher than that from PLLA. The tensile strength, tensile modulus and elongation deduced from the stress-strain curves were shown in Figs. 1-26(b) and 1-26(c), respectively. For pure PLLA, the tensile strength, tensile modulus and elongation were relatively low, with only (15. 40 ± 2. 80) MPa, (1. 39 ± 0. 03) GPa and 2. 06% ± 0. 52% , respectively. As nMgO increased up to 3% , the tensile strength, tensile modulus and elongation were gradually enhanced to (21.27 ±2.12) MPa, (1.73 ±0.17) GPa and 3.17% ±0.51%. However, after adding 5% nMgO, the upward trend stopped, with tensile strength, tensile modulus and elongation reducing to (18.52 ±0.71) MPa, (1.62 ±0.08) GPa and 2.28% ±0.31%, respectively.

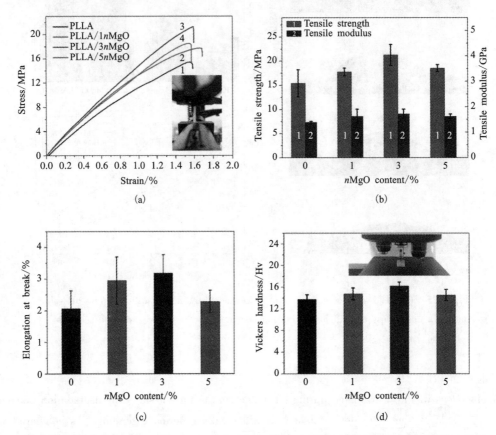

Fig. 1-26 (a) Typical tensile stress-strain curves; (b) tensile strength and tensile modulus, (c) elongation deduced from the tensile stress-strain curves; (d) the Vickers hardness obtained by indentation tests. The values were expressed as mean ± errors, $n = 3$.

The Vickers hardness of PLLA and PLLA/nMgO obtained by indentation tests were shown in Fig. 1-26(d). Pure PLLA exhibited a low Vickers hardness of (13.75 ±0.82) Hv. With nMgO increasing up to 3% and 5%, the Vickers hardness reached (15.15 ±0.71) Hv and (14.55 ± 1.02) Hv, respectively, which indicating that the incorporated nMgO effectively enhanced the hardness of PLLA matrix.

The tensile fracture morphologies of PLLA and PLLA/nMgO were presented in Fig. 1-27. PLLA presented a smooth fracture surface, indicating its brittle characteristics. PLLA/nMgO showed a relative rough fracture surface, reveedig their enhanced toughness. For PLLA/$3n$MgO, a large amount of dimple-shaped cavities were observed on the fracture surface. It was considered that the incorporated nMgO obstructed the development of cracks and resulted in uneven surfaces.

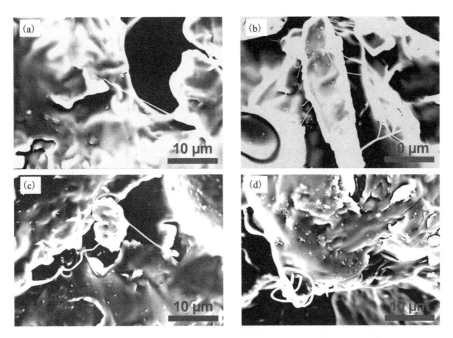

Fig. 1-27　The tensile fracture morphologies of（a）PLLA,（b）PLLA/1nMgO,（c）PLLA/3nMgO and（d）PLLA/5nMgO.

Regarding the tensile and indentation tests, the incorporation of MgO significantly enhanced the strength and hardness. The increased crystallinity was considered to be the major contributor to the improved strength and hardness. On one hand, the improved crystallinity of PLLA/3nMgO was favorable to an improvement of its mechanical stability. On the other hand, the particle reinforcement effect of the homogeneously distributed nMgO in PLLA matrix, should also be taken into consideration. The homogeneously distributed MgO particles with higher hardness could act as a strengthening agent by load transmitting and crack deflection, thus improving the resistance of PLLA matrix to external force. Meanwhile, the elongation was enhanced from 2.06 ± 0.52% to 3.17 ± 0.51%. Usually, the increased crystallinity resulted in a poor toughness with reduced elongation, because the orderly arranged molecular chains would increase the interaction forces between molecule chains and thus limit their movements. Nevertheless, the incorporated MgO nanoparticles overshadowed the effect of increased crystallinity on toughness. Particularly, the rigid MgO nanoparticles could produce stress concentration effect as the matrix was impacted by external force, which could easily stimulate microcracks in the surrounding matrix and absorb certain deformation energy. In this case, the interface between matrix and MgO nanoparticles produced yield and plastic deformations. In addition, the MgO nanoparticles hindered the crack growth of the matrix, so as not to develop into breakage. Thus, the toughness of PLLA/3MgO was slightly higher than PLLA. It should be noted that excessive MgO reduced the tensile properties of PLLA. As presented in Fig. 1-21, such an excessive nMgO led to aggregation in PLLA matrix and resultantly reduced the crystallinity. Previous studies reported that the agglomeration of reinforcing phases not only affected the ordered arrangement of crystallization and integrity of the PLLA matrix, but also caused the formation of interfacial defects. All the phenomena mentioned above would deteriorate the tensile properties of PLLA matrix.

1.3.3.5　Cell Response

Fluorescence images of MG-63 cells cultured on PLLA and PLLA/$3n$MgO scaffolds for 1, 4, 7 days were presented in Fig. 1-28 (a). Live cells were stained in green, whereas dead cells were stained in red. Obviously, almost no dead cells appeared on the scaffolds during cell culture. Particularly, MG-63 cells presented classical fusiform shape after 1 day culture, indicating their normal cell development. After culture for 4 and 7 days, cells began to form filopodia, and secreted a large amount of extracellular matrix. Meanwhile, live cell number increased considerably with culture period gradually extending to 7 days, which suggested that both PLLA and PLLA/$3n$MgO scaffolds facilitated normal cell proliferation. It was worth noting that the cells density on PLLA/$3n$MgO scaffold was higher than that on PLLA scaffold, indicating that PLLA/$3n$MgO scaffold was more beneficial to cell growth.

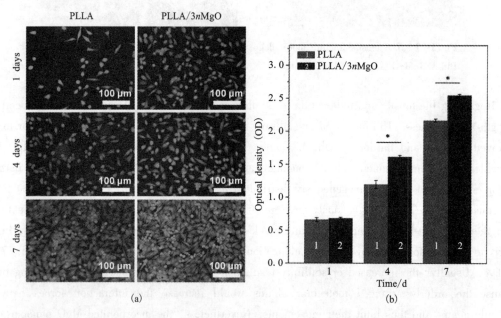

Fig. 1-28　(a) Fluorescence images of MG-63 cells and (b) Optical density obtained by the CCK-8 assays. The values were expressed as mean ± errors, $n = 3$, $^*p < 0.05$.

CCK-8 assays were used to quantitatively assess the cell viability, with results shown in Fig. 1-28(b). Clearly, the cell viability on both PLLA and PLLA/$3n$MgO scaffolds increased with incubation time increasing. After 7 days' culture, the OD value increased from 0.66 to 2.16 for PLLA scaffold, while it increased from 0.68 to 2.55 for PLLA/$3n$MgO scaffold. More importantly, PLLA/$3n$MgO scaffold exhibited higher cell activity compared with PLLA scaffold at the same culture time. These results confirmed that nMgO promoted cell proliferation.

The ALP activity of MG-63 cells cultured on PLLA and PLLA/3nMgO scaffolds were investigated, as shown in Fig. 1-29. With the increase of cell culture days, the ALP activity of MG63 cells increased. The cells cultured on the PLLA/3nMgO scaffold exhibited more intensive ALP staining than PLLA scaffold under the same cell culture time. Moreover, the cells cultured on the PLLA/3nMgO scaffold presented affluent filopodia which extended to the adjacent cells, indicating the improved proliferation and differentiation of cells.

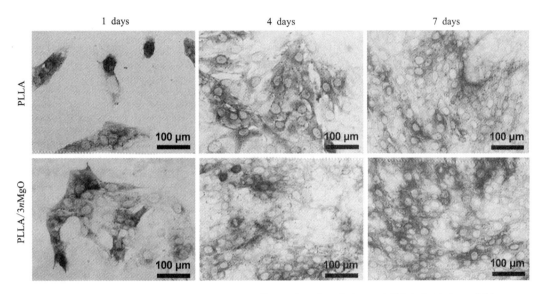

Fig. 1-29   ALP staining images of MG-63 cells incubated on PLLA and PLLA/3nMgO scaffolds

For bone scaffolds, beneficial cell behaviors including cell proliferation and cell differentiation played key roles for the realization of bone repair and regeneration. In present study, the incorporated nMgO clearly improved cell behavior. Improved cell behavior of PLLA/3nMgO was partly ascribed to the increased pH caused by the incorporation of nMgO. As PLLA scaffold degraded, a large amount of acidic degradation products formed in culture medium and resultantly reduced the pH value. The immersion tests revealed that the pH value decreased to 6.7 after immersion for 4 weeks. It was reported that a pH value ranging from 7.6 to 8.5 was more favorable to normal cell growth. A pH too high or too low should give rise to negative effects on cell proliferation. As for PLLA/3nMgO scaffold, the degradation of nMgO effectively neutralized the acid products and resulted in a near-physiological environment with suitable pH value for cell growth. On the other hand, the degradation of nMgO should result in a release of Mg^{2+} into the culture medium, which also might do a favor to the improved cell behavior. Mg is a necessary nutrient element, with a daily intake of ~350 mg for adult. Previous studies confirmed that Mg element involved in the synthesis of various enzymes and could effectively promote the growth and proliferation of bone cells.

1.3.4　Conclusions

In this chapter, PLLA/nMgO scaffolds were successfully prepared by SLS. The incorporated nMgO not only caused the reinforcing effect, but also enhanced the crystallinity of PLLA, thus improving the mechanical stability of PLLA/nMgO scaffolds. The results showed that the tensile strength, tensile modulus and Vickers hardness were increased by 38%, 24% and 11%, respectively. Moreover, as an alkalineoxide, nMgO effectively neutralized the acidic product formed by the degradation of PLLA, resulting in a more favorable physiological environment for cell proliferation and differentiation. All these positive results suggested that SLS-processed PLLA/$3n$MgO scaffold was of great potential for bone repair.

Chapter 2

Regulation of Degradation Rate

Grain micro-nanocrystallization is an important method to overcome the degradation rate of bio-magnesium alloys at present. However, the recrystallized grains are easy to be coarsened during the long time and high temperature processing of conventional processes. It is believed that laser rapid solidification can refine the grain size, reduce the composition segregation, and extend the solid solubility, thus showing a great potential in improving the corrosion resistance of bio-magnesium alloys.

2.1　3D Honeycomb Nanostructure-encapsulate Magnesium Alloys with Superior Corrosion Resistance and Mechanical Properties

2.1.1　Introduction

Magnesium (Mg) and its alloys have received much attention by virtues of good biocompatibility and biodegradability. Their densities and elastic modulus are also close to those of human bone, which can reduce the undesirable stress shielding effect. In addition, Mg is an essential element with osteogenic potential and participates in many metabolic reactions and biological mechanisms. However, Mg alloys are highly susceptible to corrosion due to its low potential (-2.37 V), especially in chlorine- or carbonate-containing solution. As a result, their degradation rates in body fluid are much higher than the requirement of bone repair, which easily results in the premature loss of structural and mechanical integrity before bone healing. Therefore, it has long been the major challenge to improve the corrosion resistance and mechanical stability of Mg alloys.

Graphene oxide (GO) is a two-dimensional nanomaterial consisting of a single layer of carbon atoms. As a derivative of graphene, the carbon atoms in GO arranged neatly in a hexagonal lattice. Moreover, the basal plane of GO is decorated with functional groups such as hydroxyl, epoxide, carbonyl, and carboxyl groups. GO has excellent physical and mechanical properties (specific surface area of 2630 $m^2 \cdot g^{-1}$ and breaking strength of 130 TPa). More importantly, it possesses outstanding anti-permeability and chemical inertia, which can impede the infiltration of gases, liquids, ions, and other corrosive medium by erecting a separation zone between the matrix and the corrosive medium, thereby blocking the charge transfer at the interface. Thus, it is expected to utilize the prominent physical shielding effect of GO to improve the corrosion resistance of Mg alloys. In addition, the oxygen-containing groups on the carbon atom plane endow GO with good ability for bone-like apatite deposition, which may also hinder the invasion of corrosive medium to Mg alloys.

In the past years, many studies have been carried out to investigate the effects of GO or graphene on Mg and its alloys. Rashad M et al. fabricated Mg alloy reinforced with graphene. It was found that graphene uniformly dispersed in the Mg matrix and improved the mechanical properties. Tong L B et al. prepared GO coating on the surface of Mg by electrophoretic deposition. The results showed that the GO coating could prevent the direct contact between the matrix and body fluids, and thus improved the corrosion resistance of Mg alloys. These studies have confirmed the positive effects of GO on Mg alloys, with a focus on either the mechanical properties (GO as the second phase) or the corrosion resistance (GO as the surface coating or coating additive). However, the GO coating can only protect the matrix from corrosion at the initial stage, and once the coating falling off, the Mg matrix will expose to the corrosion medium and still undergo rapid degradation. Recently, the only study on the degrade resistance of Mg alloys by adding a small amount of GO as dispersed second phase was reported. The results showed aggravated galvanic corrosion and degradation as a result of the simultaneous exposure of GO and Mg matrix to the corrosion medium. Therefore, new strategies should be explored to utilize the excellent anti-permeability of GO while inhibit its galvanic corrosion with the matrix, thereby improving the corrosion resistance and mechanical properties of Mg alloys.

In this work, GO was incorporated into AZ61 alloy via selective laser melting (SLM) to fabricate three-dimensional (3D) honeycomb nanostructure-encapsulated Mg alloys: the honeycomb nanostructure was constructed by GO as a second phase and Mg grains were encapsulated in the honeycomb unit, aiming to improve the corrosion resistance and mechanical properties. The microstructure and mechanical properties of the AZ61 – GO alloys were investigated. Emphasis was put on the corrosion behavior and corresponding mechanisms. And the factors affecting the formation of honeycomb nanostructure were revealed and discussed. Moreover, the biocompatibilities of the alloys with and without GO were also evaluated.

2.1.2　Materials and Methods

2.1.2.1　Materials and Processing

The AZ61 powders were supplied by Tangshan Weihao Magnesium Powder Co., Ltd. It was produced by gas atomization technique with particle sizes ranging from 55 μm to 80 μm. GO (diameter 8 – 15 μm; purity >98%) was obtained from Chengdu Organic Chemicals Co., Ltd., Chinese Academy of Sciences. Herein, semi powder method was used to obtain the mixed powders of AZ61 and GO. In order to prevent agglomeration, GO was firstly ultrasonic shaking in ethanol for 1 h to break the Van der Waals force by using an ultrasonic cleaner machine (Changzhou Ronghua instrument manufacturing Co., Ltd.). At the same time, the AZ61 powders were separately ultrasonic shaking in ethanol for 1 h. Subsequently, the two solutions were mixed together and mechanically stirred at 2000 r/min for 2 h with assisted ultrasonic shaking. The resulting AZ61 – GO solution was then vacuum distilled and dried in an atmosphere-controlled furnace at 60 ℃ for 6 h to remove the residual ethanol. Finally, the mixed powders with different GO contents (denoted as AZ61 – xGO, where x = 0%, 0.2%, 0.4%, 0.6%, 0.8%, 1.0%, 1.2%, mass fraction, respectively) were obtained and used for alloy preparation. The preparation process was conducted in argon atmosphere on a homemade SLM system (laser power of 80 W, scanning speed of 15 mm/ s, laser spot size 50 μm).

2.1.2.2　Microstructural Characterizations

The prepared AZ61 – xGO samples for microstructural observation were polished into a mirrorlike surface. Subsequently, the samples were observed under an optical microscope(DM2500, Leica, Germany) and a scanning electron microscope (SEM, Phenom pure, Phenom-World BV, Netherlands) equipped with an energy dispersive spectrometer. Before optical microscope analysis, acetic-picral solution was prepared with 1.5 g picral acetic (purity 99.2%), 100 mL ethanol (purity 99.7%), 6 mL acetic acid (purity 99.6%), and 10 mL distilled water, and then it was used to etch the polished samples for 20 s.

2.1.2.3　Immersion and Electrochemical Tests

Electrochemical tests were conducted on a CHI604D electrochemical workstation (CH Instrument, China) to evaluate the corrosion behaviors of the AZ61 – xGO alloys. So far, many media, including simulated body fluid (SBF), CO_2-bicarbonate buffer, etc., have been developed to evaluate the corrosion of Mg alloys. Because SBF has similar compositions to human body fluids, it has been widely used to simulate the corrosion behavior of Mg-based bone implant materials. Therefore, in this work, SBF was used as the corrosive medium to study the corrosion behavior of AZ61 – xGO alloys. The SBF contained 8.035 g/L NaCl, 0.335 g/L $NaHCO_3$, 0.225 g/L KCl, 0.231 g/L $K_2HPO_4 \cdot 3H_2O$, 0.311 g/L $MgCl_2 \cdot 6H_2O$, 0.292 g/L $CaCl_2$, 0.072 g/L Na_2SO_4 and 6.228 g/L Tris ($HOCH_2)_3CNH_2$, following the preparation procedure of Gu et al. And a three-electrode configuration was used with 250 mL SBF solution as the electrolyte, AZ61 – xGO samples as the working electrode, a saturated calomel electrode (SCE) as the reference electrode, and a platinum electrode as the counter electrode. Before the electrochemical tests, all the AZ61 – xGO samples were mounted in epoxy resin with an exposed area of 0.45 cm^2. Afterwards, the mounted samples were immersed in electrolyte to obtain the open circuit potential (OCP) and the potential dynamic polarization curves were recorded with a sweep rate of 0.5 mV/s at 37 ℃. Finally, corrosion potentials (E_{corr}) and corrosion current densities (I_{corr}) were obtained by the Tafel extrapolation method from the polarization curves and the corrosion rates (P_i) were calculated. All the tests were normally repeated five times under the same conditions to check their reproducibilities.

Immersion tests were carried out to investigate the long-term corrosion behavior in terms of hydrogen evolution and weight loss. For hydrogen evolution tests, the AZ61 – xGO samples were immersed in SBF solution for 360 h at 37℃. And the evolved hydrogen originating from the corrosion of the samples was collected during the immersion. Later, the volume of hydrogen was recorded accordingly. Moreover, the presence of corrosion morphologies and corrosion products were characterized using SEM and the elemental compositions in different phases were confirmed using EDS. For weight loss tests, the samples were immersed in SBF for 360 h at 37℃ by water bath. Before the tests, the samples were ground on progressively finer grades of emery papers up to 4000 grit and then weighed. All immersion tests were carried out without agitation or circulation. In order to remove the corrosion products with minimal dissolution of the base alloy, chemical cleaning of the corroded sample was carried out in boiling 15% CrO_3 + 1% $AgCrO_4$ solution for 1 min, followed by acetone washing. Finally, the weight loss for each sample was measured and used for the calculation of the corrosion rate. Each test was repeated three times to obtain the repeatable results.

2.1.2.4　Mechanical Characterization

The hardness (HV) of the AZ61 − xGO alloys was determined by a hardness tester (HXD-1000TM/LCD, Shanghai Taiming Optiacal Instrument Co., Ltd., China). The samples were subjected to a load of 1.96 N for 15 s. Six different locations were tested for each sample and six samples were tested for each group. Whereafter, the compression yield strengths of the AZ61 − xGO alloys were obtained on a universal testing machine (Instron, USA) in compression mode with a loading speed of 0.5 mm/min. The stress-strain curves were recorded, from which the corresponding compression yield strengths were calculated. And six tests were performed for each group.

2.1.2.5　Cell Culture Tests

Human osteosarcoma MG-63 cells were used to study the in vitro cell response of the AZ61 − xGO alloys. MG-63 cells were incubated in Dulbecco's modified Eagle's medium (DMEM) (Gibco, Grand Island, USA) supplemented with 10% fetal bovine serum (FBS) (Gibco, Grand Island, USA), 100 U · mL^{-1} penicillin, and 100 mg · mL^{-1} streptomycin (BI, Kibbutz Beit-Haemek, Israel) at 37℃ in humidified atmosphere with 5% CO_2. Laser melted AZ61 − GO samples were separately soaked in DMEM with a surface area to extraction volume ratio of 1.25 cm^2 · mL^{-1} and then the extracts were collected. For Cell Counting Kit-8 (CCK-8) assay, the extracts were diluted at concentrations of 10%, 50%, and 100%, respectively, and the MG-63 cells were then incubated in the above diluted extracts for 1, 3, and 5 days. After incubation, the cells were digested and seeded in 96 − well plates with 1000 cells per well. After 6 h culture at 37℃ in 5% CO_2 incubator, the cells were incubated with 10 μL CCK-8 (5 mg/mL, Sigma-Aldrich, USA) for 2 h at 37℃, then the absorbance was measured at 450 nm by Paradigm Detection Platform (Beckman Coulter, USA). For cell viability, the MG-63 cells were incubated in the 100% extracts for 1, 3, and 5 days, and then cells were digested and seeded upon glass slide in 6 − well plates (5 × 10^3 cells per 100 mL). Afterwards, the cells upon glass slide were stained with Calcein-AM and Ethidium homodimer at 25℃ for 30 min and then visualized by a fluorescence microscope (BX50, Olympus, Japan). For morphological analysis, the AZ61 − GO samples were settled in 6 − well plates and 1 mL MG-63 cells suspensions were added in each well. After being cultured for 6 h, the samples were fixed with 2.5% glutaraldehyde for 1 h at room temperature, followed by washing twice in PBS solution and dehydrating in a graded series of ethanol (75% , 80% , 95% , and 100%). The samples were then dried with CO_2 and observed by SEM.

2. 1. 2. 6　Statistical Analysis

The experimental data were averaged from independent experiments and analyzed by using SPSS 19. 0 software. And Student's t-tests were carried out between different groups to calculate the values of p , which were significant when $p < 0.05$.

2. 1. 3　Results and Discussion

2. 1. 3. 1　Morphologies and Compositions

The morphologies and compositions of as-received and mixed powders were analyzed by SEM/ EDS (Fig. 2-1). It can be seen that the AZ61 powder presented uniform spherical particles with an average diameter of approximately 60 μm [Fig. 2-1 (b)]. The as-received GO in Fig. 2-1 (c) showed a thin and wrinkled texture with large surface area, which was beneficial for the formation of wrapping effect. The corresponding element composition [Fig. 2-1 (d)] indicated a C content of 67. 71% and a O content of 32. 29% , which were close to that of GO in many other studies. As for the mixed AZ61 – 1. 0GO powder [Fig. 2-1 (e)], GO was found to almost uniformly distributed among the AZ61 particles. It can be observed from the enlarged image in Fig. 2-1 (f) that GO were unbound and closely wrapped the AZ61 particles. The close and full wrapping implied a favorable affinity and effective protection of GO to AZ61 alloys. The GO wrapped AZ61 powder was further demonstrated by EDS line-scan analysis [Fig. 2-1 (g)] , which showed that the contents of C and O gradually decreased while that of Mg increased, as the scan path moved from GO to AZ61. These results demonstrated that GO could be uniformly dispersed and closely wrapped AZ61 particles in the mixed powders.

In order to investigate the distribution state of GO in the matrix after SLM, we studied the surface morphology of AZ61 – 1. 0GO alloy [Fig. 2-2 (a)]. And it can be seen that there were bright and dark phases on the surface as marked by red arrows. In order to reveal their compositions, detailed SEM-EDS studies were carried out to determine the element distribution across the interface (Line A and point B). There were gradual increases in both the C and O contents and a gradual decrease in the Mg content across the interface [Figs. 2-2 (b) and 2-2 (c)] , which suggested that the bright region was Mg phase and the dark region corresponded to GO. Moreover, good interfacial bonding was observed between GO and the Mg matrix without the formation of gaps or voids. To gain a global view of GO distribution, element map analysis [Figs. 2-2 (d)-2 (f)] was further conducted on the whole surface in Fig. 2-2 (a). It can be seen that C elements (referring to GO) mainly distributed at the dark area and Mg elements (referring to Mg matrix) at the bright area. More interestingly, C elements formed a honeycomb structure with Mg elements distributing in the honeycomb units. All of these findings indicated that GO wrapped the α- Mg grains along grain boundaries and formed a honeycomb nanostructure with a-Mg grains encapsulated in the honeycomb units after the SLM process.

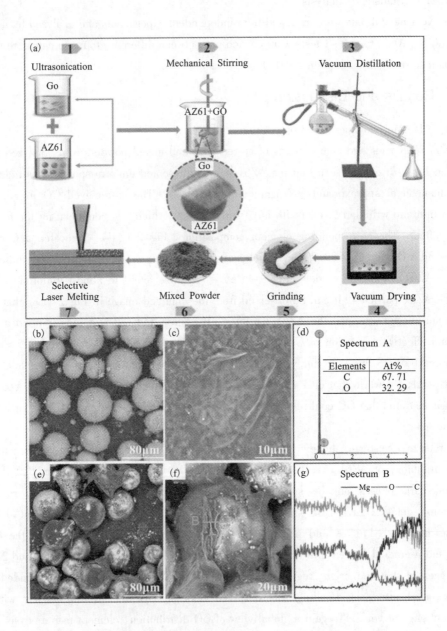

Fig. 2-1 (a) Schematic for the synthesis of AZ61 – xGO alloys, SEM images of (b) as-received AZ61 powder, (c) as-received GO, AZ61 – 1.0GO powder at (e) low-magnification and (f) high-magnification, the EDS results of (d) point A and (g) line B.

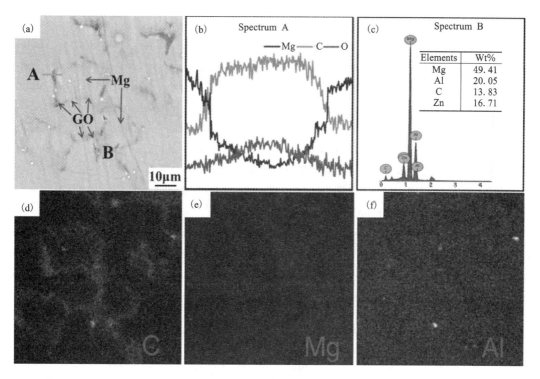

Fig. 2-2 (a) SEM image of the surface morphology of AZ61 – 1. 0GO alloy after SLM, EDS spectra of (b) line A and (c) point B, element maps of (d) C, (e) Mg, and (f) Al.

2.1.3.2   Corrosion Behavior

Given the outstanding anti-permeability of GO, the unique honeycomb nanostructure might play a very important role in improving the corrosion resistance of AZ61 alloys and a hypothetical schematic diagram was proposed in Figs. 2-3(a) – (c). For AZ61 alloys, the degradation process in SBF usually occurs via electrochemical reactions. On the one hand, α-Mg matrix reacts with the corrosion medium accompanying by hydrogen evolution [Fig. 2-3(a)]. And the reaction is shown in Equation (2-1):

$$\text{Mg} + 2\text{H}_2\text{O} \longrightarrow \text{Mg(OH)}_2 + \text{H}_2 \uparrow \qquad (2\text{-}1)$$

As a result, α-Mg is transferred into Mg(OH)_2 film [Fig. 2-3(b)]. However, the Mg(OH)_2 film is loose and porous, which is easily to fall off and can not hinder the continued infiltration of body fluids. On the other hand, the OH^- originating from Mg degradation can react with the HPO_4^{2-} in SBF according to Equation (2-2), resulting in the formation of PO_4^{3-}.

$$\text{HPO}_4^{2-} + \text{OH}^- \longrightarrow \text{PO}_4^{3-} + \text{H}_2\text{O} \qquad (2\text{-}2)$$

Afterwards, the PO_4^{3-} will bond with the Ca^{2+} in SBF or Mg^{2+} to form the compounds of hydroxyapatite or magnesium phosphate on the surface. However, the deposited compounds are not enough to construct a dense protective layer on the matrix surface. As the soaking continued, the body fluids can easily infiltrate the corrosion product layer and invade the fresh α-Mg matrix [Fig. 2-3(c)]. Therefore, these corrosion reactions will periodically continue and inevitably lead to the rapid degradation of AZ61 alloys.

For the honeycomb nanostructure encapsulated AZ61 – GO alloys, GO could play important roles in heterogeneous nucleation and grain refinement of α-Mg [Fig. 2-3(d)], which was bound to a better corrosion resistance than AZ61 alloy. As a result, the progress of α-Mg corrosion can be hindered by less generation of Mg(OH)$_2$ and hydrogen. Moreover, the rich oxygen-containing groups on GO can promote apatite deposition on the Mg matrix by providing beneficial sites for hydroxyapatite nucleation, which may lead to a dense apatite layer and hinder the further invasion of body fluids. More importantly, the GO in the corrosion layer and apatite layer can act as a reinforcement to impede them from falling off the matrix [(Fig. 2-3(e)]. After a tough fight, the corrosion layer and apatite layer will eventually fall off and the body fluids encounter the honeycomb nanostructure. It is known that the dense and stable honeycomb nanostructure can act as a protective shield to effectively isolate Mg matrix from the body fluids by virtue of the outstanding anti-permeability of GO [Fig. 2-3(f)]. Through the above synergetic mechanisms, the honeycomb nanostructure encapsulated AZ61 – GO alloys can be effectively protected against corrosion, leading to a step-by-step degradation process.

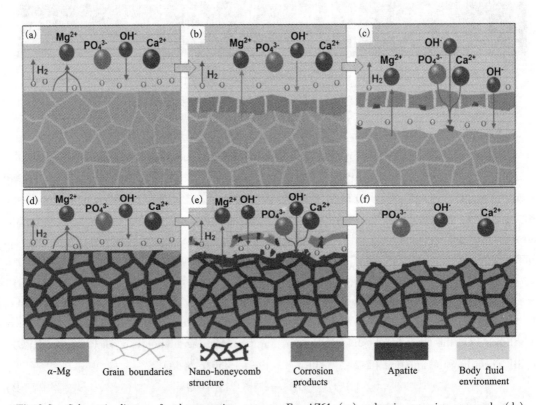

Fig. 2-3 Schematic diagram for the corrosion process: For AZ61 (a) galvanic corrosion occurred, (b) corrosion product formed on the surface, (c) solution invaded the inner fresh Mg matrix. For the honeycomb nanostructure encapsulated AZ61 – 1.0GO alloy: (d) galvanic corrosion occurred, (e) corrosion product and apatite formed on the surface, (f) GO acted as a tight protective fence covering α-Mg matrix.

In order to verify the hypothesis above, degradation tests were carried out to investigate the degradation properties of AZ61 and AZ61 –1.0GO alloys. Firstly, electrochemical tests were applied to investigate their degradation behaviors. The polarization curves were presented in Fig. 2-4 (a) and the E_{corr} and I_{corr} were calculated based on electrochemical curve were listed in Tab. 2-1. It can be seen that AZ61 –1.0GO alloy exhibited a slight shift in potential $[(-1.56 \pm 0.03)$ V] and a much lower current density $[(35 \pm 3)$ μA/cm^2] compared with those of AZ61 alloy $[-1.54 \pm 0.02)$ V and (50 ± 4) μA/cm^2, respectively]. And the P_i of AZ61 – GO alloys were calculated from electrochemical test curves using Tafel extrapolation. AZ61 –1.0GO alloy exhibited a much lower corrosion rate (0.76 mm/a) compared with those of AZ61 alloy (1.21 mm/a).

It was reported that the corrosion rates obtained by electrochemical tests were not in agreement with hydrogen evolution experiments. In order to better reveal the corrosion behavior of this magnesium alloy, immersion tests were also applied to investigate the long-term degradation behavior in terms of hydrogen evolution and weight loss tests (Fig. 2-4). For hydrogen evolution test, at the initial stage of immersion, many bubbles were observed arising from the surface of AZ61 alloy while little bubbles on AZ61 –1.0GO alloy. And furthermore, it could be seen that the total hydrogen evolution volume of AZ61 –1.0GO alloy at 360 h was 15.3 mL/cm^2, which was almost one half of that of AZ61 alloy (30.5 mL/cm^2), indicating a slower corrosion rate for AZ61 –1.0GO alloy. Moreover, the corrosion rates of the AZ61 and AZ61 –1.0GO alloys were also obtained according to weight loss test [Fig. 2-4(c)]. The results showed that AZ61 –1.0GO alloy exhibited the lower degradation rate (1.14 mm/a) than AZ61 alloy (1.65 mm/a).

In addition, the degradation morphology of AZ61 and AZ61 – 1.0GO alloys were also characterized by SEM/EDS, after immersion for 2 days. In general, AZ61 alloy presented a loose surface feature with many corrosion cracks in different sizes [Fig. 2-4(d)] while AZ61 –1.0GO alloy showed less corrosion cracks on the corrosion surface [Fig. 2-4(e)]. From the enlarged images [Figs. 2-4(f) and 2-4(g)], it could be seen that the cracks on the surface of AZ61 – 1.0GO alloy were narrower and deeper than those on AZ61 alloy. This phenomenon indicated more corrosion product formation and severer corrosion of AZ61 alloy than with AZ61 – 1.0GO alloy. More interestingly, a thin GO sheet (point C) was found to distribute across several cracks [Fig. 2-4(g)], indicating that GO could bridge the cracks in the corrosion layer and prevent it falling off the matrix. Moreover, there were many crystals on the surfaces of the two alloys, especially AZ61 – 1.0GO alloy [Figs. 2-4(d) and 2-4(e)]. EDS analysis at point A and B [Fig. 2-4(h)] showed the presence of Ca, P, and O elements and their atomic ratios on AZ61 –1.0GO alloy were higher than that on AZ61 alloy. This could ascribe to the rich oxygen-containing functional groups on GO, which promoted the deposition of apatite on AZ61 –1.0GO alloy and protected α-Mg matrix from the invasion of body fluids to some extents, thus the corrosion rate slowing down. In a word, all these results verified the proposed hypothesis of the honeycomb nanostructure in improving the corrosion resistance of AZ61 alloy.

In order to study the effect of GO content on the degradation behavior of AZ61 alloy, degradation tests were also carried out on AZ61 – xGO alloys. The resultant polarization curves and

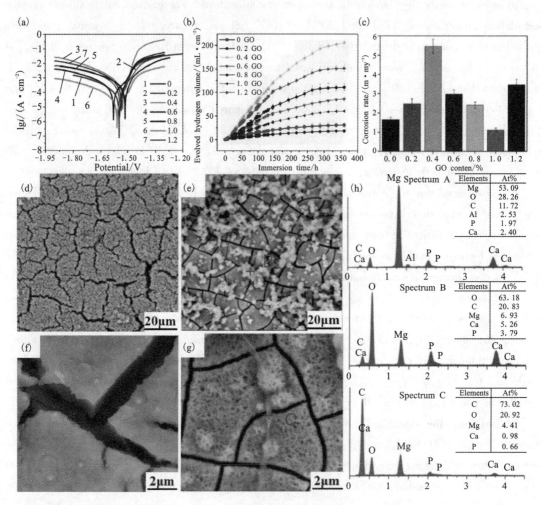

Fig. 2-4 (a) Polarization curves of AZ61 − xGO alloys by electrochemical tests; (b) Hydrogen evolution volume of AZ61 − xGO alloys by immersion tests; (c) Weight loss rate of AZ61 − xGO alloys after immersion in SBF solution for 360 h; The corrosion surfaces of (d), (f) AZ61 and (e), (g) AZ61 − 1.0GO alloys after immersion for 2 days; (h) EDS analysis of point A, B, and C.

electrochemical parameters were shown in Fig. 2-4 and Tab. 2-1, respectively. It was obvious that the corrosion current density of AZ61 − xGO alloys significantly increased from 50 to 212 μA/cm^2 with GO content increasing from 0 to 0.4%. However, with GO content further increasing, the corrosion current density gradually decreased and reached the lowest value 35 μA/cm^2 with GO content of 1.0%. Interestingly, with a further increase of GO content to 1.2%, the corrosion current density again increased to 135.16 μA/cm^2. And the corrosion rates of AZ61 − xGO alloys were calculated from electrochemical test curves using Tafel extrapolation (Tab. 2-1). The results showed that AZ61 − 1.0GO alloy exhibited the lowest degradation rate (0.76 mm/a) compared with those of AZ61 − xGO alloys. Moreover, the hydrogen evolution analysis also revealed similar phenomenon in the corrosion rates of AZ61 − xGO alloys. Specifically, the corrosion rates remarkably increased from 31.03 mL/cm^2 for AZ61 alloy to 205.23 mL/cm^2 for AZ61 − 0.4GO alloy, then gradually decreased to 15.03 mL/cm^2 for AZ61 − 1.0GO alloy, but increased again to 65.25 mL/cm^2 for AZ61 − 1.2GO alloy. The corrosion rates of the AZ61 − xGO alloys were also obtained according to weight loss test [Fig. 2-4(c)]. It could be seen that the values of corrosion rate were different between the electrochemical tests, which was also reported by Song G et al. But the corrosion rates showed basically the same trend with the variation of GO content in the two tests. These results demonstrated that, despite the improvement in corrosion resistance by the honeycomb nanostructure, GO content had an important influence on the degradation behaviors of AZ61 − xGO alloys.

Tab. 2-1　Corrosion parameters from the polarization curves

Composion	E_{corr}(V vs. SCE)	$I_{corr}/(\mu A \cdot cm^{-2})$	$P_i/(mm \cdot a^{-1})$
AZ61	− 1.54 ± 0.02	50 ± 4	1.21 ± 0.09
AZ61 − 0.2GO	− 1.54 ± 0.02	89 ± 12	2.03 ± 0.27
AZ61 − 0.4GO	− 1.52 ± 0.03	212 ± 16	4.84 ± 0.36
AZ61 − 0.6GO	− 1.57 ± 0.02	118 ± 13	2.67 ± 0.30
AZ61 − 0.8GO	− 1.51 ± 0.02	85 ± 6	1.94 ± 0.14
AZ61 − 1.0GO	− 1.56 ± 0.03	35 ± 3	0.76 ± 0.07
AZ61 − 1.2GO	− 1.53 ± 0.02	135 ± 15	3.08 ± 0.34

In order to reveal the reasons for the changes of degradation rates at different GO contents, the surface morphologies of AZ61 − xGO alloys were studied by SEM (Fig. 2-5). It could be seen that island-like phases homogeneously distributed in AZ61 alloy [Fig. 2-5 (a)] and EDS results demonstrated that they were Mg-Al intermetallic phases [Fig. 2-5(h)]. As for AZ61 − GO alloys (Figs. 5b-5g), GO was found to locate at the grain boundaries of the matrix, which have been confirmed in Fig. 2-2. As a result, severe galvanic corrosion would occur between α-Mg grains and the GO at grain boundaries. Thus, the degradation rates of AZ61 − 0.2GO and AZ61 − 0.4GO alloys compared with AZ61 alloy. As GO content increased, GO gradually wrapped a-Mg grains and impeded the contact between the matrix and body fluid to some extent, partially reducing the effects of galvanic corrosion and further the degradation rates of AZ61 − 0.6GO and 0.8GO alloys in comparison with AZ61 − 0.4GO alloy. A honeycomb nanostructure wrapping the α-Mg grains was presented with GO content of 1.0% [Fig. 2-5(f)]. This honeycomb nanostructure may play a vital role in preventing the permeation of body fluid and the galvanic corrosion between GO and the matrix. Therefore, the slowest degradation rate was obtained for the honeycomb nanostructure-encapsulated AZ61 alloy. With further increasing GO content to 1.2%, GO agglomerates were observed at the grain boundaries, which can be ascribed to the high surface area and van der waals force in GO [Fig. 2-5 (g)]. This inevitably caused structural damage to the honeycomb

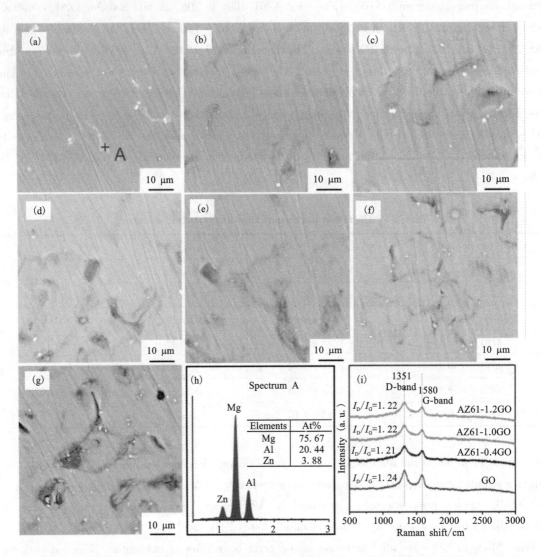

Fig. 2-5 SEM images of the surface morphologies of (a) AZ61 alloy, (b) AZ61 – 0.2GO alloy, (c) AZ61 – 0.4GO alloy, (d) AZ61 – 0.6GO alloy, (e) AZ61 – 0.8GO alloy, (f) AZ61 – 1.0GO alloy, and (g) AZ61 – 1.2GO alloy, respectively, (h) EDS results of point A, (i) Raman spectra of the as-received GO and AZ61 – xGO alloys.

nanostructure and accelerated the permeation of body fluid and galvanic corrosion. To investigate the structural changes of GO during SLM, Raman spectra were recorded on the as-received GO and AZ61 – xGO alloys. As shown in Fig. 2-5(i), the as-received GO exhibited two typical peaks at 1351 cm^{-1} and 1580 cm^{-1}, which corresponded to the vibration of carbon atoms with dangling bonds at the in-plane terminations of disordered graphite (D-band) and the sp^2 bonded carbon atoms in the 2D hexagonal lattice (G-band) of GO, respectively. After SLM, it could be observed that these two bands in the spectra of AZ61 – xGO alloys with no shifting, indicating the existence of GO in the alloys. It is well known that the relative intensity ratio of D-band to G-band (I_D/I_G) can provide information regarding the internal quality of GO. Therefore, the I_D/I_C values of AZ61 − xGO alloys were calculated and the results showed little changes, implying the structural integrity of GO after the SLM process. These findings demonstrated that GO could survive in the SLM process and GO content played an important role in the distribution and subsequent formation of honeycomb nanostructure in Mg matrix. And only at a critical value, the honeycomb nanostructure-encapsulated AZ61 alloys could be obtained.

2.1.3.3　Mechanical Properties

In addition, the grain structure of AZ61 − xGO alloys was also studied by optical microscopy after polishing and etching (Fig. 2-6). It could be seen that AZ61 − xGO alloys consisted of primary

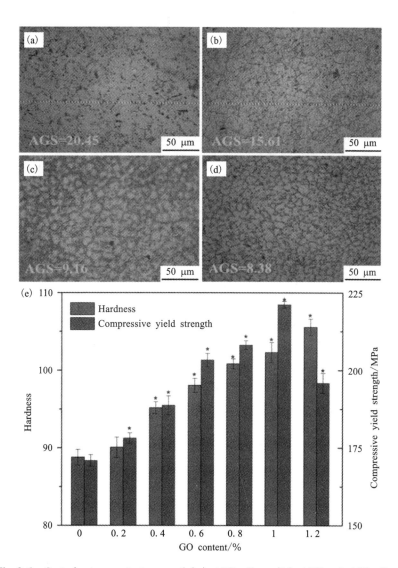

Fig. 2-6　Optical microscopic images of (a) AZ61 alloy, (b) AZ61 − 0.4GO alloy, (c) AZ61 − 1.0GO alloy, and (d) AZ61 − 1.2GO alloy. (e) The hardness and compressive yield strength of AZ61 − xGO alloys. $^*p < 0.05$.

α-Mg matrix and the grain size gradually decreased with GO content increasing. The average grain size (AGS) of AZ61 – xGO alloys was further determined by the linear intercept method. And it clearly showed that the AGS rapidly decreased from 20.45 μm for AZ61 alloy to 9.16 μm for AZ61 – 1.0GO and slightly decreased to 8.38 μm for AZ61 – 1.2GO alloy (Figs. 2-6(a) – 2-6(d)), indicating the grain refining effect of GO on AZ61 alloys.

Furthermore, hardness and compressive yield strength were tested to study the effect of GO on the mechanical properties of AZ61 – xGO alloys [Fig. 2-6(e)]. The hardness of AZ61 – xGO alloys was found to increase from 88.78 to 108.52 with GO content increasing to 1.2%, which might be ascribed to the grain refining effect and high strength of GO. In addition, it was obvious that the compressive yield strength enhanced gradually with GO content increasing from 0 to 1.0%. Subsequently, the strength declined when GO content further increased to 1.2% and achieved the peak value with 1.0% GO. The maximum compressive yield strength reached 221.05 MPa for AZ61 – 1.0GO alloy, which increased by 30% compared with those of AZ61 alloy without GO. The mechanical improvement could be attributed to the grain refinement and stress transfer from the Mg matrix to GO. It was reported that a refined grain structure was beneficial for the mechanical improvement of Mg alloys. Moreover, the SEM/EDS analysis had revealed good and sufficient interfacial bonding between GO and Mg matrix due to the favorable affinity and large specific surface area. As a result, the stress could be transferred from the matrix to GO under loading. The high-stress region would be released and transferred to other regions, thereby enhancing the loading resistance of the alloys. On the other hand, excessive GO was difficult to disperse uniformly and might form agglomerate structure and/or some inner flaws in the matrix. This would inevitably weaken the interface bonding between GO and the matrix and cause stress concentration, resulting in the impairment of the mechanical properties of AZ61 – xGO alloys.

2.1.3.4　Cell Response

To further evaluate the cell response of AZ61 – 1.0GO alloy, in vitro cell culture experiments were conducted by using MG-63 cells and AZ61 alloy served as a control [Fig. 2-7(a)]. It was worth noting that, MG-63 cells attached and spread out on the alloy surfaces, and the MG-63 cells on AZ61 – 1.0 alloy presented more flattened morphology and pseudopodia compared with those on AZ61 alloy. The better adhesion state can be ascribed to the slower corrosion and subsequent slower pH increase, which was believed to have a great influence on cell adhesion and growth. In addition, MG-63 cells were cultured in 100% extracts of these two alloys for 1, 3, and 5 days, respectively, and characterized by fluorescent staining [Fig. 2-7(b)]. It could be seen that the live cells were fusiform shape on both of AZ61 – 1.0GO and AZ61 alloys at 1st day, suggesting normal cell growth. After 3 days' culture, the cells in AZ61 – 1.0GO extract developed abundant filopodia and more cells were observed compared with those in AZ61 extract. As the culture time extended to 5 days, a larger number of cells were observed in AZ61 – 1.0GO extract than AZ61 extract due to active cell proliferation. The cell morphology and fluorescence images indicated that GO incorporation could improve the adhesion and growth of MG-63 cells on AZ61 alloy. To quantitatively evaluate the cell viability, CCK-8 assay was also carried out in different extracts [Fig. 2-7(c)]. In the 100%

extracts, a higher optic density was observed in AZ61 – 1.0GO extract compared with AZ61 extract. Moreover, the optic density increased as the culture time extended from 1 day to 5 days, which revealed that MG-63 cells proliferated in culture. Meanwhile, the extracts were diluted to 50% and 10% and increased cell viability and similar trends were obtained in comparison with the results in 100% extracts after dilution. These results indicated that the cell response of AZ61 alloy was improved with the incorporation of GO.

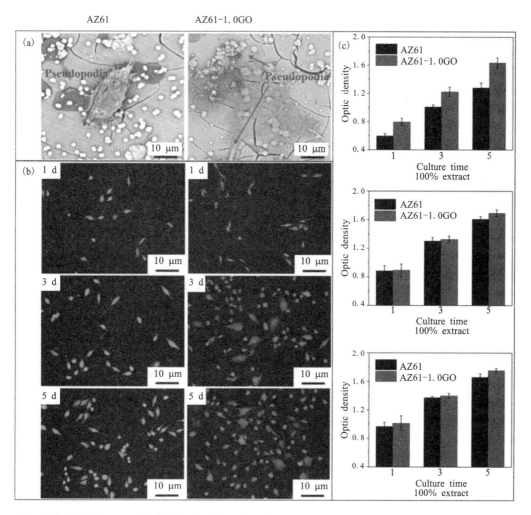

Fig. 2-7　SEM images of (a) MG-63 cells cultured on AZ61 and AZ61 – 1.0GO alloys for 6 h, (b) Fluorescent images of MG-63 cells cultured in 100% extracts for 1, 3, and 5 days, (c) Cell viability in different extracts for 1, 3, and 5 days by CCK-8 assay.

2.1.4　Conclusions

GO was incorporated into AZ61 alloy to fabricate honeycomb nanostructure-encapsulated Mg alloys.

（1）GO was found to distribute at the grain boundaries and gradually wrapped the α-Mg grains. And a honeycomb nanostructure was formed with α-Mg grains encapsulated in the honeycomb units with GO content of 1.0%.

（2）GO existing in the corrosion layer prevented it falling off the Mg matrix by bridging effect. The oxygen-containing groups on GO promoted the deposition of apatite and impeded the intrusion of corrosive medium.

（3）Compared with AZ61 alloy, the AZ61 – xGO alloys generally showed accelerated corrosion, except for the AZ61 – 1.0GO alloy which exhibited a slower corrosion due to the effective protection of the honeycomb nanostructure.

（4）The hardness of AZ61 – xGO alloys was found to increase with GO content increasing and the compressive yield strength reached a maximum value of 221.05 MPa for AZ61 – 1.0GO alloy.

（5）MG-63 cells were found to adhere and spread well on AZ61 – 1.0GO alloy and showed better cytocompatibility in comparison with AZ61 alloy.

2.2　Regulating Degradation Behavior by Incorporating Mesoporous Silica for Mg Bone Implants

2.2.1　Introduction

Mg and its alloys have been proposed as promising bone implant materials because of their natural biodegradability, good biocompatibility, and suitable mechanical properties. Mg can degrade in the human body in the form of corrosion, thus avoiding the second surgery. Meanwhile, Mg is necessary element in human body with a daily intake of $250 \sim 300$ mg and is naturally stored in the bones. Furthermore, Mg and its alloys possess similar Young's modulus of ($41 \sim 55$ GPa) and density ($1.7 \sim 1.9$ g/cm^3) to these of human bone ($15 \sim 25$ GPa and $1.8 \sim 2.1$ g/cm^3), which effectively prevents the stress shielding effect. Nevertheless, Mg alloys urgently demand an adjustable degradation to meet the requirement for bone repairing application, because their degradation rates are too rapid to provide enough time for bone healing (at least 12 weeks).

The main reasons for the rapid degradation of Mg alloys can be ascribe to (1) the low corrosion potential (standard corrosion potential -2.37 V) which makes it extremely easy to be corroded in the physiological environment; (2) the incompact corrosion product layer mainly consisted of $Mg(OH)_2$ which results in continuous corrosion. To address these issues, extensive efforts have been done to enhance the corrosion resistance of Mg by alloying with inert noble elements or surface modifications. However, most of the alloying elements have very limit solid solution in α-Mg and their intermetallic compounds prefer to form negative galvanic corrosion against α-Mg. On the other hand, surface modification only offer a solution for delaying the start of corrosion and rapid corrosion usually takes place once the modified surface breaks down.

Recently, mesoporous silica (MS) has received intensive attentions in bone tissue engineering because of its unique intrinsic structure with large specific surface area and pore volume. Previous studies revealed that increasing the specific surface area and pore volume significantly accelerated the kinetic process of apatite deposition. This motivates us to hypothesize that an enhanced apatite deposition rate may be achieved if MS was incorporated into Mg alloys. And the apatite layer covered on Mg matrix may offer more effective protections as compared with $Mg(OH)_2$ layer. On the other hand, it is possible to enhance the surface passivation through compositing Mg alloys with electrochemical inactive MS. Furthermore, silicon is a necessary element in human body. It plays a key role in aiding the bone healing process, as well as the construction of the immune system.

In this work, for the first time, MS was incorporated in Mg-6Zn-0.5Zr (ZK60) alloy by using selective laser melting (SLM) technology. SLM was a typical additive manufacturing technology, which could fabricate complicated parts that was difficult to produce using traditional manufacturing process. Meanwhile, SLM involved a rapid cooling rate over 1×10^5 K/s during solidification, thus preventing the growth of grains and reducing the composition segregation. And the finer grains and homogeneous microstructure were believed to be favorable for enhancing the mechanical properties and degradation resistance. ZK60 was selected basing on its excellent mechanical strength and good cytocompatibility. The degradation behavior, microstructures evolution and in vitro cell responses of SLM processed Mg-based composites were studied in depth.

2.2.2　Materials and Methods

2.2.2.1　Material and Sample Fabrication

The original materials included spherical ZK60 powder ($30 \sim 60$ μm, 99.9% purity) and the stick shaped MS ($1 \sim 5$ μm). ZK60 powder was purchased from Tangshan Weihao Materials Co., Ltd. (Tangshan, China). And MS with pore diameter of $5 \sim 10$ nm and specific surface area of $550 \sim 600$ m^2/g was obtained from Nanjing XFNANO Materials Tech Co., Ltd. (Nanjing, China). These two kinds of powder were mixed homogeneously using a ball mill at a rotation speed of 260 rpm for 4 h. Ar gas was used during milling to avoid the oxidation.

The homemade SLM system consisted of a fiber laser with a maximal power of 500 W, a spot diameter of 50 μm, a working platform and a computer system. The samples were fabricated by a layer-by-layer method. As a layer was deposited via high-energy laser melting, another layer was created just on top of the previous one. The SLM process parameters including laser power and scanning rate determined the laser energy density. And too high laser energy density caused the burning of Mg, whereas low laser energy caused the partial melting of the Mg powder, thus reducing the density of the fabricated samples. Moreover, laser beam spot and hatch spacing had a significant effect on the accuracy of the fabricated samples. Therefore, it was important to get the optimal parameters. After a series of preliminary experiments, cubic samples (6 mm ×6 mm ×6 mm) were fabricated using the SLM system with optimal processing parameters: laser power of 120 W, spot size of 50 μm, layer thickness of 100 μm, hatch spacing of 40 μm, and scan speed of 20 mm/s. Ar gas was used to provide a protective atmosphere during SLM. The SLM processed Mg-based composites in this study had a nominal MS contents with 4%, 8%, or 12%. These composites were designated as ZK60/4MS, ZK60/8MS, and ZK60/12MS, respectively, with MS content increasing.

2.2.2.2　Microstructural Characterizations

The SLM processed samples were polished with SiC abrasive paper and chemically etched using a picric acid solution. Then the microstructures were observed utilizing an optical microscope (Leica DM500, Germany) and a scanning electron microscopy (SEM, QUANTA FEG250, USA) equipped with energy dispersive spectroscopy (EDS, JSM-5910LV, Japan). The relative density of the SLM samples was investigated by measuring the porosity.

The phase compositions were analyzed by an X-ray diffractometer (XRD, D8 Advance, Bruker AXS Inc., Germany) in a small angle range from 0 to 6° with a scan rate 2°/min. Surface hydrophilicity of SLM processed ZK60/MS was investigated using a contact angle analyzer (DSA100, Germany).

2.2.2.3　Electrochemical Tests

The electrochemical properties of SLM processed ZK60/MS in simulated body fluid (SBF, 37℃, pH 7.4) were investigated using an electrochemical workstation (CHI604D, China). The SBF consisted of 8.035 g/L NaCl, 0.355 g/L NaHCO$_3$, 0.225 g/L KCl, 0.231 g/L K$_2$HPO$_4$ · 3H$_2$O, 0.311 g/L MgCl$_2$ · 6H$_2$O, and 0.292 g/L CaCl$_2$. A flat cell and ZK60/MS samples were used as the standard setup and working electrode, respectively. While a platinum sheet and Ag/AgCl electrode (in saturated KCl) were used as counter electrode and reference electrode, respectively. An open circuit potential of ZK60/MS samples was achieved before recording the potential dynamic polarization curves. Three repetitions were tested for each group.

2.2.2.4　Immersion Tests

Immersion tests were performed in SBF (37℃, pH 7.4) at a surface area to volume ratio of 0.1 cm^2/mL without changing the SBF. At specific immersion time, soaked specimens were removed from SBF and the corresponding ion concentrations (Ca, P) in SBF were determined utilizing inductively coupled plasma-atomic emission spectroscopy (ICP-AES, Thermo Elemental, USA). Meanwhile, the pH values of the SBF were detected during immersion. Meanwhile, the corrosion surfaces were studied by SEM after soaking for 1 week.

Weight loss method was used to quantitatively assess the corrosion rate. After immersion for 1 week, samples were removed from SBF. The weight losses were measured after removing the corrosion products. The corrosion rates were calculated by (2-3):

$$C = W/(DAt) \tag{2-1}$$

Where C referred to the corrosion rate (mm/a), W was the weight loss of the samples (g), D denoted to the standard density (g/mm^3), A indicated the exposure area (mm^2), and t was the soaking time (year).

2.2.2.5　In Vitro Cell Tests

Human osteoblast-like MG-63 cells (ATCC, Rockville, MD, USA) were used for the in vitro cell tests. DMEM supplemented with 10% fetal bovine serum, 100 U/mL penicillin and 100 mg/mL streptomycin was used as culture medium. SLM processed ZK60/MS composites were soaked in culture medium for 3 days to prepare the extracts with the exposure area to solution volume ratio of 1.25 cm^2/mL.

An indirect contact method was used to study the cell viability. MG-63 cells were seeded in a 96 – well plate at a density of 5×10^3 cells/mL with 100 μL of culture medium for each well and then cultured for 24 h. The culture medium was then substituted with 100 μL of prepared extracts. After culture for 1, 3, and 5 days, respectively, 10 μL of Cell Counting Kit-8 (CCK-8) solution was added to each well and incubated for 2 h at 37℃. Afterward, the absorbance was determined at 450 nm by a paradigm detection platform (BECK MAN, CA).

Direct Cell Adhesion Assay. MG-63 cells were directly seeded on the specimens, which were set in 24 – well plates, with a density of 1×10^4 cells per well. Then the cells were cultured for 6 h, 1 and 3 days, respectively. Subsequently, the cells were rinsed gently with phosphate buffered solution (PBS, Grand Island Biological Co., USA) and then stained using Calcein-AM and Ethidium homodimer-1 reagents for 15 min. Afterward, the samples were rinsed gently with PBS twice, and then fixed on glass slides to observe the cell morphology using a fluorescence microscopy (BX60, Olympus, Japan).

2.2.2.6　Statistical Analysis

Each group of experiments was repeated at least three times. And the obtained data were expressed as the mean ± standard error. Student's t test was utilized to determine the level of significance. Differences were considered significanly with a $p < 0.05$.

2.2.3　Results and Discussion

2.2.3.1　Microstructure Evolutions

The surfaces of the SLM processed ZK60/MS samples were grinded and corroded, and then the microstructure was observed by an optical microscope, as presented in Fig. 2-8. SLM-processed ZK60 consisted of fine equiaxed grains, with few MgZn second phase precipitated at grain boundaries. For ZK60/4MS and ZK60/8MS, a small amount of irregular reinforced particles with a size of $1 \sim 3$ μm, as marked by red arrows in Fig. 2-8(b), (c), uniformly distributed within Mg matrix. Nevertheless, with MS increasing to 12%, a fraction of reinforced particles aggregated into clusters in local areas in the Mg matrix. And some small-sized pores appeared in the matrix, as indicated in Fig. 2-8(d), leading to a visible decrease in density. Such an agglomeration of reinforced particles also occurred in other Mg based composites processed by powder metallurgy and casting.

For SLM processed Mg-based parts, the densification rate was a key factor which influenced the degradation behaviors and mechanical properties. Therefore, the relative density of SLM processed ZK60/MS composites was studied by measuring the porosity, with results depicted in Fig. 2-9. SLM processed ZK60 obtained a nearly full density of 98.3% ± 0.8%. After the incorporation of MS particles, ZK60/4MS and ZK60/8MS still maintained a high-level relative density of 97.2% ± 1.4% and 96.4% ±2.4%, respectively. But a dramatic reduce of relative density to 81.5 ±7.1% occurred with MS content increasing to 12%, which was significantly lower than that of ZK60. It was suggested that excessive incorporation of MS deteriorated the densification behavior of SLM processed ZK60/MS composites, which was consistent with the previous analysis of optical

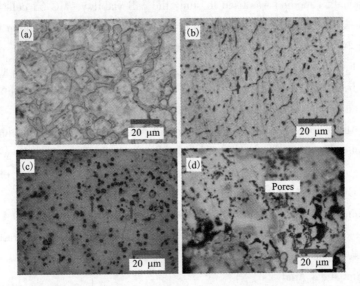

Fig. 2-8 Typical optical microstructures of the SLMed ZK60 composited with different nominal MS contents. (a) ZK60, (b) ZK60/4MS, (c) ZK60/8MS and (d) ZK60/12MS. As the addition amounts of MS reached 12%, segregation occurred, resulting in the formation of pores in matrix.

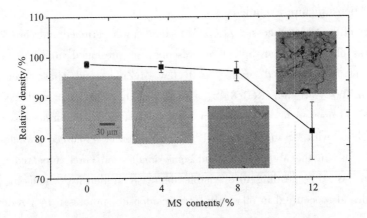

Fig. 2-9 Measured relative density of SLMed ZK60/MS composites plotted against MS contents. Insets shown the cross-section microstructure of ZK60/MS obtained by SEM. The scale bar represented 30 μm for all the insets. Values were expressed as mean ± error, $n = 3$.

microstructures. In general, during SLM process, the metal particles (ZK60) fully melt into liquid phase, whereas the incorporated MS particles with a relative high melting point maintained in solid phase. Nevertheless, excessive solid particles tended to gathered together and limited the flow of liquid phase to a certain extent, thus reducing the densification rate of Mg matrix.

On the other hand, the particle distribution state in Mg matrix also exerted a great effect on the overall performance for SLM processed ZK60/MS. Therefore, the microstructure of the SLM processed ZK60/8MS composite was further investigated by using both optical microscope and backscatter electron (BSE) imaging, with results presented in Fig. 2-10. Lamellar particles with relatively bright gray scale were observed homogeneously distributed in Mg matrix [Fig. 2-10(b)]. The corresponding EDS elemental mapping demonstrated that these particles were rich in Si element. EDS analysis of over five regions on the lamellar particles revealed that the average atomic ratio of the particles was close to that of silica, which confirmed that the homogeneously distributed lamellar particles were MS. Meanwhile, the EDS analysis revealed that 3.42% Zn dissolved in α-Mg matrix with only few MgZn precipitation, developing a super saturated solid solution. Furthermore, there were no obvious gaps and cracks at the two-phase interface, indicating a formation of compact bonding interface between α-Mg matrix and MS particles, as shown in Fig. 2-10(b4). A compact bonding interface was believed to be favorable for the mechanical behavior of the composite. Gu et al. revealed that a steep temperature gradient and a sufficient flowability within the molten pool during SLM process resulted in Marangoni convection, which in turn led to the movement and

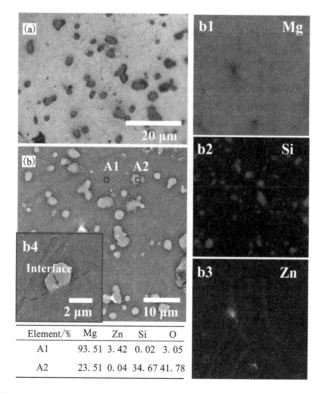

Element/%	Mg	Zn	Si	O
A1	93.51	3.42	0.02	3.05
A2	23.51	0.04	34.67	41.78

Fig. 2-10   Optical microscopy and BSE micrographs of the SLMed ZK60/8MS: (a) optical micrograph and (b) corresponding BSE image showing the distribution state of MS particles in Mg matrix; (b1 – b3) EDS mapping of element distribution for Mg, Si and Zn, respectively. (b4) compact bonding interface formed between the MS particle and α-Mg matrix.

rearrangement of solid reinforced particles. Under this circumstance, the reinforced particles were fully wetted by the liquid phase, and resultantly distributed uniformly within molten pool. Subsequently, the molten pool underwent a rapid solidification and maintained the homogeneous dispersion state of solid particles, as well as a compact bonding interface.

2.2.3.2　Phase Composition and Surface Hydrophilicity

The small-angle XRD patterns of ZK60 powder, MS powder, ZK60/8MS mixed powders, and SLM-processed ZK60/8MS composite were obtained, as depicted in Fig. 2-11. The insets in Fig. 2-11 showed the morphologies of ZK60 and MS powders. Clearly, no diffraction peaks were detected in ZK60 powder. While a strong characteristic peak at about 1.1° (100), as well as relative weak peaks at about 1.6° (110) and 1.8° (120) were detected in MS powder, which revealed that MS possessed a highly ordered mesoporous structure. For ZK60/8MS mixed powders, the diffraction peak at 1.1° (110) turned weak due to a low content of MS. More importantly, the characteristic peak (100) at 1.1° still presented in SLM processed ZK60/8MS composite and maintained the peak intensity as compared with ZK60/8MS mixed powders. These results indicated that SLM process with a rapid melting and rapid solidification had not wrecked the ordered mesoporous structure of the incorporated MS.

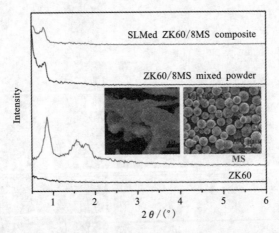

Fig. 2-11　Small angle XRD patterns of ZK60, MS, ZK60/8MS
mixed powder and SLMed ZK60/8MS composite.

The surface hydrophilicity of SLM-processed ZK60/MS composites was studied using contact angle measurement, with results depicted in Fig. 2-12. The water contact angle of SLM processed ZK60 was 81.6° ±2.4°, which was very close to that of the previously reported Mg alloys. And the water contact angle on ZK60/MS composites was gradually reduced to 50.8° ±4.1° and 41.2° ± 8.4° with MS content increasing to 8% and 12%, respectively, indicating that incorporating MS improved the surface hydrophilicity. Surface hydrophilicity depended on surface chemical composition and surface microtexture. After the incorporation of MS, a large amount of MS particles were homogeneously exposed to the surface (Fig. 2-8), which clearly altered the surface chemical composition and surface micro texture. Specifically, the exposed MS particles with high specific surface area and pore volume were beneficial to absorb water. On the other hand, the silanol functional groups exposed on MS particles could attract water molecules by hydrogen bonding. For biomaterials, an improved surface hydrophilicity was useful for them to absorb nutrients and bioactive factors as implanted in vivo, thus potentially aiding bone healing as implants.

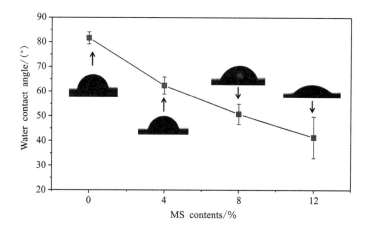

Fig. 2-12　Water contact angle on surface of SLMed ZK60/MS, which significantly decreased with MS content increasing. Insets were the typical water contact photograph for ZK60/MS samples. Values were expressed as mean ± error, $n = 3$.

2.2.3.3　Degradation Behavior

Electrochemical tests were conducted to investigate the surface passivation of SLM processed ZK60/MS samples. The potentiodynamic polarization curves of polished ZK60/MS samples in SBF at 37℃ were depicted in Fig. 2-13(a). And the corresponding electrochemical parameters obtained from Tafel extrapolation of the potentiodynamic polarization curves were presented in Fig. 2-13(b). SLM processed ZK60 exhibited a relative low corrosion potential (Ecorr) of (−1.59 ±0.04) V. After incorporating with MS, the Ecorr was enhanced to −1.52 to −1.40 V. And the Ecorr values of ZK60/MS samples changed positively with MS content increasing. Furthermore, the corrosion current densities (I_{corr}) of the ZK60/4MS [(21.86 ±2.42) $\mu A/cm^2$] and ZK60/8MS [(14.63 ± 3.95) $\mu A/cm^2$] were considerably smaller than that of ZK60 [(31.24 ±4.21) $\mu A/cm^2$]. In general, an enhanced Ecorr indicated an improved corrosion resistance of the surface. And a decreased I_{corr} represented a reduced corrosion rate once the surface was broken down by pitting corrosion. Thus, it was reasonable to deduce that ZK60/8MS possessed an improved anticorrosion ability, basing on a comprehensive consideration of its more positive Ecorr and smaller I_{corr}. Similar enhanced surface passivation of Mg-based composites was also found in the investigation of the electrochemical properties of Mg-Zn-Mn alloy and β-TCP reinforced Mg-Zn-Mn metal matrix composite.

Immersion experiments were carried out to investigate the corrosion behavior in vitro in term of a

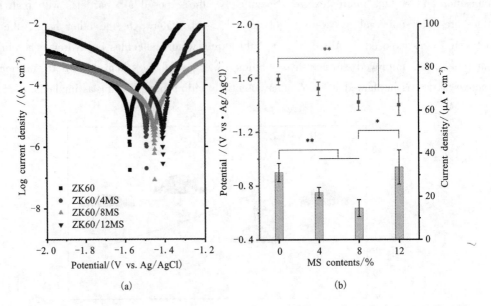

Fig. 2-13　Electrochemical testing results of SLMed ZK60/MS samples. (a) potentiodynamic polarization curves; (b) Ecorr and I_{corr} derived from Tafel extrapolation of potentiodynamic polarization curves; values were expressed as mean ± error, $n = 3$, $^*p < 0.05$, $^{**}p < 0.01$.

long period. The variations of pH values in the SBF were depicted in Fig. 2-14(a), after soaking ZK60/MS for various periods. For all the samples, the pH of SBF rose rapidly in the initial 2 days, then slowly rose and eventually stabilized. Clearly, the rapid degradation of Mg matrix and resultant release of OH⁻ ions should be responsible for the rapidly increased pH value. With the degradation proceeding, much corrosion products covered on the surface, which in turn prevented the degradation as a protective layer. Thus, the change rate of pH value slowed down after a period. It should be noted that the pH value obtained from ZK60/8MS stabilized at 8.6 after 7 days' immersion, which was a statistically significant lower pH value ($p < 0.01$) than ZK60. Furthermore, weight loss method was used for a quantitative analysis of the degradation rate. ZK60/8MS exhibited a significantly reduced degradation rate of (0.67 ±0.15) mm/a, as compared with ZK60 with a degradation rate of (1.57 ±0.21) mm/a [Fig. 2-14(b)]. These results indicated that an incorporation of moderate amount of MS (8%) into ZK60 effectively improved corrosion behavior with a reduced degradation rate. One had to, however, note that the corrosion rate of ZK60/MS composite was sharply increased to (2.21 ±0.38) mm/a with MS increasing up to 12%, because the negative effect of poor densification rate on corrosion behavior gained the upper hand.

According to the above results, ZK60/8MS exhibited an optimal degradation behavior. Thus, the variations of ion concentrations in SBF soaking ZK60/8MS and ZK60 (as control) were further investigated by ICP experiments, in order to have a deep understanding of the degradation characteristics. Results showed that both Ca and P ion concentrations reduced as soaking time extending, as shown in Fig. 2-14 (c). Similarly, at the initial 2 days, the Ca and P ion

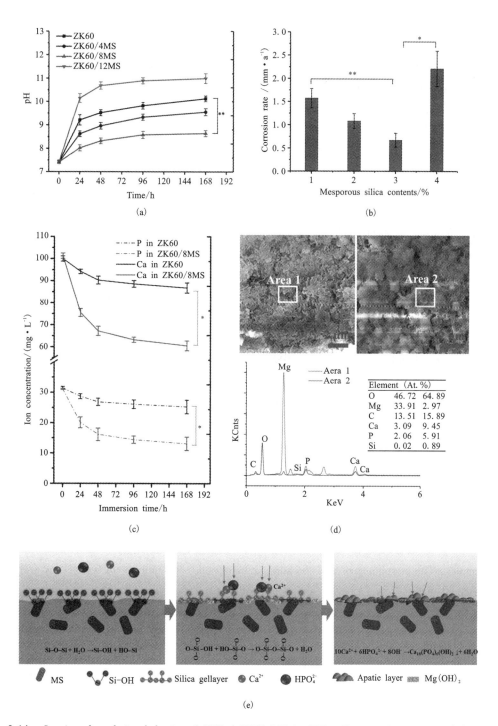

Fig. 2-14　In vitro degradation behavior of SLMed ZK60/MS in SBF. Changes of pH values (a) and ion concentrations (c) in SBF during immersion of ZK60/MS for 7 days; (b) the degradation rate obtained by weight loss method; Values were expressed as mean ± error, $n = 3$, $^{*}p < 0.05$, $^{**}p < 0.01$. (d) the surface of soaked ZK60 and ZK60/8MS in SBF after 7 days, and corresponding EDS results showing the compositions of the degradation products; (e) schematic diagram showed the deposition of apatite on ZK60/MS.

concentrations decreased fast. The they decreased slowly and eventually stabilized at a specific value. Remarkably, the Ca and P ion concentrations in SBF of ZK60/8MS exhibited a faster decrease rate than ZK60. The surface morphologies of ZK60/8MS and ZK60 after immersion in SBF for 7 days were presented in Fig. 2-14(d). For ZK60, the surface was covered by much $Mg(OH)_2$ with a typically rough and loose structure, indicating that it experienced a serious corrosion. Distinctively, ZK60/8MS sample was covered by many deposits with needle-shape, which was a typical morphology of bone-like apatite. The corresponding EDS results also revealed that the deposits were mainly composites of O, C, Ca and P with a Ca/P ratio of -1.6, also indicating the formation of bone-like apatite. Combining the changes of Ca and P ion concentrations and surface morphology, it was reasonable to conclude that the incorporation of MS particles facilitated the apatite formation on the ZK60/MS surface.

The schematic diagram of the deposition of apatite layer on ZK60/MS was depicted in Fig. 2-14 (e). Initially, soluble silica dissolved along with the cleavage of Si—O—Si bond, which led to the formation of silanols (Si—OH) on the MS/solution interface. Then the silanols underwent condensation and formed a silica gel layer on the surface. In alkaline environment, the silica-rich gel layer was charged negatively. Thus, Ca^{2+} and HPO_4^{2-} were attracted to the silica-rich gel layer in turn. Such a migration of Ca^{2+} and HPO_4^{2-} groups to the silica-rich gel layer facilitated the formation of amorphous calcium phosphate layer, which subsequently crystallized into bone-like apatite layer. Significantly, the apatite layer exhibited a denser structure than $Mg(OH)_2$, as shown in Fig. 2-14(d). Thus, a reduced corrosion rate was obtained for ZK60/8MS, because the compact apatite layer acted as a more protective surface film, effectively hindering the continuous corrosion of inner Mg matrix. Moreover, the accelerated dynamic of apatite deposition on ZK60/8MS was believed to be beneficial to form interfacial bonds with bone tissue, thus promoting bone healing in vivo.

2.2.3.4 In Vitro Cell Responses

Direct cell adhesion assays of MG-63 cells were carried out on SLM processed ZK60/8MS and ZK60 samples. The morphologies and spreading state of cells after culture for 6 h, 1 day and 3 days were presented in Fig. 1-8a. And the statistical results of live cell density on samples were presented in Fig. 1-8b. It could be seen that very few dead cells were adhered on surface for all the specimens. Moreover, the cells adhered on surface increased with the culture time extending. More importantly, the adherent cells on the ZK60/8MS were considerably more than those on ZK60 over the whole culture period, revealing an improved cytocompatibility of ZK60/8MS. Furthermore, MG-63 cells on ZK60 exhibited a roundish and poor spreading morphology after 3 days' culture, while cells cultured on ZK60/8MS appeared well spread out with affluent pseudopods after culture for 1 and 3 days. The enhanced cell adhesion and growth of ZK60/8MS were believed to be closely related with the surface morphology and microstructure. It was believed that the incorporated MS with highly ordered mesopores offered an abundance of opportunities for the interactions between cells and the culture medium, thus promoting cell adhesion and proliferation.

The viability of cells, incubated in the extracts of SLM processed ZK60/8MS and ZK60 for 1,

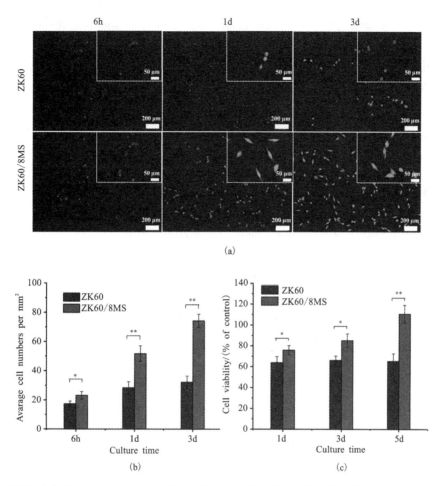

(a)

(b)   (c)

Fig. 2-15 (a) Fluorescence images of the adherent cells subjected to Live/Dead staining and (b) statistical analysis of adherent cell density of MG-63 cells on ZK60/8MS and ZK60, respectively. High magnification images were inserted to better describe the cells spreading state; (c) Viability of MG-63 cells incubated in the extracts of ZK60/8MS and ZK60. Values were expressed as mean ± error, $n = 3$, $^{*}p < 0.05$, $^{**}p < 0.01$.

3, and 5 days, was investigated via CCK-8 assay [Fig. 2-15 (c)]. For ZK60, it exhibited -63.8% cell viability at 1st day, -66.1% at 3th day, and -65.5% at 5th day, respectively; whereas for ZK60/8MS, it achieved 75.8% cell viability at 1st day, -88.5% at 3th day, and even an enhancement of -110.8% at 5th day, respectively. Clearly, ZK60/8MS showed excellent cell viability in comparison to ZK60, indicating that the incorporation of MS could induce no cytotoxicity to MG-63 cells but rather promote the cell growth. An improved biocompatibility of ZK60/8MS could partly ascribe to the reduced degradation rate caused by compositing with MS. During the degradation of Mg based materials, the resultant rise of OH^- concentration as well as the osmotic pressure in culture medium might exert minor negative effects on osteoblast cell proliferation. For ZK60/8MS, the released Mg^{2+} and OH^- in extracts were significantly reduced comparing with ZK60, causing a near-physiological condition with adequate pH, concentration and osmolality for cell survival. On the other hand, the released Si ion into the culture medium accompanied by the degradation of ZK60/8MS might also contribute to the improved biocompatibility. As a necessary nutrient element for the human body, Si element also aids the growth of bone tissue. Briefly, the ZK60/8MS with improved biocompatibility could promote cell adhesion and proliferation, which might contribute to accelerating the bone healing process.

2.2.4 Conclusions

In this research, MS was incorporated into ZK60 to improve the degradation behavior via SLM technology. MS particles dispersed homogeneously within Mg matrix and formed a good interface binding, due to the fast heating and cooling by SLM. The incorporated MS increased the surface passivation of the Mg matrix with a more positive corrosion potential. On the other hand, MS with mesoporous structure and excellent bioactivity effectively promoted the deposition of apatite layer, which acted as an effective protection layer hindering the continuous corrosion of Mg matrix. Both of these contributed to the improvement of the degradation behavior of ZK60, resulting in a 57% reduction in the degradation rate. Furthermore, the incorporation of MS into ZK60 could promote the cell adhesion and proliferation. It was suggested that SLM-processed ZK60/8MS was a promising bone repair material.

2.3 Uniform Degradation Mode and Enhanced Degradation Resistance of Mg Alloy via a Long Period Stacking Ordered Phase in the Grain Interior

2.3.1 Introduction

As a potential bone implant material, Mg alloys have attracted widespread attention due to their biodegradability, biocompatibility, and proper mechanical property. Their elastic modulus (the range from 40 to 45 GPa) is near to that of natural bone (the range from 10 to 40 GPa), which can avoid the stress-shielding effect. Besides, Mg is one of the most important bivalent ions in the formation of biological apatite and also a key factor for bone metabolism. In addition, as a highly electronegative metal, Mg can degrade gradually in the human physiological environment, which can avoid the second surgical operation for removing. However, too rapid degradation rate and non-uniform degradation mode of Mg alloys in physiological environment will result in mechanical integrity losing prematurely, which limit their practical application. Therefore, it is necessary to enhance degradation resistance and transform the degradation mode from non-uniform to uniform.

The microstructure is a vital factor to determine the degradation behaviors of Mg alloys. Most Mg alloys are multi-phase alloy and their degradation behaviors are influenced by the distribution of the second phase because of the formation of galvanic corrosion between the Mg matrix and the second phase. Furthermore, the second phase distributed along grain boundaries is the main cause of the non-uniform degradation. Thus, a second phase distributed in the grain interior is expected to enhance the degradation resistance and form uniform degradation mode of Mg alloys. As a kind of second phase, long period stacking ordered (LPSO) phase is distributed in the grain interior. Besides, it has parallel lamellar shape in the grain interior, which may inhibit the degradation extending to the neighboring grains. In addition, long period stacking ordered phase is an unstable fault phase. It may preferentially degrade and then form compact degradation product film, displaying a protection effect on the Mg matrix.

Of course, the formation of LPSO phase in Mg alloys depends on their chemical composition. Recently, a criterion for the formation of LPSO phase in Mg-Zn-rare earth element alloys was proposed by Kawamura and Yamasaki. Rare earth elements should have a hexagonal close-packed (hcp) structure as well as a large solid solubility limits (> 3.75%) in Mg-rare earth element alloys. In addition, the atomic size of the rare earth elements should be larger than that of Mg (0.160 nm) by 8.4% – 11.9%. Gadolinium (Gd), as a rare earth element, has a hcp structure, large solid solubility limit (4.53%) in binary Mg-Gd alloy and the atomic size of 0.180 nm, which well satisfied the criteria for the formation of LPSO phase ($Mg_{12}ZnGd$). Furthermore, it also exhibits acceptable biocompatibility as an alloying element in biodegradable Mg alloys.

In this work, Mg-3Zn-0.5Zr-xGd (mass fraction) (ZK30 – xGd) alloys were prepared by laser melting method. The microstructure was studied using scanning electron microscopy (SEM) with energy dispersed spectroscopy (EDS) and the phase composition was studied using X-ray diffraction (XRD). The degradation properties were investigated by electrochemical techniques and immersion tests in simulated body fluid. The cell culture was performed to evaluate the biocompatibility.

2.3.2   Experimental Procedures

2.3.2.1   Materials

The initial Mg-3Zn-0.5Zr (mass fraction) (ZK30) powder was spherical with average particle size of 50 μm and the initial Gadolinium (Gd) powder was irregular in shape with average particle size of 5 μm. The two powders were blended at a rate of 100 r/min for 10 h using a ball grinder under argon atmosphere.

The ZK30 – xGd (x = 0%, 5%, 10%, 15%, and 20%, denoted as ZK30, ZK30 – 5Gd, ZK30 – 10Gd, ZK30 – 15Gd, ZK30 – 20Gd, respectively) alloys were prepared through laser rapid melting the powder mixture of ZK30 powder and Gd powder on the homemade laser rapid melting machine. The machine was composed of the fiber laser, the optical focusing system and the control system. The maximum output power and wavelength of the fiber laser were 500 W and 1064 nm, respectively. The laser beams could be focused into a minimum spot size of 50 μm. The parameters were as follows: the laser spot diameter, the laser power, the scanning speed and the hatch spacing kept constant at 150 μm, 60 W, 600 mm/min, and 100 μm, respectively. During laser rapid melting process, the whole building chamber was protected by high purity argon atmosphere to prevent oxidation. The cubic alloy samples with a size of 10 mm × 10 mm × 10 mm were built by laser melting metal powder in a layer-by-layer method.

2.3.2.2　Microstructure

For microstructural observation, alloys were polished and etched using an acetic-picral solution. Scanning electron microscope (SEM) equipment with an energy dispersed spectroscopy (EDS) was employed to study the composition distribution of the alloys. An X-ray diffraction (XRD) analysis was conducted using a Bruker D8 Advance spectrometer with scattering angles ranging from $10°$ to $80°$ to characterize the phase composition.

2.3.2.3　Degradation Properties

The electrochemical tests of the alloys were performed on the electrochemical workstation (CHI660C) in the simulated body fluid (SBF) at $37℃$. For the electrochemical tests, the alloys were sealed with paraffin with an exposed area of 1 cm^2. In order to obtain a stable open circuit potential, the alloys were immersed in the SBF for 5 min. Then, the measurement was conducted in potential ranging from -300 mV to $+300$ mV compared to the open circuit potential. The scan rate for the test was 1 mV/s. The Tafel extrapolation method was employed to evaluate the corrosion potential and current of the alloys.

Immersion tests were carried out in SBF at $37℃$. Before the test, the alloys were polished with 1 μm diamond suspension, cleaned with acetone and then dried. The measurement of hydrogen evolution was employed using a gas burette to evaluate the degradation rate of alloys. After immersing for 168 h in SBF, the alloys were removed, gently washed with deionized water, and subsequently dried using warm air. The morphology and composition of degradation products were analyzed using the SEM and X-ray photoelectron spectroscopy (XPS), respectively. The degradation products of alloys were removed using the chromic acid as cleaning solution (20 g chromic oxide, 1 g silver nitrate and 100 mL deionized water) for 10 min, and then surface morphologies of the alloys were investigated using SEM.

2.3.2.4　Cytocompatibility

The cytocompatibility of the alloys was assessed using human osteoblast-like MG63 cells. The MG63 cells were cultured in Dulbecco's modified Eagle's medium (DMEM). Cells were incubated in a humidified atmosphere of 5% CO_2 and 95% air at $37℃$. In order to prepare extraction, alloys were immersed in DMEM with the surface area/extraction volume 1.25 cm^2/mL. After immersing for 120 h ($37℃$, humidified atmosphere and 5% CO_2), the supernatant fluid was withdrawed after centrifugation to prepare the extraction. Cells cultured in DMEM medium were served as negative control. MG63 cells were cultured in 96 - well cell plates at 5×10^3 cells/100 μL for 24 h to allow attachment. The culture medium was then substituted with 100 μL of extraction. After incubating for 1, 3 and 5 d, 10 μL cell counting kit-8 solution was introduced to every specimen, incubating for another 2 h at $37℃$. The optical density was read using a spectrophotometer (BIO-RAD 680) at wavelength of 490 nm.

MG63 cells (5×10^3 cells/100 μL) were cultured in 96 - well cell plates for 24 h to allow attachment. The culture medium was then substituted with 100 μL of extraction. After incubating for 5 d, 5% glutaric dialdehyde diluent was used to fix the cells at $4℃$ for 20 min. Afterward, the fixed cells were rinsed with phosphate buffer saline (PBS) solution, followed by permeabilizing with

0.2% Triton X-100 for 15 min at 4℃. After rinsing with PBS solution for three times, the cells were stained with rhodamine phalloidin for 1 h following by three times rinses with PBS solution, and further stained with hoechst fluorescent dyes for 5 min, and then observed using a fluorescence microscope a digital camera.

2.3.2.5   Statistical Analysis

The quantitative data were obtained from six independent experiments and presented as mean ± standard deviation. Statistical analysis was conducted using SPSS 19.0 software to assess the difference. In all analyses, it was considered to be significant when the value of p was less than 0.05 (significance level).

2.3.3   Results and Discussion

2.3.3.1   Microstructure

The SEM and EDS analysis of the alloys were presented in Fig. 2-16. The ZK30 alloy consisted of equiaxed grains and a few of granular shaped precipitates distributed at grain boundaries [Fig. 2-16(a)]. Network precipitates were formed at grain boundaries of the ZK30 – 5Gd alloy [Fig. 2-16(b)]. Lamellar precipitates were distributed in the grain interior of the ZK30 – 10Gd alloy. When the Gd content was further increased, the lamellar precipitates gradually transformed to block-shape precipitates and the volume fraction of block-shape precipitates increased with the Gd content

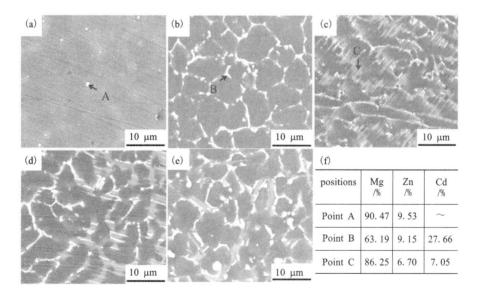

positions	Mg /%	Zn /%	Cd /%
Point A	90.47	9.53	~
Point B	63.19	9.15	27.66
Point C	86.25	6.70	7.05

Fig. 2-16   Microstructure of the alloys (a) ZK30, (b) ZK30 – 5Gd, (c) ZK30 – 10Gd, (d) ZK30 – 15Gd, (e) ZK30 – 20Gd, (f) EDS results of the precipitates. The ZK30 alloy consisted of equiaxed grains and a few of granular shaped precipitates distributed at grain boundaries. Network precipitates were distributed at grain boundaries of the ZK30 – 5Gd alloy. Lamellar precipitates were distributed in the grain interior of the ZK30 – 10Gd alloy. When the Gd content increased further, the lamellar precipitates transformed to block-shape precipitates.

increasing. The EDS analysis revealed that the granular shaped precipitates [point A in Fig. 2-16 (a)] were comprised of Mg (90.47%) and Zn (9.53%). The network precipitates [point B in Fig. 2-16(b)] were comprised of Mg (63.19%), Zn (9.15%) and Gd (27.66%). The lamellar precipitates [point C in Fig. 2-16(c)] were comprised of Mg (86.25%), Zn (6.70%) and Gd (7.05%).

The XRD spectra of the alloys and the local magnification of the XRD characteristic peaks (2θ: $30° \sim 40°$) were presented in Fig. 2-17. The ZK30 alloy was composed of α-Mg phase as well as MgZn phase. When alloying 5% (mass fraction) Gd to ZK30 alloy, a new (Mg, Zn)$_3$Gd phase was detected. When ZK30 alloying with 10% Gd, another new Mg$_{12}$ZnGd phase appeared, which possessed a long-period stacking ordered (LPSO) structure. As the Gd content increased continuously to 20% (mass fraction), the main phases were the same as those of the ZK30 − 10Gd alloy. Combined with the results of SEM and EDS, the granular shaped precipitates, the network precipitates and the lamellar precipitates were suggested to be MgZn phase, (Mg, Zn)$_3$Gd phase and LPSO phase, respectively.

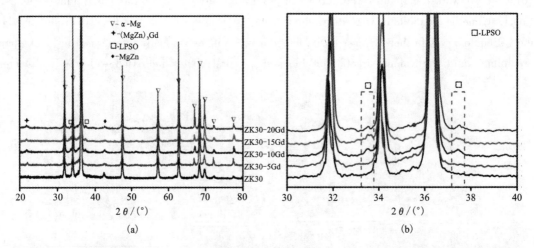

Fig. 2-17 (a) The XRD spectra of the ZK30 − Gd alloy and (b) the local magnification of the XRD characteristic peaks (2θ: $30° \sim 40°$). The peak of (Mg, Zn)3Gd phase appeared in ZK30 −5Gd alloy. When the Gd content increased further, the peak of long period stacking ordered (LPSO) phase (Mg$_{12}$ZnGd) appeared.

2.3.3.2 Degradation Properties

The electrochemical polarization curves of the alloys immersed in SBF were presented in Fig. 2-17(a). The current densities of the alloys were shown as follows: (80.91 ± 6.8) μA/cm^2(ZK30), (49.88 ± 6.2) μA/cm^2(ZK30 −5Gd), (26.73 ± 5.9) μA/cm^2(ZK30 − 10Gd), (55.46 ± 6.2) μA/cm^2(ZK30 − 15Gd) and (145.55 ± 7.3) μA/cm^2(ZK30 − 20Gd). The ZK30 − 10Gd alloy had the lowest current density, which suggested that it had the best degradation resistance. The polarization curves of the ZK30 − 10Gd alloy after immersing for in SBF different times were shown in Fig. 2-18(b). Results showed that the corrosion potential of the alloy increased and its corrosion current density decreased with the immersion time increasing, which indicated that the degradation resistance gradually enhanced with the immersion time increasing. In other word, a stable and compact degradation product film formed gradually on the ZK30 – 10Gd alloy during the immersion.

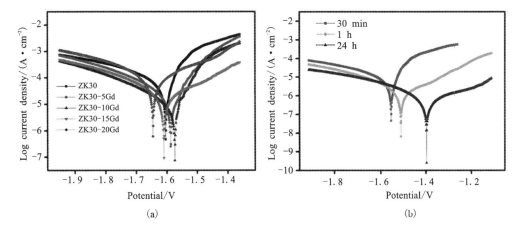

Fig. 2-18　(a) Polarization curves of the alloys immersed in SBF. The ZK30 – 10Gd alloy had the lowest current density; (b) Polarization curves of the alloy for different immersion times in SBF. The corrosion potential of the alloy increased and its corrosion current density decreased with the immersion time increasing.

The hydrogen volume evolutions of the alloys immersed in SBF were recorded, and the results were presented in Fig. 2-19(a). It indicated that the hydrogen evolution volume of ZK30 – 10Gd alloy was (16.84 ± 1.02) mL/cm^2 after immersion for 168 h, which was lower than those of ZK30 $[(29.15 \pm 1.17)$ mL/cm$^2]$, ZK30 – 5Gd $[(20.86 \pm 1.02)$ mL/cm$^2]$, ZK30 – 15Gd $[(25.31 \pm 1.17)$ mL/cm$^2]$ and ZK30 – 20Gd $[(36.56 \pm 1.25)$ mL/cm$^2]$. The degradation rates of the ZK30

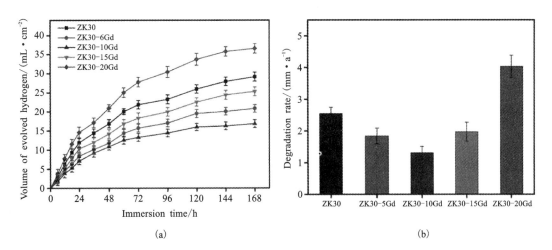

Fig. 2-19　(a) Hydrogen evolution volume curves as a function of the immersion time in SBF and (b) degradation rates calculated from the mass loss test.

– Gd alloy calculated according to mass loss test [Fig. 2-19(b)]: respectively based on polarization test, hydrogen evolution and weight loss, were summarized in Tab. 2-2. As could be seen, although the values of the degradation rate were different based on these various assessment methods, the variation trends of the degradation rate were consistent, which showed that ZK30 – 10Gd alloy exhibited the lowest degradation rate [(1.31 ±0.21) mm/a].

Tab. 2-2 Degradation rates of ZK30 and ZK30 – Gd alloys in SBF. P_i was calculated based on polarization test; P_h was calculated based on H_2 evolution; P_w was calculated based on weight loss.

Samples	$I_{corr}/$ ($\mu A \cdot cm^{-2}$)	$P_i/$ ($mm \cdot a^{-1}$)	$V_h/$ ($mL \cdot cm^{-2} \cdot d^{-1}$)	$P_h/$ ($mm \cdot a^{-1}$)	$\Delta W/$ ($mg \cdot cm^{-2} \cdot d^{-1}$)	$P_w/$ ($mm \cdot a^{-1}$)
ZK30	80.91 ±6.8	1.85 ±0.16	4.16 ±0.17	9.48 ±0.39	1.21 ±0.11	2.55 ±0.21
ZK30 – 5Gd	49.88 ±6.2	1.14 ±0.14	2.98 ±0.15	6.79 ±0.34	0.88 ±0.12	1.84 ±0.25
ZK30 – 10Gd	26.73 ±5.9	0.61 ±0.13	2.41 ±0.15	5.49 ±0.34	0.63 ±0.11	1.31 ±0.21
ZK30 – 15Gd	55.46 ±6.2	1.28 ±0.14	3.62 ±0.17	8.25 ±0.39	0.94 ±0.15	1.97 ±0.31
ZK30 – 20Gd	145.55 ±7.3	3.33 ±0.17	5.22 ±0.18	11.9 ±0.41	1.92 ±0.17	4.03 ±0.35

The degradation product films on ZK30 – Gd alloy, were exhibited in Fig. 2-20 after immersing in SBF at 37℃ for 168 h. In general, the insoluble degradation products formed on the surface of the alloys could play a protection role. The degradation product film of the ZK30 alloy exhibited a peeled-off surface characteristic and plenty of wide cracks [Fig. 2-20(a)]. The degradation product film of the ZK30 – 5Gd alloy presented relatively shallow cracks. Significantly, a relatively integrated degradation product film formed on ZK30 – 10Gd alloy [Fig. 2-20(c)]. With the Gd content increasing further, the width of the cracks on the degradation product film gradually increased [Figs. 2-20(d) and 2-20(e)]. The results showed that degradation product film of the ZK30 – 10Gd alloy had the best protection effect.

The XPS analysis was carried out to define the composition of the degradation product film on ZK30 – Gd alloy after immersion for 168 h. The Mg, O and Gd elements were observed in survey spectrum [Fig. 2-21(a)]. In order to get more detailed information about the chemical bonding states of the elements, the high resolution spectra of Mg1s, O1s and Gd3d were acquired. The spectrum of Mg1s was shown in Fig. 2-21(b), which could be resolved into two components centered at 1302.7 eV and 1303.2 eV. Binding energy at 1302.7 eV was attributed to Mg hydroxyl stretching (Mg-OH). The O1s peak could be resolved into two components centered at 531.7 eV and 532.7 eV, which were in accordance with the O^{2-} and OH^-, respectively [Fig. 2-21(c)]. The Gd3d peak position corresponded to the standard binding energy peak position of Gd_2O_3, indicating that the Gd in the degradation products was in the form of Gd_2O_3. According to the analysis of the XPS spectra, the degradation film on ZK30 – Gd alloy was mainly composed of Mg $(OH)_2$ and Gd_2O_3.

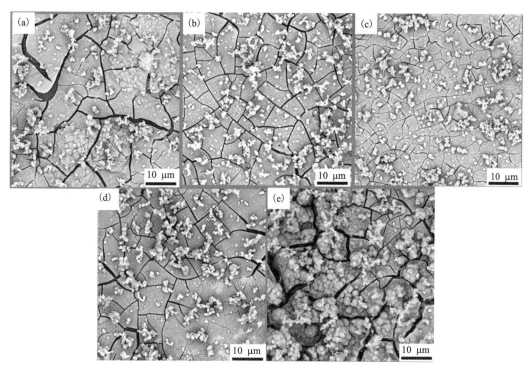

Fig. 2-20　The degradation product films after immersion in SBF at 37℃ for 168 h (a) ZK30, (b) ZK30 −5Gd, (c) ZK30−10Gd, (d) ZK30−15Gd, (e) ZK30−20Gd. The degradation product film of the ZK30 alloy exhibited a peeled-off characteristic and plenty of wide cracks. The degradation product film of the ZK30−5Gd alloy presented relatively shallow cracks. The relatively integrated degradation product film formed on ZK30−10Gd alloy. With the Gd content increasing further, the width of the cracks on the degradation product film gradually increased.

The morphologies of ZK30 − Gd alloy after removing the degradation product were shown in Fig. 2-22. Many degradation pits were observed on ZK30 and ZK30 − 5Gd alloys [Figs. 2-22(a) and 2-22(b)]. And the size of the degradation pits matched with the grain size of α-Mg in the alloys. Clearly, the degradation mode of ZK30 and ZK30 − 5Gd alloys was pit corrosion, which was a non-uniform degradation mode. With Gd content (mass fraction) increasing to 10%, the morphology of the ZK30 − 10Gd alloy turned smooth and uniform [Fig. 2-22(c)], indicating a uniform degradation mode. However, some corrosion ditches appeared on the surface of ZK30 − 15Gd and ZK30 − 20Gd alloys, suggesting that the degradation mode changed to non-uniform degradation mode as the Gd content increasing further.

The high degradation resistance and uniform degradation mode of the ZK30 − Gd alloy were closely associated with its microstructure and degradation product film. In ZK30 alloy, micro-galvanic coupling formed between the cathode intermetallic compound phase and the anodic Mg matrix because of their potential differences, resulting in severe pitting degradation. This was the common degradation mode of Mg alloys when the intermetallic compound phase distributed at the

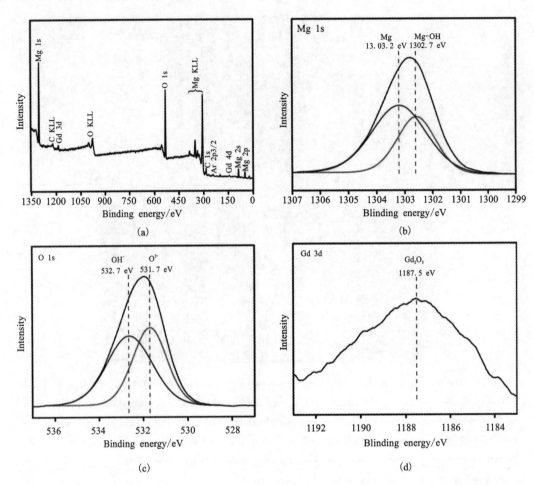

Fig. 2-21 XPS spectra of the degradation product film of ZK30 – Gd alloy after immersion for 168 h: (a) XPS survey spectrum. The Mg, O and Gd elements were observed in survey spectrum. (b) High resolution Mg1s spectrum. The spectrum of Mg1s could be resolved into two components centered at 1302.7 eV (Mg-OH) and 1303.2 eV (Mg). (c) High resolution O1s spectrum. The O1s peak could be resolved into two components centered at 531.7 eV (O^{2-}) and 532.7 eV (OH^-). (d) High resolution Gd3d spectrum. The Gd3d peak position corresponded to the standard binding energy peak position of Gd_2O_3.

grain boundaries. However, the degradation mode was fundamentally different in ZK30 – Gd alloy with LPSO phase distributed in the grain interior. LPSO phase was a precipitate with a long periodic stacking fault structure, whose energy and activity were higher than those of Mg matrix. Therefore, compared with the Mg matrix, LPSO phase acted as anode rather than cathode in the micro-galvanic corrosion, which preferentially degraded to form compact degradation product films along with the degradation of the LPSO phase. It should be noted that the Pilling-Bedworth ratio of Gd (1.29) was greater than 1. Thus, the formation of Gd_2O_3 in the degradation product film of ZK30 – Gd alloy was beneficial to increase the relative density of the degradation product film, which could enhance capacity to resist the penetration of aggressive solution. In addition, the incorporation of high content

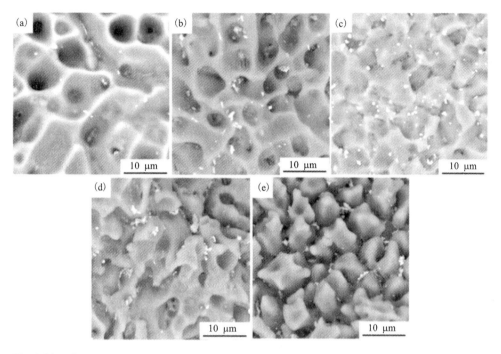

Fig. 2-22 The morphology of ZK30 – Gd alloy after immersion in SBF for 168 h and then removing the degradation product: (a) ZK30 alloy, (b) ZK30 – 5Gd alloy, (c) ZK30 – 10Gd alloy, (d) ZK30 – 15Gd alloy, (e) ZK30 – 20Gd alloy. Many degradation pits were observed on ZK30 and ZK30 – 5Gd alloys and the size of the degradation pits matched with the grain size of α-Mg in the alloys. As the Gd content (mass fraction) increased to 10%, the morphology of the ZK30 – 10Gd was smooth and uniform. However, there were corrosion ditches on both ZK30 – 15Gd and ZK30 – 20Gd alloys.

Gd^{3+} in the degradation product film could increase the positive charge of the degradation product film, which could prevent the osmosis of aggressive anions (Cl^-) through the degradation product film by adsorbing anions, thus further inhibited the degradation. Furthermore, as a kind of second phase in Mg alloys, LPSO phase was the lamellar-shape and distributed in the grain interior, which could inhibit the degradation extending to the neighboring grains.

LPSO phase was conducive to slow down the degradation rate, whilst the $(Mg, Zn)_3 Gd$ phase was stable intermetallic, which could act as the cathode in the micro-galvanic corrosion between the Mg matrix accelerating degradation. As a consequence, the degradation rate was determined by the factor which played a major role. The content of LPSO or $(Mg, Zn)_3 Gd$ phase in ZK30 – Gd was determined by the content of Gd. For ZK30 – 10Gd, LPSO phase was a major secondary phase and only little $(Mg, Zn)_3 Gd$ phase distributed at the grain boundaries. The positive influence of LPSO phase on inhibition of degradation was greater than the negative influence of the $(Mg, Zn)_3 Gd$ phase, so the degradation rate of ZK30 – 10Gd slowed down. As the Gd content (mass fraction) increased to 15% (ZK30 – 15Gd) or 20% (ZK30 – 20Gd), the number of $(Mg, Zn)_3 Gd$ phase increased dramatically and that of LPSO phase increased not obviously. The increased $(Mg, Zn)_3$

Gd phase in ZK30 – 15Gd and ZK30 – 20Gd resulted in a rapid degradation rate due to the microgalvanic corrosion, which could not be offset by the positive influence on degradation resistance caused by LPSO phase. Therefore, the degradation rate increased apparently with Gd content increasing.

2.3.3.3 Cytocompatibility

It is essential to have an acceptable cytocompatibility for biomaterials using as human implants. Thus, the cell viability assay was carried out to evaluate the cytocompatibility of ZK30 – 10Gd alloy, due to its optimal degradation behavior. And ZK30 was used as the control. The viability of MG63 cells after culture in extracts of ZK30 – 10Gd alloy and the ZK30 alloy for 1, 3 and 5 d were shown in Fig. 2-23. The results showed that viability of cells after culture in ZK30 – 10Gd and ZK30 alloys extraction were higher than that of the negative control groups. Moreover, the cell viability of the ZK30 – 10Gd alloy was better than that of ZK30 alloy. The enhanced cytocompatibility of the ZK30 – 10Gd alloy was attributed to the improvement of its degradation resistance. It was well known that Mg alloys could degrade gradually in the culture medium and release metallic ions and hydroxyl ions. And high concentrations of metallic ions and hydroxyl ions caused high osmolality and pH value which exerted slightly inhibitory effects on cell growth. Compared with ZK30, ZK30 – 10Gd alloy possessed high degradation resistance, which reduced metallic ions and hydroxyl ions to release to the culture medium, forming a approximate physiological environment for cells growth.

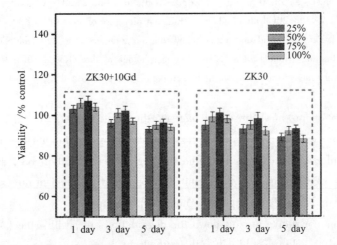

Fig. 2-23 Viability of MG63 cells after culture in the ZK30 – 10Gd and ZK30 alloy extraction with 25%, 50%, 75% and 100% concentrations after 1, 3 and 5 d.

The fluorescence microscopy images of the MG63 cells cultured in ZK30 – 10Gd and ZK30 alloy extractions for 5 d were shown in Fig. 2-24. The results showed that MG63 cells after culture in ZK30 – 10Gd and ZK30 alloy extractions with different concentrations exhibited round and spindle shapes, which was the normal morphology of the cells. The cell viability assay and fluorescence imaging of the cells suggested that the ZK30 – 10Gd alloy had good cytocompatibility. The result of cytocompatibility evaluations for ZK30 – 10Gd alloy was in agreement with that of previous reports, which stated that Mg alloys with high solubility rare earth elements exhibited cytocompatibility.

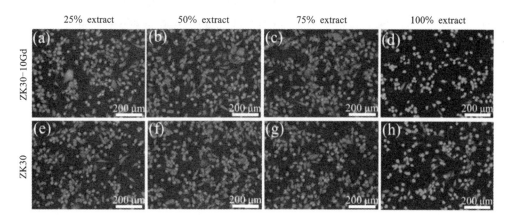

Fig. 2-24   Fluorescence images of MG63 cells cultured for 5 d for the ZK30 – 10Gd alloy in (a) 25%, (b) 50%, (c) 75% and (d) 100% extractions and ZK30 alloy in (e) 25%, (f) 50%, (g) 75% and (h) 100% extractions.

2.3.4   Conclusions

ZK30 – Gd alloy was fabricated by selective laser melting. A long period stacking ordered (LPSO) phase ($Mg_{12}ZnGd$) formed in ZK30 – Gd alloy and distributed in the grain interior. ZK30 – Gd alloy showed higher degradation resistance than ZK30 alloy, and ZK30 – 10Gd alloy possessed the lowest degradation rate (1. 31 mm/a). Moreover, the degradation mode of the alloy was transformed from non-uniform degradation to uniform degradation. These could be ascribed to the preferential degradation of the LPSO phase, the formation of compact degradation product films and the inhibition of the parallel lamellar structure in the grain interior on the extension of degradation. However, as the Gd content increased to 15% (ZK30 – 15Gd) or 20% (ZK30 – 20Gd), the degradation rate increased apparently with Gd content increasing, due to that the accelerating degradation effect caused by (Mg, Zn)$_3$Gd phase could not be offset by the positive influence on degradation resistance caused by LPSO phase. In addition, the ZK30 – Gd alloy exhibited good cytocompatibility.

2.4   Positive Feedback Effects of Mg on the Hydrolysis of Poly-L-lactic Acid (PLLA): Promoted Degradation of PLLA Scaffolds

2.4.1   Introduction

Poly-L-lactic acid (PLLA), as bone scaffold material, possesses good biocompatibility. It can be degraded to lactic acid and then decomposed to carbohydrate in physiological environments, being absorbed ultimately in the body by metabolism. Nevertheless, the too slow degradation rate of PLLA scaffolds dosen't match the growth rate of bone, which severely impedes the formation of new bone. Introducing a material with faster degradation is a common method to accelerate the degradation of PLLA scaffolds. Zhang et al introduced silk fibroin into PLLA scaffolds and found that the degradation of the scaffolds was accelerated, but the tensile strength decreased. A. Vieira et al added PCL to PLLA scaffolds and found that the weight loss of the scaffolds increased, and acid products of PCL further decreased the pH, which was adverse for cellular response. Furthermore, they accelerated the degradation of scaffolds only due to the fast degradation of themselves, rather than the degradation of PLLA was promoted.

One of key factors slow the degradation rate of PLLA is that the acid degraded products inhibit the hydrolysis of PLLA. Therefore, adding a material to consume the acid degraded products may accelerate the degradation of the PLLA. Mg, as a alkali metal material, can degrade and produce $Mg(OH)_2$ in the physiological environment. $Mg(OH)_2$ could neutralize the acid degraded products of PLLA. Hence, introducing of Mg into PLLA may be an effective strategy to accelerate the degradation. Besides, Mg has high strength and hardness, and can be used as particle strengthening phase in polymer matrix. In addition, Mg is one of the essential trace elements in human body, which is beneficial for cell response. There are several studies on the composites of PLLA and Mg in the current reports. Some researches utilized Mg as reinforced phase to improve the mechanical and thermal properties of PLLA, and others utilized PLLA as a coating to increase the corrosion resistance of Mg. Nevertheless, few studies focused on the effect of Mg on the degradation behavior of PLLA, in the form of porous scaffold.

In this work, Mg was introduced into PLLA to increase its degradation rate. PLLA/Mg scaffolds were fabricated via selective laser sintering (SLS). The effects of Mg on the degradation behavior of the scaffolds were studied based on the measurements of pH value and weight loss as well as characterization of degradation morphology. Meanwhile, the degradation mechanism of the PLLA/Mg scaffolds was analyzed. Besides, the mechanical properties of the scaffolds were tested. In addition, the cytocompatibility and thermal properties were assessed.

2.4.2　Materials and Methods

2.4.2.1　Materials

PLLA powder, with the particle size about 1 μm, the viscosity of 1.46 dL/g and the melting temperature of 175℃ ~ 185℃, was obtained from Shenzhen Polymtek Biomaterial Co., Ltd. (Shenzhen, China). Mg powder (> 99.9%) with average particle sizes about 500 nm was obtained from Shanghai Pantian nano Materials Co., Ltd., China. The pH of phosphate buffer solution (PBS) was 7.4.

2.4.2.2　Porous Scaffolds

PLLA/Mg powders were obtained as follows: PLLA and Mg powders first were weighted according to the weight ratios(100:0, 99:1, 97:3, 95:5, and 93:7). Then two kinds of powder were blended into beakers containing 20 ml anhydrous alcohol, with dispersing for 20 min by ultrasonic and magnetic stir, respectively. Afterwards the mixed powders were obtained by filtration and put into an electrothermal blowing dry cabinet for drying at 55℃ for 6 hours. Eventually the PLLA/Mg powders were prepared.

PLLA/Mg porous scaffolds were fabricated by SLS system, it was consisted of a CO_2 laser, control system, sintering platform and three-dimensional lifting platform. Laser sintering power of 2. 3 W and laser scanning speed of 120 mm/min were choseas technological parameters to fabricate the porous scaffolds. The specific sintering process could be described as follows: (1) The powders were spreaded flatly on the sintering platform. (2) The spreaded layer was sintered selectively according to designed scaffold model. (3) The lifting platform dropped a height equivalenting to previous spreaded layer thickness. (4) Steps (1) ~ (3) were repeated until porous scaffolds were obtained utterly. (5) The porous scaffolds were brushed off by an air compressor to get rid of residuary powders.

2.4.2.3   Characterization

Phenom scanning electron microscopy (FEI Co. , USA) was used to observe the distribution state of the Mg in the scaffolds. Element contents of specimens' surface were examined by energy-dispersive spectroscopy (EDS). The phase analysis of the porous scaffolds was tested by an X-ray diffraction machine (Karlsruhe, Germany) at a scanning rate of 8°/min from 10° ~ 80° of scattering angles.

2.4.2.4   Thermal Properties

The DSC and TGA of the scaffolds were carried out on asynchronous thermal analyzer (STA-200, China). These scaffolds were ground into powders and taken into ceramic crucible, heating from 30℃ to 600℃ with heating speed of 20 ℃/min under nitrogen atmosphere. Melting point temperature of DSC and remaining mass percentage of TGA at 600℃ were identified from the testing curves.

2.4.2.5   Degradation Performance

The degradation performance of the scaffolds was evaluated in PBS solution (pH 7. 4): Four samples per group were weighted as initial weight (W_i), then each sample (10 mm × 10 mm × 3 mm) was put into sealed tube containing 10 ml PBS solution and fixed on a shaker at 37℃ in order to simulate the natural human physiological environment. After degradation of 1, 2, 3 and 4 weeks, samples were fetched and then dried at 50℃ on an electrothermal blowing dry box until the weight did not change anymore, each sample was weighted as ultima weight (W_u). The weightloss percentage (W_L) of the scaffolds was calculated according to the following formula: $W_L = (W_i - W_u)/W_i \times 100\%$. Moreover, a pH-meter was used to measure the pH value of the immersion medium and morphologies of the degraded scaffolds were obtained by SEM.

2.4.2.6   Mechanical Properties

Compression tests were performed on a Mechanical tester (WD-D1, LTD, China) with a specimen size of 10 mm × 10 mm × 5 mm at a cross-head rate of 1 mm/min. The compression load was applied on scaffolds until the scaffolds were completely crushed and the stress-strain curves were recorded through compressive tests. Then compression strength was calculated by dividing the peak load by the cross-sectional area of the scaffolds. The compressive modulus was obtained from the slopes in the initial elastic region of the stress-strain curves. The Vickers hardness of the scaffold specimens (4 mm ×4 mm ×2 mm) was measured by hardness tester. A test force of 2. 94 N was applied on the surface of specimens to induce rhombicindentations with a loading time of 15 s at the room temperature. The Vickers hardness could be calculated by the Equation (2-3):

$$HV = 0.102 \frac{F}{S} = 0.102 \frac{2F \cdot \sin\left(\frac{\theta}{2}\right)}{d^2} = 0.1891 \frac{F}{d^2} \tag{2-3}$$

where HV represented Vickers hardness value; F represented test force; S represented the indentation cross-sectional area (mm^2); θ represented the angle between the opposite sides of the indenter, the value was taken as 136°; d represented arithmetic mean of two diagonal lengths of indentation (mm). The tests were carried out in sextuplicate.

2.4.2.7 Cytocompatibility

The MG-63 cells (Cellular Biology Institute, Shanghai, China) were used to investigate the cell adhesion on the PLLA and PLLA/Mg scaffolds with 5% Mg. The scaffolds firstly were sterilized with ultraviolet ray, afterwards rinsed twice in PBS, followed by exposure to ultraviolet light 15 min. The MG-63 cells were cultured on Dulbecco's modifed Eagle's medium (DMEM, HyClone, USA) under normal situation. Besides, 10% fetal bovine serum and gentamicin were added into DMEM. The MG-63 cells were cultured on scaffolds for 1 and 3 days in condition of 5% CO$_2$ at human body temperature (37℃). The solution was changed every second day.

Cell proliferation on the PLLA and PLLA/Mg scaffolds with 5% Mg was tested by MTT assay for 1, 3 and 5 days, respectively. At each time point, adding MTT solutions into scaffolds and incubating at human body temperature.

2.4.2.8 Statistical Analysis

Experimental data were presented in the form of mean ± standard deviation (SD). " * " represented a significant difference, and " * * " represented a very significant difference.

2.4.3 Results and Discussion

2.4.3.1 Microstructure

The distribution state of the Mg in the scaffolds was shown in Fig. 2-25. Mg particles began to appear in the matrix and dispersed evenly in the surface of scaffolds [Fig. 2-25(a)-(d)] when its content increased to 5%. There were agglomeration been observed when the content of Mg further increased [Fig. 2-25(e)], due to the large surface energy and distance of Mg particles decreasing. Two cross points S1 and S2 [Fig. 2-25(e)] were chosen to analyze the element compositions of the scaffolds with EDS, which confirmed that white dots were Mg by comparing S1 and S2 [Fig. 2-25 (f)].

2.4.3.2 Thermal Properties

The thermal properties of the scaffolds were studied by DSC and TGA tests to explore the effect of Mg on the melting and decomposing points of the scaffolds (Fig. 2-26). The PLLA scaffolds

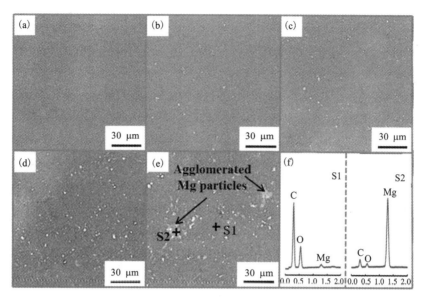

Fig. 2-25   Morphologies of the PLLA and PLLA/Mg scaffolds with 1%, 3%, 5% and 7% Mg and EDS spectra (f) S1, S2. Mg dispersed evenly on the surface of scaffolds when its contents increased until 5%, while some aggregates appeared when the content of Mg further increased.

displayed a endothermic peak locating at 184.9 ℃ [Fig. 2-26(a)], which coincided with the melting point of PLLA. the melting point of PLLA increased gradually with the increase of Mg content and it shifted about 5 ℃ when Mg content was 7%. The cause might be attributed to two aspects: on one hand, Mg acted as a nucleation site and caused the crystallization to take place at higher temperature, which lead the PLLA/Mg scaffolds to melt at a higher temperature. On the other hand, Mg had a higher melting point than PLLA and it would absorb some heat during heating process, which delayed the melt of PLLA and thus brought about a higher melting temperature of PLLA/Mg scaffolds than PLLA scaffold. Inversely, the decomposition points and decomposition temperatures interval of PLLA/Mg scaffolds decreased gradually with the increment of Mg content [Fig. 2-26(b)]. This may be accounted for the grenter amount of water PLLA, which could be absorbed with the increment of Mg content, meanwhile Mg could be regarded as a decomposition catalysts due to acting as active sites in the matrix.

2.4.3.3   Scaffolds and Composition Analysis

A representative PLLA/Mg scaffold was prepared by SLS (Fig. 2-27). Its overall size was 13 mm × 13 mm × 11 mm (length × width × height) and the pore size was approximately 500 μm, The scaffold was integrity and presented interconnected porous structure, which was beneficial to cellular adhesion, proliferation and exchange metabolites. Hollister et al. fabricated porous scaffold and discovered that porous structure could promote new bone grow. The interfacial reaction between PLLA and Mg was studied through XRD analysis, which was shown in Fig. 2-27(d). It revealed

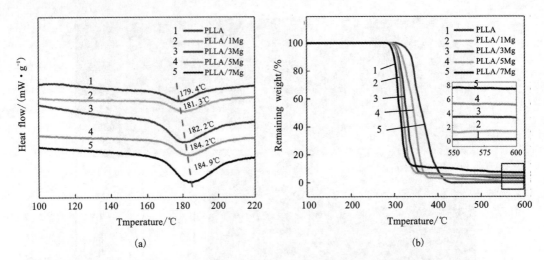

(a)   (b)

Fig. 2-26 DSC (a) and TGA (b)thermograms of PLLA and PLLA/Mg scaffolds with 1%, 3%, 5% and 7% Mg. The melting point of PLLA shifted towards high temperature and decomposition point and decomposition temperatures intervals decreased with the increment of Mg content.

that there was no interaction between PLLA and Mg. This could be evidenced by a comparison with the JCPDS card for PLLA and Mg by MDI Jade 6. The XRD pattern of PLLA scaffolds showed two characteristic diffraction peeks at $2\theta = 16.3°$, $19.6°$, which were corresponding to (101) [or (200)] and (113) [or (204)] planes, respectively. Meanwhile, there were three main peaks at $2\theta = 32.0°$, $34.1°$ and $36.4°$ for Mg and the peak intensities constantly increased with the addition of Mg.

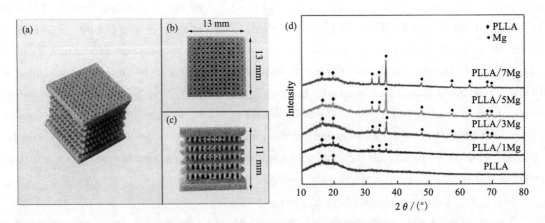

Fig. 2-27 A representative PLLA/Mg scaffold fabricated by SLS: (a) isometric view, (b) vertical view, (c) lateral view and (d) XRD diffractograms of PLLA and PLLA/Mg scaffolds with 1%, 3%, 5% and 7% Mg. The diffraction intensity of Mg increased with the addition of Mg.

2.4.3.4 Degradation Property

The morphologies of PLLA and PLLA/Mg scaffolds, immersed in PBS after 4 weeks, were visualized in Fig. 2-28. The morphology of PLLA scaffolds remained similar to the one immersed before [Fig. 2-28(a)]. Conversely, the PLLA/Mg scaffolds with 1% Mg displayed a rough surface relatively and appeared some micropores [Fig. 2-28(b)]. A more microporous structure was observed on the surface of the PLLA/Mg scaffolds and the size of pores also increased gradually with the content of Mg increased to 5% [Fig. 2-28(c), (d)]. There were some pits observed when the content of Mg further increased, due to the effect of Mg accelerate of the degradation of PLLA and then hydrolysis products of PLLA dissolved in the solution, ultimately leaving some pits on the surface of the scaffolds. Base on the analysis above, we could conclude that the addition of Mg accelerated the degradation of the scaffolds. Moreover, the higher the proportion of Mg in the PLLA matrix was, the faster the degradation rate of the scaffolds was.

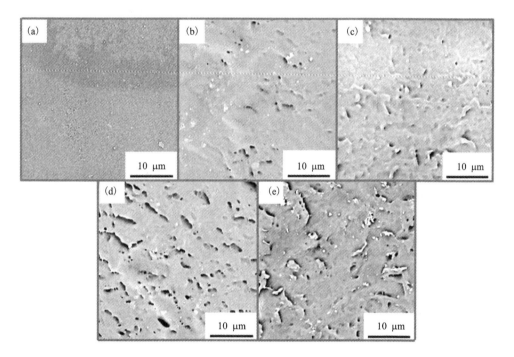

Fig. 2-28   The morphologies of PLLA and PLLA/Mg scaffolds with 1%, 3%, 5% and 7% Mg after degradation in PBS for 4 weeks.

The pH values were monitored during 4 weeks' immersion [Fig. 2-29(a)]. The pH value of degradation medium of PLLA declined constantly with the increment of immersion time, due to the acid degradation products, and decreased to 6.9 after 4 weeks' immersion. The pH tendency of the PLLA/Mg was different from that of PLLA. With the degradation of Mg in PBS solution, the pH value raised to a high value after the first week. With the increment of immersion time, the pH value of degradation medium gradually decreased owing to the degraded acid products of PLLA. The pH value after 4 weeks increased with the increment of Mg content, ascribed to the production of Mg $(OH)_2$ from the degradation of Mg. Thus, the introduction of Mg into PLLA matrix produced a local alkaline circumstance and showed a higher pH value in comparison with PLLA. The weight loss of

PLLA/Mg scaffolds with immersion of 4 weeks was recorded in Fig. 2-29 (b). All the samples presented weight loss. Among them it could be seen that the weight loss of PLLA scaffolds was the lowest at every time point and changed little after 4 weeks. But PLLA/Mg scaffolds experienced much higher weight loss than PLLA scaffolds, and the weight loss increased with the addition of Mg, indicating that Mg accelerated the degradation of scaffolds.

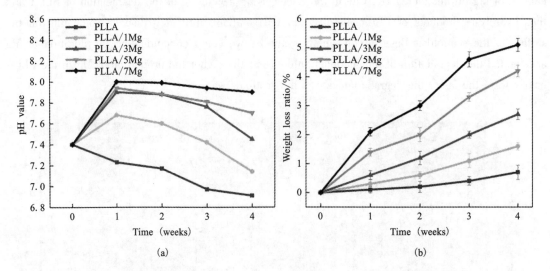

Fig. 2-29 pH value (a) and weight loss ratio (b) curves of PLLA and PLLA/Mg scaffolds with 1%, 3%, 5% and 7% Mg after 4 weeks immersion in PBS solution. Mg elevated the pH of the degradation medium and accelerated the weight loss of the scaffolds.

The mechanism of Mg accelerating the degradation of scaffolds was summarized in Fig. 2-30. Firstly more water uptake happened to the PLLA/Mg scaffolds due to easily invade of the PBS solution from the interface between Mg particles and PLLA matrix, while water penetrating into the PLLA scaffold was difficult due to its hydrophobicity. Then two reactions would occur simultaneously as follous. On one hand, PLLA would hydrolyze by break of the ester bonds to produce acid products [Equation (2-4)]:

$$PLLA \longrightarrow R_1 - COOH + R_2 - OH \tag{2-4}$$

On the other hand, Mg was highly susceptible to degradation under PBS solution to produce $Mg(OH)_2$ [Equation (2-5)]:

$$Mg + H_2O \longrightarrow Mg(OH)_2 + H_2 \uparrow \tag{2-5}$$

Afterwards, $Mg(OH)_2$ could consume the acid degraded products of PLLA, promoting the hydrolysis [Equation (2-6)]; meanwhile, the acid degraded products of PLLA could consume the alkaline product $Mg(OH)_2$, promoting the degradation of Mg.

$$Mg(OH)_2 + 2R_1 - COOH \longrightarrow (R_1COO)_2Mg + 2H_2O \tag{2-6}$$

So more acid degraded products of PLLA and $Mg(OH)_2$ were produced, and then consumption by neutralization, forming a positive feedback on the degradation of the scaffolds.

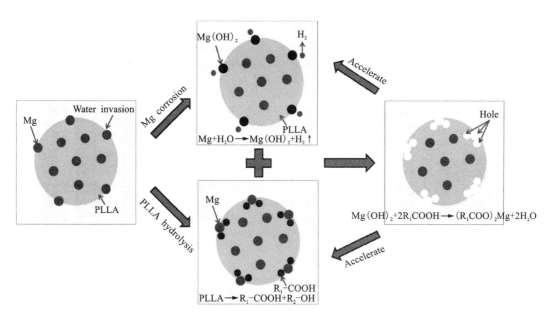

Fig. 2-30　The mechanism of the Mg accelerates the degradation of scaffolds. Firstly more water penetrated into the PLLA/Mg scaffolds. Then two reactions would occur simultaneously: PLLA hydrolyzed to produce acid products; Mg degraded to produce Mg(OH)$_2$. Afterwards, Mg(OH)$_2$ could consume the acid products of PLLA to promote the hydrolysis of PLLA; Meanwhile, the acid products of PLLA could consume Mg(OH)$_2$ and promote the degradation of Mg. Finally, this could form a positive feedback on the degradation of the scaffolds.

2.4.3.5　Mechanical Properties

Compressive strength and compressive modulus of the scaffolds were shown in Fig. 2-31(a). The compressive strength and compressive modulus of PLLA scaffolds were 22.9 MPa and 2.8 GPa, respectively, which reached peak value when the Mg content increased to 5%: increasing by 114.5% and 85.7%, respectively. This could attribute to that Mg played a role of particle strengthening phase, nevertheless, appeared detrimental effect with further increment of Mg due to agglomeration, which was consistent with Fig. 2-25(e). The Vickers hardness of PLLA scaffolds containing different Mg contents presented in Fig. 2-31(b). The Vickers hardness of the PLLA/Mg scaffolds with 5% Mg was 118.4 MPa and increased by 73.9% compared to PLLA scaffolds. Although the Vickers hardness of the PLLA/Mg scaffolds with 5% Mg was near to that with 7% Mg, the compressive strength and modulus of scaffolds with 5% were higher than that with 7% Mg. Considering synthetically the degradation and mechanical experiments, the scaffold with 5% Mg was selected to further evaluate cytocompatibility.

2.4.3.6　Cytocompatibility

The morphologies of MG63 cells, after 1 d and 3 d of incubation on the PLLA and PLLA/Mg scaffolds with 5% Mg, were shown in Fig. 2-32. After 1 d, MG63 cells on the surfaces of the PLLA scaffolds presented fusiform shape and didn't appear filopodia [Fig. 2-32(a)], and the cells

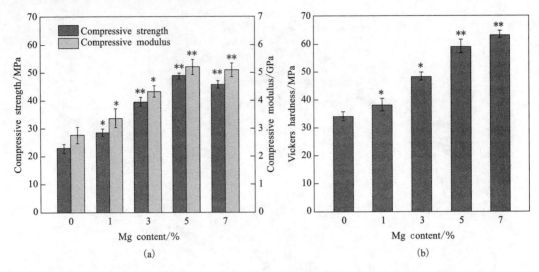

Fig. 2-31　Compressive strength and compressive modulus (a), and Vickers hardness (b) of the PLLA and PLLA/Mg scaffolds with 1%, 3%, 5% and 7% Mg. Compressive strength and compressive modulus of PLLA/Mg scaffolds increased when Mg content increased to 5%, nevertheless appeared detrimental effect with further increment of Mg. The Vickers hardness increased with the addition of Mg.

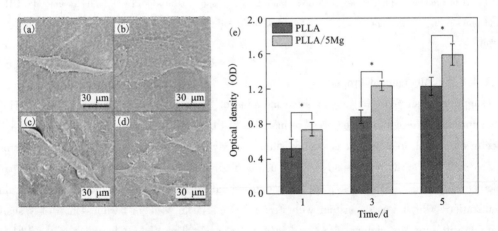

Fig. 2-32　The morphologies of MG63 cells cultivated on PLLA and PLLA/Mg scaffolds with 5% Mg for different time: (a) and (c) 1 day, (b) and (d) 3 days and MTT assay (e) for the scaffolds cultured for 1, 3, and 5 days. MG63 cells cultivated on the PLLA/Mg scaffolds presented better adhesion, spread and proliferation compared with the PLLA scaffolds.

presented clintheriform when the cells were cultured for 3 d [Fig. 2-32(b)]. In comparison, MG63 cells emerged much filopodia anchoring on the surfaces of the PLLA/Mg scaffolds with 5% Mg after 1 d [Fig. 2-32(c)], and grew and stretched to clintheriform obviously after 3 d [Fig. 2-32(d)], which suggested the addition of Mg was conducive to cellular adhesion and spread. The proliferation of MG63 cells cultured on the PLLA and PLLA/Mg scaffolds with 5% Mg, was shown in Fig. 2-32

(e) by MTT assay. The number of cells of PLLA/Mg scaffolds with 5% Mg increased and showed a significant difference after culturing for 1 day compared with the PLLA scaffolds. Meanwhile, the number of MG63 cells also increased as culture time. The result indicated that the introduction of Mg promoted the proliferation of MG63 cells and demonstrated a good cytocompatibility.

2.4.4   Conclusions

In this study, Mg was introduced into PLLA scaffolds to increase their degradation rates. The PLLA/Mg scaffolds were fabricated via SLS, and showed a three-dimensional interconnected porous structure. The introduction of Mg elevated the pH value of the degradation medium and increased the weight loss of the scaffolds. These could be attributed to the alkaline product $Mg(OH)_2$ from the degradation of Mg. It neutralized the acid degraded products of PLLA to promote the hydrolysis of PLLA. Meanwhile, the acid degradation products of PLLA could consume the $Mg(OH)_2$ and promoted the degradation. The mutual neutralization between PLLA and Mg gave a positive feedback on the degradation of the scaffolds. Besides, the compressive strength, compressive modulus and Vickers hardness of the scaffolds were also increased due to the particle strengthening effect of Mg. In addition, the scaffolds showed good cytocompatibility. This study suggested the PLLA/Mg scaffolds may be a potential candidate of bone implants.

Chapter 3

Endow of Anti-bacterial Function

Silver nanoparticles have good antimicrobial properties. In this chapter, silver was successfully introduced into bone implants by in situ growth and ion exchange technology, which endowed polymer scaffolds with durable and stable antimicrobial activity. At the same time, mesoporous material was used to achieve the slow release of silver ions, as well as long-term effective antimicrobial efficacy.

3.1 Antibacterial Polymer Scaffold Based on Mesoporous Bioactive Glass Loaded with in Situ Grown Silver

3.1.1 Introduction

Bacterial infection is a serious problem during orthopedic treatment and often leads to the failure of bone implant. The use of antibiotics is currently the usual method of preventing bacterial infection, while long-term medication may cause bacterial resistance. Recently, silver (Ag) nanoparticle has been considered as an effective antibacterial agent owing to their strong bactericidal activity and broad bactericidal spectrum, as well as no bacterial resistance. Nevertheless, the application of Ag-based antibacterial materials still faces some problems need to be solved, such as the aggregation of Ag nanoparticles in the matrices and the burst release of silver ions (Ag^+) after implant.

It is known that a carrier to load Ag nanoparticles is an effective method to address the aforementioned problems. Serving as a carrier, mesoporous bioactive glass (MBG) has unique advantages: their high specific surface area (up to 750 m^2/g) and large pore volume (about 1 cm^3/g). The silanol enriched mesoporous surface can promote the entry of Ag^+ into the mesoporous channel via electrostatic adsorption. The huge pore volume supplies a large amount of space for Ag loading and the order mesoporous channel provide a "leak-free" function for well control of Ag release. Additionally, the degradation of MBG releases active elements (silicon and calcium) that could up-regulate gene expression levels and induce osteoblast differentiation. Hence, MBG may be a promising carrier for Ag loading to prevent bacterial infections in bone repair. It is worth noting that the method of loading Ag into the mesoporous channel of the MBG is still an urgent problem to address.

In order to obtain Ag nanoparticles in/on a carrier, the redox reaction has been widely employed. For example, Pant et al. prepared Ag nanoparticles on reduced graphene sheets by hydrazine redox reaction and confirmed its effective antibacterial activity. Bhaduri et al. prepared an $Ag-Fe_3O_4$-carbon nanotube composite using sodium borohydride as a reducing agent and found that the composite had high catalytic and antibacterial activity. Compared with these reducing agents, polydopamine is a green reducing agent with plenty of catechol groups and amine groups and exhibits excellent adhesion properties and cytocompatibility. More importantly, its catechol groups are capable of adsorbing Ag^+ into the mesoporous channel via the coordination reaction, and then reducing it into metallic Ag by the redox reaction. Subsequently, metallic Ag acts as nucleation sites, thereby promoting in situ growth of Ag nanoparticles in mesoporous channel. More interestingly, the size of silver nanoparticles can be regulated by adjusting the concentration of Ag^+ ions and the amount of polydopamine. Therefore, polydopamine maybe an ideal reducing agent for obtaining Ag nanoparticles in the mesoporous channel of MBG.

Herein, MBG was used as a carrier and modified with polydopamine (denoted as pMBG). Then, pMBG was further used to capture Ag^+ within silver nitrate ($AgNO_3$) solution and in situ reduce them to metallic Ag. Finally, the Ag-loaded pMBG (Ag@pMBG) was introduced to polymer matrices (poly-l-lactic acid and poly-glycolic acid blends, the mass ratio is 1 : 1) to develop a composite scaffold by additive manufacturing technology. The morphology, structure and chemical composition of Ag@pMBG were analyzed. Moreover, the overall performance of the composite scaffold was evaluated, including antibacterial activity against E. coli, cytocompatibility of osteoblasts, Ag^+ release profile and mechanical properties. Besides, a possible antibacterial mechanism of the composite scaffold was proposed.

3.1.2   Materials and methods

3.1.2.1   Materials

Polyglycolic acid (PGA) with number-average molecular weight (Mn) of 100 kDa and poly-l-lactic acid (PLLA) with Mn of 150 kDa were obtained from Shenzhen Polymtek Biomaterial Co., Ltd. (Shenzhen, China). Dopamine hydrochloride and Tris-HCl (pH = 8.5, 99%) were bought from Sigma (Shanghai, China). Silver nitrate ($AgNO_3$) was bought from Sinopharm Chemical Reagent Co., Ltd. All of the above raw materials were used as received.

Mesoporous bioactive glass (MBG) was obtained by a traditional sol-gel method process, according to a reported research with minor change. Briefly, 3.0 g amphiphilic block copolymer $EO_{20}PO_{70}EO_{20}$ (P123) and 240 mL HCl (2 mol/L) were added to 30 mL of distilled water in a 40℃ water bath with stirring until the solution became clarify. Then, 8.5 g tetraethyl orthosilicate (TEOS), 0.98 g triethyl phosphate (TEP) and 5.94 g $Ca(NO_3)_2 \cdot 4H_2O$ were added to the solution. Subsequently, the mixture was stirred at room temperature for 24 h, and then the resulting precipitate was directly dried in air at 100℃ for 20 h. After that, the synthesized powder was calcined in air at 600℃ for 6 h at a heating rate of 1 ℃/min to completely remove the surfactant template and prepare the final MBG powder.

The preparation of polydopamine-modified MBG was based on our previous study with some modifications. Typically, 4 g of MBG was mixed with 2 g of dopamine hydrochloride in 1000 mL of 10 mmol/L Tris-HCl buffer solution (pH 8.5) using magnetic stirring. During the process, the mixture's color gradually turned to dark brown due to the formation of polydopamine. After 6 h of incubation, the mixture was centrifuged at 6000 r/min for 15 min. Subsequently, the precipitate was washed with deionized water to remove unattached polydopamine and unreacted dopamine. Finally, the precipitate was dried prior to the experiment and denoted as pMBG.

3.1.2.2 In Situ Grown Ag Nanoparticles on pMBG

The strategy used to in situ grown Ag nanoparticles on pMBG powder (denoted as Ag@pMBG) was illustrated in Fig. 3-1 (a). Firstly, various concentrations (20-80 mmol/L) of Ag^+ aqueous solutions were prepared via dissolving $AgNO_3$ particles into deionized water. Subsequently, 1 g of pMBG powder was added to 250 mL of freshly prepared Ag^+ aqueous solutions and magnetic stirring was performed at room temperature at 100 r/min for 5 h. In this process, Ag^+ was first adsorbed on the mesoporous wall via the coordination reaction between Ag^+ and catechol groups. These Ag^+ adsorbed on the pMBG were then in situ reduced to metallic Ag by redox activity of catechol groups, and finally these metallic Ag was in situ grown in the mesoporous channel to form nanoparticles. Ag@pMBG powder was repeatedly washed with excess deionized water for several times, collected by centrifugation, and followed by drying in a vacuum oven for 12 h. The obtained powder was designated as xAg@pMBG, where x represented the initial $AgNO_3$ concentration (x = 2, 4, 6, and 8, respectively).

3.1.2.3 Scaffold Preparation

It is well known that PLLA has a slow rate of biodegradation, while the PGA has a very fast one. Studies have shown that mixtures or copolymers of different ratios of PLLA and PGA may achieve a regulatable degradation rate. Therefore, in the present study, PLLA and PGA were mixed at a mass ratio of 1 : 1 as the matrix material for preparing a scaffold. Prior to the preparation of scaffold, the mixed powder was prepared. Briefly, 0.75g Ag@pMBG or pMBG powder was dispersed in 15ml of absolute ethanol under sonicate for 30 min. Then, the suspension was homogeneously mixed into 85 mL PLLA-PGA solution in ethanol (0.05 g/mL), in which the Ag@pMBG or pMBG was fixed at 15 wt.% in reference to the total weight. The above mixture solution was subjected to ultrasonic vibration, magnetic stirring, filtration, vacuum drying, and mechanical milling in order to obtain the mixed powder for scaffold preparation. The selective laser sintering process was applied to prepare composite scaffold, as shown in Fig. 3-1 (b). Typically, the laser beam scanned the powder bed comply with the construction of scaffold. The laser energy caused the scanned powder to rapidly warm up to the melting point of the polymer matrix, which made the matrix powder to melt and solidify rapidly. At this point, MBG still retained its inherent morphology and structure without being affected due to its significantly stable thermal properties relative to the

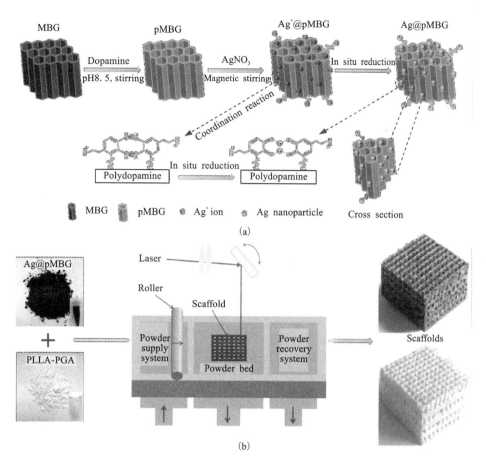

Fig. 3-1　(a) Schematic of Ag@ pMBG preparation, i. e. , in situ reduction of Ag^+ to Ag nanoparticles on the inner and outer surfaces of mesoporous channel of MBG by redox activity of catechol groups. (b) Schematic for preparation of porous composite scaffolds by selective laser sintering. The macroscopic morphology (optical images) of the typical porous scaffolds (PLLA-PGA/Ag@ pMBG and PLLA-PGA/ MBG) demonstrated a uniform pore and strut structure.

substrate. Subsequently, the powder bed dropped a single powder layer thickness (0. 1 mm) and repeated the sintering process until the scaffold was obtained. Throughout the whole sintering process, laser power, scan rate and scan line spacing were maintained at 2. 3 W, 100 mm/s and 1 mm, respectively. Typical porous scaffolds (PLLA-PGA/Ag@ pMBG and PLLA-PGA/MBG) were shown in the Fig. 3-1(b).

3. 1. 2. 4　Characterization

The chemical compositions of Ag @ pMBG, pMBG and MBG were determined by X-ray photoelectron spectroscopy(XPS, ThermoFisher-VG Scientific, USA). Phase composition of these powders was characterized by wide-angle X-ray diffraction (XRD) at rate of 8°/min from 10° to 80° using X-ray diffractometer (D8 Advance, German Bruker Co. , Karlsruhe, Germany) equipped with a Cu Ka radiation. Meanwhile, the order mesoporous structure of the three powders was also evaluated by small angle XRD at rate of 2°/min from 0. 3° to 10°. The nitrogen adsorption-desorption isotherms were acquired on a sorption analyzer (3H-2000PS2, Beshide, China). The specific surface area (S_{BET}) was determined from the adsorption branch with a relative pressure range between 0. 04 and 0. 32, according to multipoint Brunauer-Emmett-Teller (BET) method. The total pore volume (V_p) and pore size distribution of samples were deduced using Barrett-Joyner-Halenda (BJH) method.

The amount of Ag nanoparticles loaded on pMBG was evaluated by thermo-gravimetric (TG) analysis using a TG analyzer. Morphological observations of powder and scaffold were conducted under scanning electron microscope (SEM, Phenom proX, Phenom-World BV, Eindhoven, Netherlands) after being sputter-coated with gold (10 mA, 20 s). Transmission electron microscopy (TEM) images were obtained on an electron microscope (JEOL-1010, Japan) operated at 200 kV. The release behavior of Ag^+ from the scaffold was monitored in deionized water. In detail, the samples were soaked in 10 mL of deionized water in darkness for different time, and the entire solution was collected at each selected interval, and fresh deionized water was refilled accordingly. The concentration of Ag^+ in the supernatant was analyzed by inductively coupled plasma atomic emission spectrometry (ICP-AES, Varian 725 – ES, US). The compressive strength of all scaffolds (including PLLA/PGA scaffold) was determined by compression test using a universal mechanical testing machine with a 100 N static compression load cell at a speed of 0. 5 mm/min. The geometry of the scaffold specimen used for the compression test was a cylinder with 5 mm in diameter and 3 mm in height. The specimen was tested according to ISO 604 (small specimen) and carried out under dry condition. The compressive strength and modulus were obtained through data analysis on the basis of the test data recorded. For ions release and mechanical properties test, each set three samples for repetition.

3.1.2.5 Antibacterial Activity Evaluation

The antibacterial activities of scaffolds with different contents of Ag nanoparticles were evaluated using Escherichia coli (E. coli, ATCC 25922). Prior to testing, all reagents, utensils and scaffold specimens (ϕ10 × 2 mm) used in the experiment were pre-sterilized with UV for 1 h.

The agar diffusion test was used to assess the release antibacterial properties of Ag-loaded scaffold. 100 μL bacterial suspensions (1 × 10^6 CFU/mL) were added into Luria-Bertani (LB) agar medium, and then scaffold specimens were placed in an agar plate and cultured for 24 h at room temperature. The percentage of bacterial inhibition was employed to quantitatively assess the antibacterial effects of the Ag-loaded scaffold. Typically, scaffold specimens were immersed in 1 × 10^5 CFU/mL bacterial suspensions for 24 h. The medium without the bacterial solution and the bacterial solution without any treatment were set as blank and negative controls, respectively. Each test was performed with three parallel samples. At each specific time, bacterial suspensions were subjected to turbidity analysis by a digital camera, and the optical density was also detected at 600 nm by using a microplate reader (SAF-6801, BAJIU Corporation, Shanghai, China). Besides, the pH values of the bacterial suspensions were also measured by a pH analyzer. The bacterial inhibition rate was calculated according to the equation.

Bacterial inhibition rate $(\%) = (B_{Control} - B_{Test})/B_{Control} \times 100\%$

where $B_{Control}$ and B_{Test} were the OD values of the negative control group and the test groups, respectively.

The bacterial morphologies on the scaffold were observed by SEM to evaluate the resistance of the scaffold to bacterial adhesion. In detail, 1×10^6 CFU/mL bacterial suspensions were inoculated on the scaffold, and the scaffold was taken out and washed with phosphate buffered solution (PBS) after 24 hours of culture. The scaffold was then fixed with glutaraldehyde, dehydrated with gradient ethanol and dried in air. Finally, the scaffold was subjected to gold sputtering for SEM observation.

3.1.2.6   Cytocompatibility

Disk scaffold samples ($\phi 10 \times 2$ mm) were selected to assess the effect of the scaffold material component on cell responses. MG-63 cells were cultivated at a density of 5×10^4 cells/scaffold in a humidified atmosphere of 5% CO_2 in DMEM (with 10% fetal bovine serum supplement). The culture medium was renewed every other day.

SEM observations were carried out to evaluate the cell adhesion morphology. The cell/scaffold constructs were extracted after cultured of 3 days and then rinsed with PBS to remove unattached cells. Whereafter, the cell/scaffold constructs were fixed with glutaraldehyde and dehydrated with gradient ethanol. Lastly, the cell/scaffold constructs dried at ambient temperature and sputtered room gold prior to morphological observation.

Fluorescence staining analysis was performed to analyze the viability of cells. In detail, the cell/scaffold constructs were withdrawn from medium and washed three times with PBS after culturing for 3 days. Then, cells were incubated in PBS containing 2 μmol/L calcein AM for 30 min. Finally, cells images were obtained under a fluorescence microscope fitted with a digital camera.

3.1.2.7   Statistical Analysis

Experimental data for all quantitative analyses were presented as means ± standard deviations. Statistical analysis was performed using either One Way ANOVA or Student's t-test if necessary. A significant difference was regarded when $p < 0.05$.

3.1.3   Results and discussion

3.1.3.1   Characterization of Ag@ pMBG

X-ray photoelectron spectroscopy (XPS) was performed to evaluate the surface elemental configurations of the prepared powder. The surface elements of Ag@ pMBG mainly included C, N, O, Si and Ag, where N and C were derived from polydopamine, as shown in Fig. 3-2(a). Clearly, the spectrum of Ag@ pMBG appeared a new peak at around 370 eV compared to pMBG and MBG, which corresponded to the signal peak of the Ag3d. For the Ag3d core level spectrum of Ag@ pMBG [Fig. 3-2(b)], the signal peaks were detected at 368.3 eV and 374.3 eV corresponding to the binding energy of $Ag3d_{5/2}$ and $Ag3d_{3/2}$, respectively, indicating that Ag was presented in the form of metallic Ag in the Ag@ pMBG powder. The wide angle X-ray diffraction (XRD) analysis was conducted for detecting the phase composition of the powder, as shown in Fig. 3-2(c). The three samples had similar XRD patterns, except that four new diffraction peaks were identified at 38.13°, 44.35°, 64.52°, and 77.44° in the pattern of Ag@pMBG. These new emerging peaks corresponded to Bragg reflections from the (111), (200), (220), and (311) crystal faces of Ag (JCPDS card number 04 – 0783), respectively, indicating the presence of cubic metallic Ag. Combined with XPS and wide angle XRD results, it could be considered that the load of Ag on the MBG was successful.

To further investigate whether the Ag loading affected the ordered mesoporous structure of MBG, small-angle XRD analysis was also performed, as shown in Fig. 3-2(d). The results demonstrated that the ordered mesoporous structure of MBG was well preserved after the modification of polydopamine. In comparison, the load of Ag led to a shift of the (100) plane peak to a larger diffraction angle and a decrease in the regularity of the mesoporous structure, indicating smaller pores or channels. A possible reason was that, during the preparation, a portion of the Ag^+ were adsorbed by the polydopamine into the mesoporous channel and then in situ reduced to the metallic Ag via the redox reaction of catechol groups. These in situ grown Ag nanoparticles occupied the space of mesoporous channel, thereby shifting the crystal face peak toward larger diffraction angles.

The N_2 adsorption-desorption isotherms and the corresponding pore size distribution of prepared powder were shown in Fig. 3-2(e) and Fig. 3-2(f). All samples exhibited typical type IV isotherms with hysteresis loops. As could be seen from Fig. 3-2(f), the pore size of these three powders gradually decreased, 5.864 nm for MBG, 5.521 nm for pMBG and 4.494 nm for Ag@pMBG, respectively. The BET surface area (S_{BET}), pore volume (V_P) and pore size (D_P) were derived from the adsorption branch, as listed in Tab. 3-1. It could be seen that the S_{BET} and V_P of Ag@pMBG were smaller than those of MBG, which might be attributed to the in situ grown Ag nanoparticles in the mesoporous channels.

Tab. 3-1　Mesoporous structure parameters of Ag@pMBG, pMBG and MBG

Samples	$S_{BET}/(m^2 \cdot g^{-1})$	$V_P/(cm^3 \cdot g^{-1})$	D_P/nm
Ag@pMBG	264	0.406	4.494
pMBG	417	0.622	5.521
MBG	618	0.726	5.864

3.1.3.2　Micromorphology of Ag@pMBG

Morphologies and elemental compositions of the Ag@pMBG were examined by SEM equipped with energy dispersive spectroscopy (EDS). As shown in Fig. 3-3(a), MBG exhibited an irregular short rod-like structure with the length of about 1 ~ 2 μm. pMBG displayed similar size and shape to the MBG [Fig. 3-3(b)], indicating the polydopamine modification did not change the surface morphology of materials. Interestingly, the catechol and hydroxyl groups of polydopamine have the ability to adsorb and in situ reduce metal ions into metallic nanoparticles, mean while oxidizing themselves to quinone and carbonyl groups respectively. In addition, the electrostatic repulsion

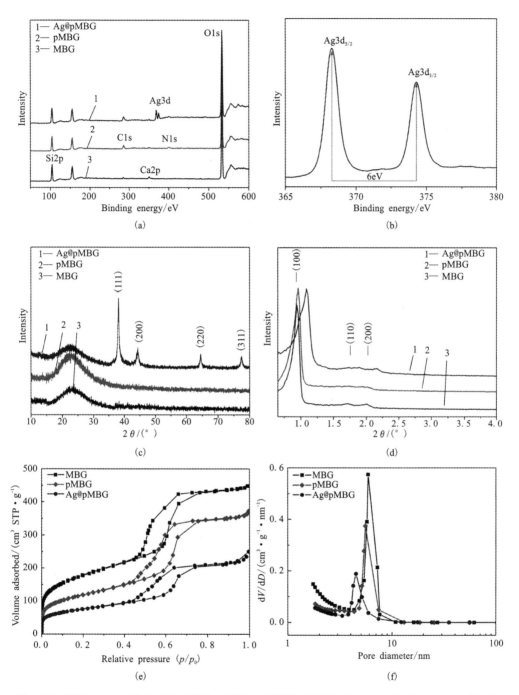

Fig. 3-2　XPS spectra of（a）Ag@ pMBG, pMBG and MBG;（b）the Ag3d core level spectrum of Ag@ pMBG;（c）Wide and（d）small angle XRD patterns of powders. These results indicated that metallic Ag nanoparticles were successfully loaded on MBG by the redox reaction of catechol groups.（e）N_2 adsorption/desorption isotherms and（f）pore size distribution from Barret-Joyner-Hallender（BJH） desorption of samples. The results of small-angle XRD and N_2 adsorption/desorption experiments indicated that in situ grown Ag nanoparticles might occupied the space of mesoporous channels.

between the Ag nanoparticles growing on pMBG was beneficial to prevent the aggregation. Hence, when pMBG powder was added in the Ag$^+$ aqueous solution, Ag nanoparticles were in situ growth on pMBG, as shown in Fig. 3-3(c) and Fig. 3-3(d).

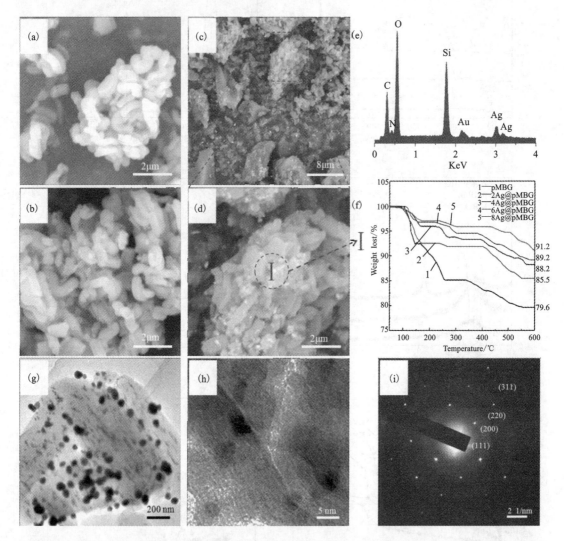

Fig. 3-3 SEM images of MBG (a), pMBG (b) and 6Ag@pMBG (c and d) powders, and EDS spectrum of 6Ag@pMBG (f). Polydopamine modification did not change the surface morphology of materials. The in situ grown Ag nanoparticles were uniformly distributed on pMBG. (e) TG curves of powders with different Ag loading. The results indicated that the amount of silver loaded on pMBG was positively correlated with the AgNO$_3$ concentration. TEM images of 6Ag@pMBG (g-i). The immobilized Ag nanoparticles were distributed on the surface of the rod-shaped MBG. Meanwhile, relatively small size Ag nanoparticles were clearly observed in the channels compared to those on the outer surface.

To further evaluate the size and distribution of Ag-nanoparticles, the morphology of the obtained material was recorded using TEM. As shown in Fig. 3-3(g), the immobilized Ag nanoparticles were distributed on the surface of the rod-shaped MBG. Meanwhile, relatively small size Ag nanoparticles (about 5 nm) were clearly observed in the channels compared to those on the outer surface, as shown in Fig. 3-3(h). In the SAED images [Fig. 3-3(i)], the lattices of (111), (200), (220), and (311) were detected, further confirming the formation of metallic Ag.

TG tests were carried out to evaluate the effect of $AgNO_3$ concentration on the loading amount of metallic Ag on pMBG and the results were shown in Fig. 3-3(e). In detail, the weight loss (mass fraction) of pMBG upon heating to 600℃ was about 20.4% due to evaporation of water and decomposition of polydopamine. Comparatively, Ag@pMBG samples showed less weight loss (approximately 8.8%) under the same conditions. Considering that under a nitrogen atmosphere, metallic Ag was stable during heating and did not cause additional weight loss. Therefore, the more Ag nanoparticles were loaded, the more residues left. According to the residual mass between pMBG and pMBG@Ag, the concentrations of Ag obtained were about 11.6%, 9.6%, 8.6%, and 5.9%, respectively. Hence, these results indicated that the amount of Ag loading on pMBG was closely related to the $AgNO_3$ concentration, which was consistent with the results reported in the literatures. In other words, the amount of Ag grown on pMBG could be adjusted by changing the concentration of $AgNO_3$ to achieve antibacterial activity, without causing side-effect on normal cells.

3.1.3.3　Antibacterial Properties

The Ag-loaded composite scaffolds were expected to exhibit potent antibacterial activity. Therefore, the qualitative and quantitative investigations about the antibacterial activity of the scaffolds were performed. Scaffold samples with diameter of 9 mm were cultured with E. coil for inhibition ring tests [Fig. 3-4(a)]. It was obviously seen that all the scaffolds had an obvious inhibition ring on agar plate except the PLLA-PGA/MBG one, indicating the antibacterial function of Ag-loaded scaffolds. The diameters of the inhibition rings were calculated and listed in Tab. 3-2. It was worth pointing out that the inhibition rings of 6Ag@pMBG and 8Ag@pMBG were 22.5 mm and 24.2 mm, respectively, suggesting the robust antibacterial activity.

To further analyze the antibacterial activity of the Ag-loaded composite scaffolds, bacterial inhibition rate and turbidity analysis tests were carried out, as shown in Fig. 3-4(b) and Fig. 3-4(c). It could be seen from Fig. 3-4(c), the turbidity of the suspension after incubation with the Ag-free scaffold (PLLA-PGA/MBG scaffold) was similar to that of the negative control group, indicating that the reproduction of the bacteria was not inhibited. In comparison, the suspension became transparent after incubating with the Ag-loaded scaffold, indicating most of the bacteria were inhibited from growing or even killed. For bacterial inhibition rate tests, the antibacterial activity of the scaffolds showed a positive correlation with the amount of Ag, as shown in Fig. 3-4(b). The composite scaffolds loaded with 6Ag@pMBG and 8Ag@pMBG exhibited high levels of bacteriostatic activity with a bacterial inhibition rate of over 99%. However, the Ag-free scaffold showed no visible antibacterial activity, demonstrating that Ag confered the antibacterial effect on the scaffolds. These results showed that the Ag-loaded scaffolds developed in this work had significant antibacterial activity.

The pH values of the medium (soaked with different scaffolds) were measured after 24 h of culture, as shown in the Tab. 3-3. It could be seen that the pH of the blank group was maintained

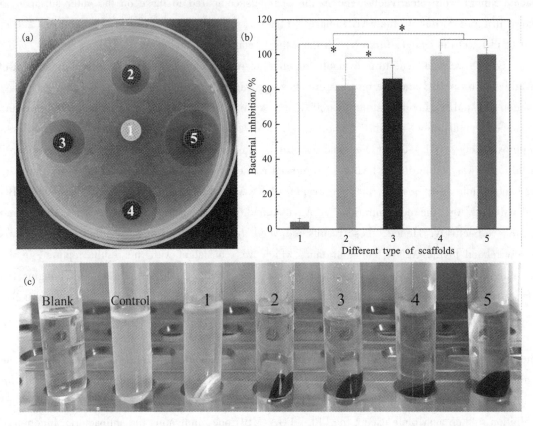

Fig. 3-4 (a) Inhibition rings formed around the different scaffold samples after 24 h culture; (b) bacterial inhibition rate and (c) turbidity analysis of E. coli in liquid medium containing different scaffolds after 24 h of culture. Numbers 1 ~ 5 indicated PLLA-PGA/MBG, PLLA-PGA/2Ag@ pMBG, PLLA-PGA/4Ag@ pMBG, PLLA-PGA/6Ag@ pMBG and PLLA-PGA/8Ag@ pMBG scaffolds, respectively. The results showed that all the scaffolds had an obvious inhibition ring on agar plate except the PLLA-PGA/MBG one, indicating the antibacterial action of Ag-loaded scaffolds. Moreover, the antibacterial activity of the scaffolds showed a positive correlation with the amount of Ag.

around the pH of the original medium (pH = 7.4). In all experimental groups, the negative control had the lowest pH of about 6.8. This might be due to the growth of bacteria causing an increase in environmental acidity (ie., a decrease in pH). In comparison, the pH of the groups immersed with scaffolds were higher than that of the control group, which might be due to the degradation of MBG could alleviate the decrease in pH. The Ag@ pMBG-containing groups had a higher pH relative to the MBG-containing group. This might be due to the presence of Ag that inhibited the proliferation of bacteria or killed bacteria, thereby limiting the pH drop off. Although PLLA-PGA/MBG and PLLA-PGA/xAg@ pMBG groups had similar pH values, PLLA-PGA/MBG group had no significant inhibition or killing effect on bacteria. These results indicated that Ag confered PLLA-PGA/Ag@ pMBG scaffold to inhibit or kill bacterial function.

The results of bacterial adhesion morphology were shown in Fig. 3-5. For Ag-free scaffold, a large number of rod-like bacterial adhered to the surface and were connected to each other [Fig. 3-5 (a)]. In contrast, the amount of adherent bacteria was significantly reduced in the presence of silver [Fig. 3-5(b) and Fig. 3-5(c)]. More importantly, the appearance of bacteria became distorted and atrophied, indicating that their cellular structures were impaired. There were almost no biofilm-like structure was observed on the surfaces of 6Ag@pMBG and 8Ag@pMBG scaffolds compared to those on Ag-free scaffold, as shown in Fig. 3-5(d) and Fig. 3-5(e). These results indicated that the Ag endowed the scaffold with a good resistance to bacterial adhesion and survival.

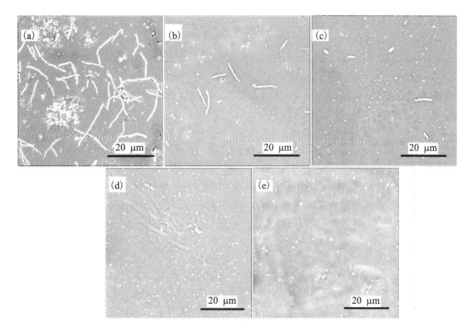

Fig. 3-5　The adhesion morphology of bacterial on different scaffolds. The letters (a)-(e) indicated PLLA-PGA/MBG, PLLA-PGA/2Ag@pMBG, PLLA-PGA/4Ag@pMBG, PLLA-PGA/6Ag@pMBG and PLLA-PGA/8Ag@pMBG scaffolds, respectively. These results indicated that the silver confered the scaffold a good resistance to bacterial adhesion and survival.

Tab. 3-2　Diameters of bacterial inhibition rings for different scaffold samples after 24 h culture.

Scaffold samples	Outer diameter/mm	Diameter difference between outer and inner diameter/mm
PLLA-PGA/8Ag@pMBG	24.2 ± 0.83	14.8 ± 0.72
PLLA-PGA/6Ag@pMBG	22.5 ± 0.78	13.1 ± 0.64
PLLA-PGA/4Ag@pMBG	17.2 ± 0.56	7.9 ± 0.43
PLLA-PGA/2Ag@pMBG	14.4 ± 0.45	5.1 ± 0.25
PLLA-PGA/MBG	—	—

Tab. 3-3 pH values of the medium of different scaffold samples after 24 h culture.

Scaffold samples	pH after 24 h with bacteria ($n = 3$)
PLLA-PGA/8Ag@ pMBG	7.8 ± 0.2
PLLA-PGA/6Ag@ pMBG	7.7 ± 0.1
PLLA-PGA/4Ag@ pMBG	7.6 ± 0.2
PLLA-PGA/2Ag@ pMBG	7.6 ± 0.1
PLLA-PGA/MBG	7.3 ± 0.2
Control	6.8 ± 0.2
Blank	7.4 ± 0.1

A possible antibacterial mechanism of Ag-loaded composite scaffolds was shown in Fig. 3-6. During the cultivation, the antibacterial active Ag^+ and Ag nanoparticles released from the composite scaffolds via the molecular diffusion and degradation behavior. The released Ag^+ bound onto negatively charged bacterial membranes by electrostatic adsorption and interaction with thiol groups (—SH) on membrane proteins, causing membrane proteins to lose respiratory and material transport functions. As a result, the interaction of Ag^+ with the bacterial membrane regulated membrane permeability and disrupted membrane integrity. Moreover, high catalytic ability of Ag and high reduction potential of Ag^+ catalyzed the single electron reduction of O_2 and damaged the respiratory chain of bacteria, thereby producing strongly oxidizing reactive oxygen species (ROS, such as OH^-, O^{2-}, H_2O_2) in the intracellular space. These highly active Ag^+ and ROS destroyed the structure and function of bacteria in the cytoplasm mainly by destroying the structure of DNA molecule through replacing hydrogen bonds, inhibiting the replication and transcription of bacterial mRNA, coagulating proteins and destroying the activity of enzymes. These attacks rapidly destroyed the proliferative capacity of the bacteria, thereby achieving the purpose of inhibition or kill. After the bacteria were lysed, Ag nanoparticles and Ag^+ were released from the corpses and involved in the next killing.

3.1.3.4 Cytocompatibility

To better evaluate the potential applications of the prepared scaffolds in tissue engineering, the cytocompatibility experiments were performed. The adhesion morphology of MG63 cells was observed by SEM after cultivated on the scaffolds for 3 days [Fig. 3-7(a)]. The cells intimately attached to PLLA-PGA scaffold, showing a flat and stretched morphology with filopodia [Fig. 3-7(a0)]. The cells cultured on the scaffold with MBG exhibited a flatter morphology [Fig. 3-7(a1)], indicating better cytocompatibility. Encouragingly, cells on PLLA-PGA/Ag@ pMBG scaffold had similar adhesion morphology to those on PLLA-PGA/MBG scaffold, as shown in Fig. 3-7(a2) ~ (a4). However, some of the cells shrank to be irregularly rounded shape on the PLLA-PGA/8Ag@ pMBG scaffold [Fig. 3-7(a5)]. The results indicated that MBG had a promoting effect on cell attachment, while excess Ag might have adverse effects, although it was generally accepted as cytocompatible.

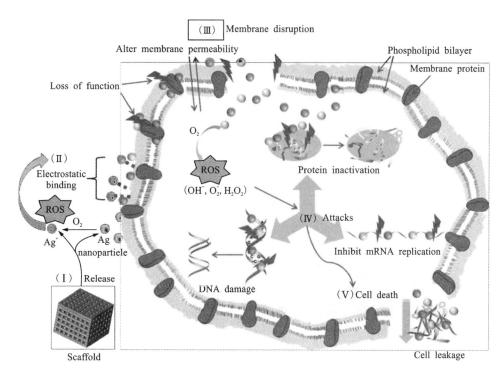

Fig. 3-6   A schematic for the antibacterial mechanism of Ag-loaded composite scaffold. (I) Release of
Ag nanoparticles and Ag$^+$. (II) Electrostatic binding: Ag$^+$ binds bound with negatively charge bacterial
membranes by electrostatic interaction. (III) Cell membrane disruption: the interaction of Ag$^+$ with the
bacterial membrane altered membrane permeability and disrupted membrane integrity. (IV) Intracellular
attacks: the structure of DNA molecule destroed by replacing hydrogen bonds, the transcription and
synthesis of mRNA inhibited and the protein to be attacked it inactivation. (V) Cell death: Ag
nanoparticles and Ag$^+$ were released from the corpses of the bacteria and involved in the next killing.

The viability of MG-63 cells was detected at 3th day by using live cell imaging, as shown in
Fig. 3-7 (b). All the scaffolds showed good cytocompatibility and were able to support cell
attachment with good diffusion morphology except the PLLA-PGA/8Ag@pMBG scaffold, which was
consistent with the results of cell adhesion. The results indicated that the incorporation of MBG into
the scaffold could increase cell viability and enhance cell proliferation to some extent. Additionally,
the enhancing effect on cell response was not reduced by loading appropriate amount of Ag in the
scaffold. The good cytocompatibility of the scaffold material might be due to the large specific surface
area of the MBG facilitating cell adhesion. The hydrophilic groups of polydopamine (such as —OH
and —NH$_2$) could regulate the surface charge of the scaffold and promote cell adhesion and
stretching . In addition, the degradation of MBG released active elements (silicon and calcium) that
could up-regulate gene expression levels and induce osteoblast differentiation. To sum up, the
antibacterial activity and cytocompatibility experiments indicated that the scaffold containing
appropriate amount of Ag exhibited significant antibacterial activity and good cytocompatibility.

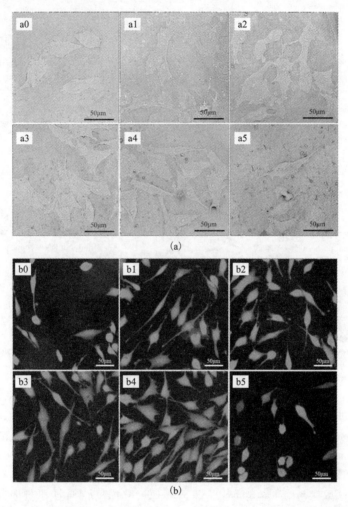

Fig. 3-7 (a) The adhesion morphology and (b) fluorescence staining of MG63
cells cultured for 3 days. Numbers 0 – 5 indicated PLLA-PGA, PLLA-PGA/
MBG, PLLA-PGA/2Ag@ pMBG, PLLA-PGA/4Ag@ pMBG, PLLA-PGA/6Ag
@ pMBG and PLLA-PGA/8Ag@ pMBG scaffolds, respectively.

3.1.3.5 Characterization of Scaffolds

Based on the balance of antibacterial activity and cytocompatibility, the PLLA-PGA/6Ag@
pMBG scaffold was selected to study the release kinetics of Ag^+. The amount of non-cumulative
Ag^+ releasing in deionized water was shown in Fig. 3-8(a). It could be seen that the release amount
of Ag^+ on the first day of soaking was 16.6 μg/ml. Subsequently, the release amount of Ag^+
decreased with the immersion time and stabilized after 7 days. Encouragingly, the release level of
Ag^+ after 28 days of soaking was still comparable to that at 7th day. Meanwhile, the cumulative
release experiments demonstrated that the release of Ag^+ showed time dependence and the release
amount remained to increase steadily after 28 days [Fig. 3-8(b)]. This sustained release properties
would help to produce long-term antibacterial effects that inhibited bacterial growth. There were

three possible factors responsible for the sustained release of Ag^+. Firstly, the Ag nanoparticles formed by in situ reduction enhanced interfacial bonding with the MBG, and thus had good stability. Secondly, the order mesoporous channel of MBG provide a "leak-free" function for well control of silver release. Thirdly, the polymer matrices provided further guarantee for the sustained release.

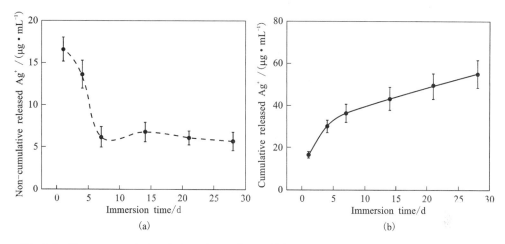

Fig. 3-8 The non-cumulative (a) and cumulative (b) silver ion release profile from the PLLA-PGA/6Ag@pMBG scaffold in deionized water. The release level of Ag^+ after 28 days of soaking was still comparable to that at 7th day. This sustained release properties would help to produce long-term antibacterial effects that inhibited bacterial growth.

The mechanical property is a key evaluation indicator for tissue engineering scaffolds. The dependence of mechanical properties of PLLA-PGA scaffold samples on Ag@pMBG contents was shown in Fig. 3-9. The addition of Ag@pMBG caused a significant increase in mechanical properties. Concretely, compressive strength and modulus were increased from (22.1±1.8) MPa and (2.2±0.1) GPa for PLLA-PGA samples to (48.2±2.2) MPa and (3.3±0.1) GPa for PLLA-PGA/MBG samples, respectively. Interestingly, for PLLA-PGA/8Ag@pMBG samples, they were further increased to (65.5±4.6) MPa and (3.8±0.2) GPa. To sum up, the compressive strength and modulus of the scaffolds with Ag@pMBG were higher than those containing the same amount of MBG. For PLLA-PGA/MBG samples, the prepared MBG powder with high surface area enhanced the reinforcing effect by filling the pores of the polymer, which had an important influence on the improvement of mechanical properties. For PLLA-PGA/Ag@pMBG samples, we speculated that the interfacial enhancement effect and particle reinforcement effect might responsible for the further improvement in mechanical properties. On one hand, the polydopamine interfacial layer improved the interfacial interaction between the inorganic filler phase and the organic polymer matrices. On the other hand, silver nanoparticles in situ grown could also be used as a particle reinforced phase to further improve mechanical properties.

The dispersion of filler in matrices is closely related to the mechanical properties of scaffold. Thereby, the top surface microstructure of the scaffolds was observed and as shown in Fig. 3-10.

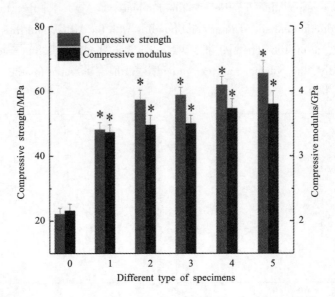

Fig. 3-9 The compressive strength and modulus of composite scaffolds samples. Numbers 0 – 5 indicated PLLA-PGA, PLLA-PGA/MBG, PLLA-PGA/2Ag@ pMBG, PLLA-PGA/4Ag@ pMBG, PLLA-PGA/6Ag@ pMBG and PLLA-PGA/8Ag@ pMBG scaffold samples, respectively. The addition of Ag@ pMBG caused a significant increase in mechanical properties. Taken together, the compressive strength and modulus of the scaffolds with Ag@ pMBG were higher than those containing the same amount of MBG. The interfacial enhancement effect of polydopamine and the particle reinforcement effect of inorganic material might be responsible for the improvement of the mechanical properties of scaffold samples.

PLLA-PGA scaffold exhibited a smooth surface [Fig. 3-10(a)]. The surface topography of PLLA-PGA/MBG became rougher and the MBG was aggregated in matrices [Fig. 3-10(b)]. In comparison, at the same level of loading (15%), Ag@ pMBG exhibited uniformly distribution in the matrix and different contents of silver did not show an adverse effect on their dispersion in the matrices, as shown in Fig. 3-10(c) ~ Fig. 3-10(f). Moreover, EDS analysis results further confirmed this conclusion, as shown in the insets of Fig. 3-10(b) and Fig. 3-10(e), respectively. The significant difference in the dispersion of Ag@ pMBG and MBG in the matrix could be attributed to polydopamine modification. Several studies have demonstrated that polydopamine modification enhances the interfacial interaction between MBG and the polymer matrix, thereby promoting its dispersibility.

3.1.4 Conclusions

In summary, novel antibacterial polymer scaffold based on mesoporous bioactive glass (MBG) loaded with in situ grown silver was constructed by additive manufacturing technology. MBG was used as a carrier for in situ grown silver to achieve sustained antibacterial activity. Polydopamine was served as a green reducing agent to adsorb Ag⁺ via coordination reaction and then reduc them in situ

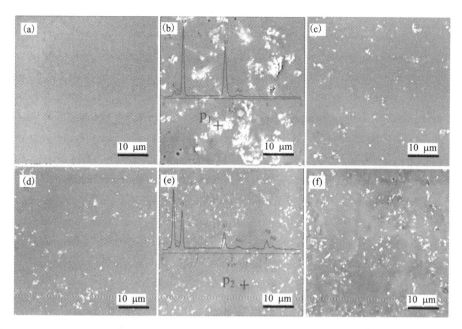

Fig. 3-10   SEM images of the top surface morphology of composite scaffolds. Letters (a)-(f) indicated PLLA-PGA, PLLA-PGA/MBG, PLLA-PGA/2Ag @ pMBG, PLLA-PGA/4Ag @ pMBG, PLLA-PGA/6Ag@ pMBG and PLLA-PGA/8Ag@ pMBG scaffolds, respectively. In comparison, at the same level of loading (15%), Ag@ pMBG exhibited uniformly distribution in the matrix and different contents of silver did not show an adverse effect on their dispersion in the matrices. The significant difference in the dispersion of Ag@ pMBG and MBG in the matrix could be attributed to polydopamine modification.

into metallic Ag nanoparticles by the redox of catechol groups. The results showed that Ag@ pMBG endowed antibacterial activity to Ag-free scaffold. The release of Ag^+ from the composite scaffold exhibited a sustained release pattern, meaning a long-term antibacterial activity. Meanwhile, the composite scaffold also had significantly enhanced mechanical properties compared to PLLA-PGA scaffolds. Taken together, the porous PLLA-PGA/Ag @ pMBG composite scaffold might be a potential candidate for the treatment of infected bone defects.

3.2   Montmorillonite with Unique Interlayer Space Imparted Polymer Scaffolds with Sustained Release of Ag^+

3.2.1   Introduction

Polyglycolic acid (PGA), a biodegradable aliphatic polyester, has received much attention as a promising scaffold material due to its excellent biocompatibility, which has been approved by US Food and Drug Administration for biomedical application. However, its poor strength and modulus are unable to provide sufficient mechanical support for bearing loads during bone repair. Besides, its degradable rate is mso fast, resulting in losing the structural and mechanical integrity earfier when applied in bone repair. Meanwhile, it is worth noticing that bacterial infection is a common problem in bone repair, which raises the failure risk of repair.

Introducing bioceramics is an effective strategy to improve the performances of polymers. Many bioceramics have been attempted, such as silicate and phosphate ceramics. Among them, Montmorillonite (MMT), an aluminum silicate ceramic, shows great potential. It has very high elastic modulus (– 170 GPa), able to act as rigid reinforcements to enhance the mechanical performances of polymers. Moreover, MMT possesses high impermeability against water, capable of acting as barriers to hinder the diffusion of water and its attack on polymer matrix, hence decreasing the permeability and slowing the degradable rate. Farida Yahiaoui et al. introduced MMT to polycaprolactone films, and found the mechanical properties and water vapor barrier properties of the films were enhanced. Ali Olad et al. prepared chitosan/gelatin/hydroxyapatite-MMT scaffolds, indicating MMT increased the mechanical properties and decreased the degradable rate of the scaffolds.

More importantly, MMT possesses unique interlayer space structure and ion exchange property. Its lattice unit consists of a central alumina octahedral sheet fused to two bilateral silica tetrahedral sheets via sharing the oxygen atoms, constructing a sandwich-like layer. The layers are regularly stacked together via Van Der Walls force, leaving gaps between the layers, which are called interlayer space. There are large amounts of negative charges in interlayer space, which are generated by the isomorphic substitutions within the layers such as the replacement of Si^{4+} in the tetrahedral by Al^{3+}. The negative charges are balanced by attracting hydrated alkaline cations such as Ca^{2+} into the interlayer space. It is worth noting that the hydrated alkaline cations only have an weak interaction with the layers, which can be easily exchanged by other cations (such as Ag^+ and Cu^{2+}) with stronger interaction. Considering that Ag^+ has good antibacterial properties and metallic Ag has higher stability, we are thinking whether a sustained Ag^+ release and long-lasting antibacterial property may be achieved if Ag can be loaded into the interlayer space of MMT via ion exchange and further chemical reduction. In this case, the impermeable layered structure of MMT may both barrier the attack of water on Ag and the diffusion of Ag^+, hence greatly lowering the release rate of Ag^+.

In this study, MMT was incorporated to PGA scaffolds to increase the mechanical properties, decrease the degradable rate, and impart them with sustained release and antibacterial properties. Three-dimensional porous scaffolds were prepared via additive manufacturing. The mechanical properties of the scaffolds were tested in terms of compressive properties and hardness. The degradable properties were evaluated with respect to mass loss, pH and morphology. More importantly, Ag^+ was loaded into the interlayer space of MMT via ion exchange, which was further chemically reduced to metallic Ag with higher stability. The Ag^+ release behaviors of the scaffolds were investigated, and the antibacterial properties were also evaluated.

3.2.2　Material and Methods

3.2.2.1　Materials and Preparation

PGA with Mw of about 100 kDa was provided by Shenzhen Polymtek Biomaterial Co. , Ltd. (Shenzhen, China). MMT with cation exchange capacity (CEC) of about 130 mmol/100 g were obtained from Chifeng Hezhengmei Chemical Industry Co. , Ltd (Chifeng, China).

PGA-MMT powders were prepared as follows: (a) certain amounts of PGA and MMT were added to two beakers with anhydrous ethanol according to the composition design, respectively; (b) the PGA and MMT suspensions were magnetically stirred for 1 h, respectively, and then ultrasonically dispersed for 1 h, respectively; (c) the MMT suspension was poured into PGA suspension, and then forth the blending suspension was magnetically stirred forth and ultrasonically dispersed respectively; (d) the PGA-MMT blending precipitate was obtained by filtering, and then was dried at 60℃ to constant weight; (e) fine PGA-MMT powders was obtained by ball willing for preparing scaffolds finally. Four formulations of PGA-MMT powders containing 2.5%, 5%, 7.5% and 10% MMT were prepared, and named as PGA-2.5% MMT, PGA-5% MMT, PGA-7.5% MMT and PGA-10% MMT, respectively.

A self-developed SLS machine, consisting mainly of a carbon dioxide laser and a 3D galvanometer scanner, was employed to fabricate scaffolds. Three-dimensional porous scaffolds were fabricated layer by layer according to the section profiles of the model: (a) a layer of the powders was spread to forming piston by a roller; (b) the spread powder layer was selectively scanned by laser beam according to the section profiles, where the powders in the scanned region were sintered together while the unscanned region remained loose; (c) the powder delivery piston ascended a height of a layer after the previous layer was finished sintering; (d) new powder layers were spread and sintered successively according to the steps (a-c) until all the layers were finished sintering. Finally, the porous scaffolds were obtained by removing the unsintered loose powders in the pores via blowing high-pressure air. The main processing parameters including laser power, scanning speed, scanning spacing and layer thickness were set as 2 W, 180 mm/s, 0.1 mm and 0.1 mm, respectively.

3.2.2.2　Microstructure and Mechanical Properties

The phase composition of the scaffolds was analyzed by X-ray diffractometer (XRD) (Bruker D8, German Bruker Co. , Karlsruhe, Germany) at 4°/min using Ni-filtered Cu Kα radiation (λ = 1.5406 Å). The identification of functional groups was performed by Fourier Transform Infrared Spectroscopy (FTIR) (Nicolet 6700, Thermo Nicolet, Madison, WI). The morphology of the scaffolds was characterized by scanning electron microscope (SEM) (Phenom ProX, Phenom-World BV, Eindhoven, Netherlands) equipped with energy disperse spectroscopy (EDS) (INCA, Oxford Instruments, UK).

The compressive properties of the scaffolds were tested with a universal testing machine (MTS Insight 30, MTS Systems Corporation, MN, USA). The loading rate was fixed at 1 mm/min. The compressive strength and modulus were determined from the automatically recorded stress-strain curves. The Vickers hardness of the scaffolds was measured with a Vickers microhardness tester (TMVS-1, Beijing Time High technology Co., Ltd, Beijing, China) at a loading force and a loading time of 2.94 N and 15 s, respectively. The values of Vickers hardness were automatically calculated and displayed.

3.2.2.3 Degradable Properties

The degradable properties of the PGA/MMT scaffolds were investigated by immersion test in PBS (pH = 7.4). The initial weight of the scaffolds prior to the test was weighed with analytical balance. The scaffolds were placed into cap-sealed centrifuge tubes containing PBS and incubated at 37℃. After incubation for scheduled time (7, 14, 21 and 28 days), the scaffolds and PBS solutions were taken out and collected, respectively. The pH values of the collected solutions were tested by a digital pH meter with 0.01 resolution. The extracted scaffolds were vacuum dried to constant weight to calculate the weight loss according to the equation (3-1):

$$\text{Weight Loss } (\%) = (W_0 - W_t)/W_0 \times 100 \tag{3-1}$$

Where W_0 and W_t represent the initial weight before immersion and the residual weight after immersion for t days, respectively. After testing the weight loss, the scaffolds were used to characterize the surface morphology by SEM to further evaluate the degradation behaviors.

3.2.2.4 Cytocompatibility

MG63 cells were used to evaluate the cytocompatibility of the scaffolds including cell adhesion, viability and differentiation. The cells were cultured in low glucose DMEM containing 10% fetal bovine serum and 1% antibiotic-antimycotic solution at 37℃ in 5% CO_2 of air atmosphere. The cells were seeded to the scaffold specimens in 48 - well plate and incubated for 1 and 3 days. The cell viability and proliferation were evaluated by fluorescence staining assay. The cells were incubated with PBS containing 4 mmol/L calcein AM for 30 min; live cells were stained green due to the calcein reaction between intracellular esterase and calcein AM. The stained cells were imaged with a light microscope. The osteogenic differentiation was assessed by ALP staining using an alkaline phosphatase color development kit(P0321, Shanghai Beyotime Biological Technology Co., Ltd, Shanghai, China) according to the instructions of the manufacturer. The stained cells were imaged with a light microscope.

3.2.2.5 Sustained Release Properties and Antibacterial Properties

Ag^+ was loaded into the interlayer space of MMT via ion exchange, and was further chemically reduced to metallic Ag with higher stability. In ion exchange, certain amounts of MMT were suspended in deionized water and magnetically stirred. Then, silver nitrate ($AgNO_3$) at a molar ratio of $AgNO_3$/CEC of MMT = 2/1 was dissolved and added into the MMT suspension. Afterwards, the suspension was kept magnetically stirring for 24 h at room temperature for sufficient ion exchange to produce MMT@ Ag^+. In chemical reduction, sodium borohydride ($NaBH_4$) at a molar ratio of $NaBH_4$/$AgNO_3$ = 2/1 was dissolved in deionized water and dropwise added into the MMT@ Ag^+ suspension with continuously magnetically stirring. After finishing adding $NaBH_4$, the suspension was kept magnetically stirring for 24 h at room temperature for sufficient chemical reduction to obtain MMT@ Ag suspension. Afterwards, the suspension was centrifuged at 10000 r/min for 10 min; the generated precipitates were washed with distilled water and then dried at 40℃ to constant weight. Finally, the dried precipitates were ball-milled for 12 h to obtain fine MMT@ Ag powders. The method to prepare PGA-MMT@ Ag powders and scaffolds was consistent with that of PGA-MMT.

The release behaviors of Ag$^+$ from the PGA-MMT@ Ag scaffolds were evaluated using deionized water immersion in cap-sealed tubes. At scheduled time intervals, the scaffold specimens were extracted from the tube and transferred to another tube containing fresh deionized water. The deionized water after immersing with the scaffold specimens was collected to detect the release amounts of Ag$^+$ using inductively coupled plasma (ICP) (ICP-OES, Spectro Blue Sop, German). The cumulative release amounts of Ag$^+$ were calculated by adding the release amounts of different time intervals(for 1, 3, 5, 7, 14, 21 and 28 days).

The antibacterial properties of the scaffolds were assessed using inhibition zone method, turbidimetry method and morphology characterization, using E. coli as testing bacteria. The bacteria were grown in lysogenic brothculture medium. They were diluted according to McFarland standard before use. Inhibition zone method was performed to assess long-lasting antibacterial properties. The bacteria/culture medium mixing suspensions at a concentration of about 1×10^6 CFU/mL were evenly spread over the plate. Subsequently, disk scaffold specimens were equidistantly placed onto the plate and incubation at 37℃. After incubating for scheduled time (1, 3, 5, 7, 14, 21 and 28 days), the inhibition zones were photographed and their diameters were measured. Turbidimetry method was performed to evaluate the antibacterial rates of the scaffolds. The scaffolds were immersed in transparent tubes containing 1×10^6 CFU/mL bacterial/culture medium mixing with suspensions and incubated in a rotary shaker at 37℃ for 24 h. After incubation, the tubes were photographed to directly observe the turbidity of the suspensions. Meanwhile, the absorbance of the suspensions was quantitatively tested with a microplate reader at 600 nm to calculate the antibacterial rates according to the equation (3-2):

$$\text{Antibacterial rate } (\%) = (A_2\text{-}A_1)/A_1 \times 100 \tag{3-2}$$

where A_2 and A_1 were the absorbance of the bacterial suspensions immersing with and without scaffolds, respectively. SEM characterization was performed to check the morphology of the bacteria after the scaffolds was treated. The scaffolds were inoculated with bacterial suspension at a concentration of 1×10^6 CFU/mL and incubated at 37℃ for 24 h. Afterwards, the cell/scaffold constructs were fixed with 2.5% glutaraldehyde for 4 h and gently washed with PBS, followed by dehydrated with a graded series of alcohol and then dred at 37℃ for 24 h. Finally, the scaffolds were gold sputtered for SEM characterization.

3.2.2.6   Statistical Analysis

The data were expressed as the mean ± standard deviation. Levene's test was used to examine the equality of variances. Statistical significance was determined by unpaired two-tailed Student's t-test, with $^*p < 0.05$ to be significantly different.

3.2.3　Results and Discussion

3.2.3.1　Characterization of PGA-MMT Scaffolds

SEM morphologies of PGA, MMT and PGA-MMT powders were shown in Fig. 3-1 (a)-Fig. 3-1 (c). It was obvious that MMT was much smaller than PGA, with sizes of several microns [Fig. 3-1 (b)] and dozens of microns [Fig. 3-1 (a)], respectively. The size difference made it easy to distinguish them in the PGA-MMT powders [Fig. 3-1 (c)]. According to the results of laser

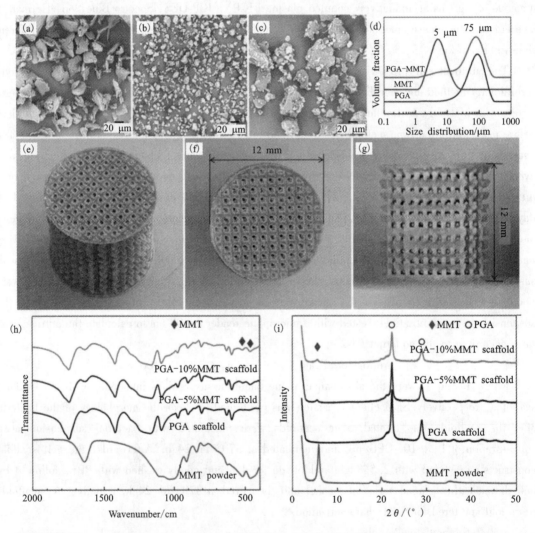

Fig. 3-11　The morphologies of (a) PGA, (b) MMT and (c) PGA-MMT powders; the size difference made it easy to distinguish PGA and MMT; (d) the size distribution of the powders; PGA-MMT powders showed two peaks belonging to PGA and MMT; (e-g) the photographs of a representative SLS-fabricated three-dimensional porous PGA-MMT scaffold from (e) isometric, (f) top and (g) left views; the porous structure was well-ordered and completely interconnected with pore size of about 400 μm; (h) the FT-IR spectra and (i) XRD patterns of scaffolds; MMT was detected in the PGA-MMT scaffolds.

particle-size distribution[Fig. 3-1(d)], the median particle diameter of PGA and MMT powders was about 75 μm and 5 μm, respectively, which were both detected in the PGA-MMT powders. A representative SLS-fabricated three-dimensional porous MMt-PGA scaffold was shown in Fig. 3-1(e)- Fig. 3-1(g). The scaffold exhibited a periodic and completely interconnected porous structure, with pore size of about 400 μm [Fig. 3-1(f)]. FT-IR and XRD were performed to verify the existence of MMT in scaffolds. In Fig. 3-1(h), MMT showed a absorption band at 1640 cm^{-1}, which was associated to H—O—H bending; the bands at 1104, 1032 and 913 cm^{-1} were related to Si—O—Si stretching; the bands at 518 and 464 cm^{-1} corresponded to Si—O and Si—O—X (where X = Mg or Al) bending, respectively. PGA scaffolds exhibited characteristic peaks at 1747 cm^{-1} and 595 cm^{-1}, which corresponded to C=O stretching; the bands at 1420 and 1091 cm^{-1} were associated to C—H bending; the band at 1175 cm^{-1} was related to C—O stretching. Compared with PGA scaffolds, PGA-MMT scaffolds showed two additional bands around 518 and 464 cm^{-1}, which indicated the existence of MMT in the scaffolds. In the XRD patterns [Fig. 3-1(i)], MMT showed a characteristic diffraction peak at 2θ = 5. 8°, which was corresponding to the (001) basal reflection. PGA exhibited peaks at 2θ = 22.3° and 29.0°, which were assigned to the (110) and (020) crystal planes, respectively. For PGA-MMT scaffolds, a diffraction peak around 5.8° was detected, verifying the existence of MMT.

3.2.3.2　Mechanical Properties

The mechanical properties of PGA-MMT scaffolds were tested in terms of compressive properties and hardness, as shown in Fig. 3-2(a) and Fig. 3-2(b), respectively. It could be seen that the compressive strength and modulus increased initially and decreased afterwards as MMT content increased, with a turning point at 7.5% [Fig. 3-2(a)]. The hardness showed a similar change trend to that of compressive strength and modulus [Fig. 3-2(b)]. At an optimal content of 7.5%, the compressive strength, modulus and hardness of the scaffolds achieved optimal values of 42.8 MPa, 3.7 GPa and 94.2 HV, which increased by 62.5%, 66.0% and 43.2%, respectively, compared with PGA scaffolds (26.3 MPa, 2.2 GPa and 65.8 HV, respectively). The distribution of MMT in the matrix was characterized by SEM-EDS, as shown in Fig. 3-2(c)-Fig. 3-2(h). PGA scaffold showed a relatively smooth cross section [Fig. 3-2(c)]. After incorporating MMT, the scaffolds showed relatively rough cross sections with MMT particles embedding in the PGA matrix; more particles exposed with more content [Fig. 3-2(d)-Fig. 3-2(g)]. It could be seen that MMT particles could be distributed relatively uniformly in the matrix when the content was no more than 7.5%, [Fig. 3-2(d)-Fig. 3-2(f)], while they became relatively aggregated when the content continued increasing [Fig. 3-2(g)]. It was well known that the distribution of reinforcement had significant effects on the final mechanical properties of polymer composites. When the content of reinforcements was lower than a certain value (7.5% in this work), they distributed relatively uniformly in the polymer matrix, effectively absorbing and transferring the stress, so the mechanical properties increased with the content increasing. However, when the content exceeded the certain value, the reinforcements easily formed serious aggregates, which became the center of defects, resulting in the stress concentration and collapse. As a result, the mechanical properties began to decrease.

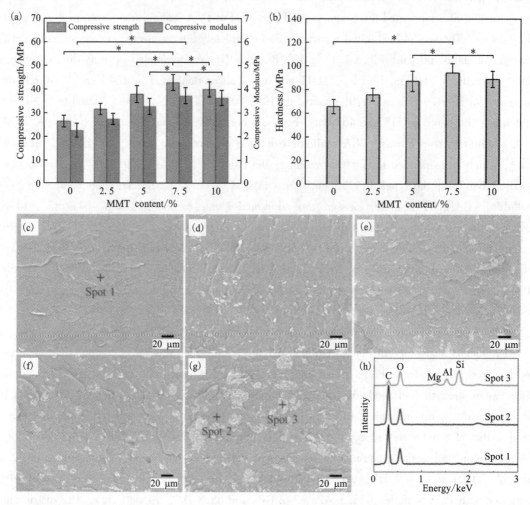

Fig. 3-12 (a) The compressive properties and (b) hardness of the scaffolds with different MMT contents; the compressive strength, modulus and hardness increased initially and decreased afterwards as MMT content increased, with a turning point at 7.5%; (c-g) cross-section morphologies showed the distribution of MMT in PGA matrix of the scaffolds containing (c) 0, (d) 2.5%, (e) 5%, (f) 7.5% and (g) 10%; (h) the EDS spectr of spots 1, 2 and 3; MMT at 2.5% ~ 7.5% was well dispersed in the scaffold matrix, while forming some obvious aggregates at 10%.

3.2.3.3 Degradable Properties

The degradable properties of PGA-MMT scaffolds were evaluated in terms of pH, mass loss and morphology after immersion in PBS, as shown in Fig. 3-3. The mass loss of the scaffolds gradually increased as the immersion time prolonged [Fig. 3-3(a)]. Moreover, it evident that incorporating MMT made the mass loss of the scaffolds decrease and the effect was enhanced with MMT content increasing. After 28 days of degradation, the mass loss of PGA, PGA-2.5% MMT, PGA-5% MMT, PGA-7.5% MMT and PGA-10% MMT scaffolds was 26.0%, 24.5%, 22.4%, 19.9% and

18.3%, respectively. The pH of PBS gradually decreased with immersion time increasing [Fig. 3-3 (b)], which resulted from the accumulation of acid degraded product of PGA. Moreover, it was noteworthy that incorporating MMT delayed the pH decrease and the effect was strengthened with MMT content increasing. After 28 days of immersion, the pH value of PBS corresponding to PGA, PGA-2.5%MMT, PGA-5%MMT, PGA-7.5%MMT and PGA-10%MMT scaffolds was 6.85, 6.91, 6.94, 6.98 and 7.05, respectively. The morphology of the scaffolds after 28 days of immersion was shown in Fig. 3-3(c)-Fig. 3-3(g). There were many pits on the surface of PGA scaffold [Fig. 3-3 (c)], which resulted from the degradation and outflow of PGA matrix. After incorporating MMT, the sizes and amounts of pits decreased, indicating MMT hindered the degradation of MMT matrix [Fig. 3-3(d-g)]. With MMT content increasing, the hindering effect enhanced. The degradation mechanism of polyesters was hydrolysis, via the attack of water and the cleavage of the ester bonds.

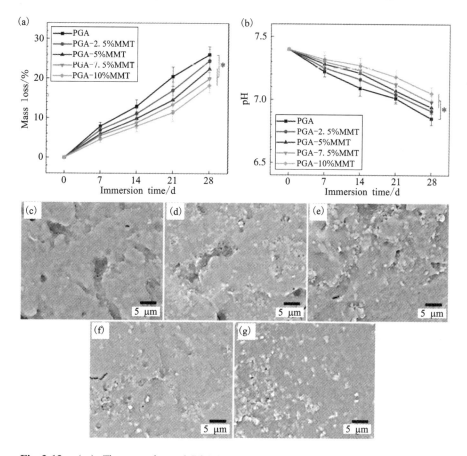

Fig. 3-13   (a) The mass loss of PGA-MMT scaffolds and (b) the pH of PBS after immersion for 7, 14, 21 and 28 days; MMT decreased the mass loss of the scaffolds and delayed the pH decrease of PBS; (c-g) surface morphology of the scaffolds containing (c) 0, (d) 2.5%, (e) 5%, (f) 7.5% and (g) 10% MMT after immersion in PBS for 28 days; MMT decreased the hydrolysis of the matrix, hindering the production of the corrosion pits.

It was noteworthy that MMT had impermeability against water. After incorporating to polymer matrix, MMT acted as impermeable barriers, hindering the diffusion of water from the surface to the bulk of the scaffolds. Meanwhile, when encountered with MMT, water must bypass it, which significantly increased the tortuosity of the diffusion path. In this case, MTT weakened the attack of water on PGA matrix, decreasing the hydrolysis. Hence, the mass losses of the scaffolds lowered and the pH decrease delayed.

3.2.3.4　Cytocompatibility

The cytocompatibility of the PGA-MMT scaffolds (selecting PGA-7.5% MMT scaffolds as a representative) was evaluated with respect to cell proliferation and osteogenic differentiation by fluorescence staining and ALP staining, respectively, as shown in Fig. 3-4(a)-Fig. 3-4(e) and Fig. 3-4(f)-Fig. 3-4(i), respectively. It could be seen that the cells increased with culture time increasing from 1 to 3 days for both of the scaffolds, indicating they had good cytocompatibility. More importantly, the cells on the PGA-MMT scaffolds were much more than those on the PGA scaffolds at the same culture time, indicating MMT promoted cell proliferation. ALP was an important marker enzyme associated with early osteogenic differentiation. It could be seen that the cells on the PGA-MMT scaffolds were stained more purple than those on the PGA scaffold, indicating MMT promoted osteogenic differentiation. The results of cell culture indicated that MMT promoted the cell behaviors on the scaffolds. It was well known that the constituents of biomaterials had significant effects on cell behaviors. Ming-You Shie et al. reported Si could actively stimulate the biological responses of MG63 cells and effectively promote the proliferation of osteoblast-like cells via the production of specific proteins. M. Magallanes-Perdomo et al. reported Si was in favorable of supporting cell adhesion and proliferation of human bone marrow cells. Wanyin Zhai et al. concluded Si played an important role in stimulating cell proliferation and osteogenic differentiation. Hence, the improvements in the cell responses on the scaffolds may be owing to the positive stimulation effects of the Si constituent in MMT.

3.2.3.5　Sustained Release Properties and Antibacterial Properties

MMT possessed unique interlayer space and ion exchange property. As shown in Fig. 3-15, its crystal lattice consists of layers where a central tetrahedral sheet of alumina is connected to two external octahedral sheet of silica via sharing the oxygen atom; the layers are stacked layer-by-layer via regular Van Der Walls force and leave gap between them called interlayer space, where exists large amounts of exchangeable Ca^{2+}. In this study, Ag was loaded into the interlayer space of MMT, and then the Ag-loaded MMT were incorporated to PGA scaffolds for imparting sustained Ag^+ release and long-lasting antibacterial properties. The synthesis of MMT@Ag included ion exchange and chemical reduction, as illustrated in Fig. 3-15. During ion exchange, Ca^{2+} in the interlayer space of MMT was exchanged by Ag^+ in aqueous solution due to the difference in the hydration energy between them:

$$Ca^{2+}-MMT + Ag^+ \longrightarrow Ag^+-MMT + Ca^{2+} \tag{3-3}$$

During chemical reduction, Ag^+ in the interlayer space and surface of the exchanged MMT was chemically reduced to metallic Ag with higher stability by BH_4^-:

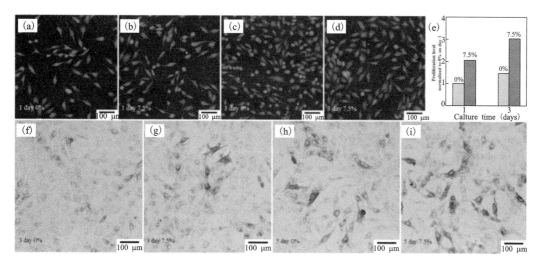

Fig. 3-14　(a-d) Fluorescence staining of MG63 cells cultured on the scaffolds containing 0 and 7.5% of MMT for 1 and 3 days, respectively; (e) the number of cells normalized to those on the scaffolds containing 0 MMT on 1st day (counted from the fluorescence staining images); (f-i) ALP staining of MG63 cells after culture on the scaffolds containing 0 and 7.5% of MMT for 3 and 7 days, respectively; MMT promoted the cell proliferation and osteogenic differentiation.

$$Ag^+ —MMT + BH_4^- + H_2O \longrightarrow Ag—MMT + B(OH)_3 + H_2 \uparrow \qquad (3\text{-}4)$$

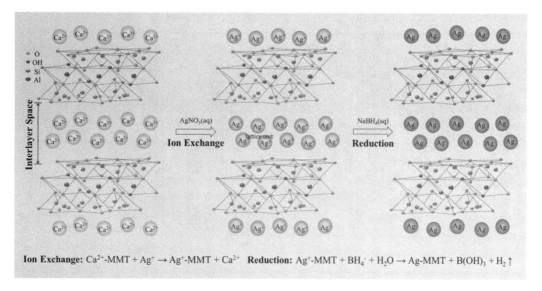

Ion Exchange: Ca²⁺-MMT + Ag⁺ → Ag⁺-MMT + Ca²⁺　**Reduction:** Ag⁺-MMT + BH₄⁻ + H₂O → Ag-MMT + B(OH)₃ + H₂↑

Fig. 3-15　The schematic diagram showing the synthesis of MMT@Ag, including ion exchange and chemical reduction; Ca^{2+} in the interlayer space of MMT was exchanged by Ag^+, which was then chemically reduced to Ag with higher stability by BH_4^-.

The XRD patterns of MMT@ Ag powders and a PGA-MMT@ Ag scaffold were shown in Fig. 3-16(a). MMT showed a characteristic diffraction peak at 5. 8°, which was associated with the interlayer space. It was noteworthy that additional diffraction peaks at 38. 4°, 44. 5°, and 64. 7° were detected in MMT@ Ag, which corresponded to the (111), (200) and (220) crystal faces of face-centered cubic Ag crystals, respectively, demonstrating the successful synthesis of Ag. Moreover, it could be obviously seen that the intensity of the characteristic peak around 5. 8° remarkably decreased and the location shifted lower, indicating Ag was synthesized into the interlayer space of MMT, which severely disturbed the ordered and periodic arrangement of the layers of MMT. All of the diffraction peaks of Ag were all detected in the PGA-7. 5% MMT@ Ag scaffold, demonstrating the presence of Ag, while the diffraction peaks of MMT were not detected due to its low crystallinity. FTIR of MMT@ Ag powder and a PGA-MMT@ Ag scaffold were shown in Fig. 3-16(b). MMT@ Ag showed no other absorption bands except MMT, indicating Ag had a high purity. Compared with the PGA scaffold, the PGA-MMT@ Ag scaffold showed two additional bands

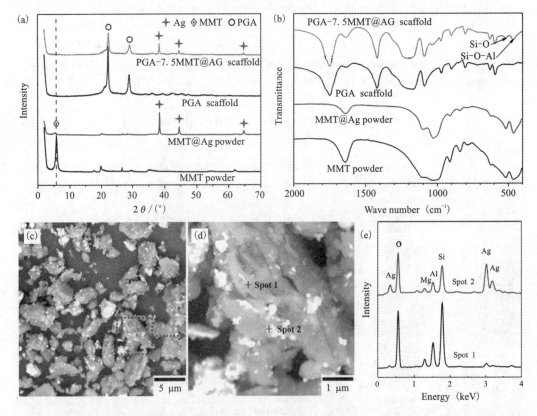

Fig. 3-16 (a) XRD patterns of MMT@ Ag powder and PGA-MMT@ Ag scaffold; there existed the diffraction peaks of Ag and MMT in the MMT@ Ag powder, and there were obvious changes in the diffraction peak intensity and position of MMT, indicating Ag was synthesized into the interlayer space of MMT; (b) FTIR of MMT@ Ag powder and PGA-MMT@ Ag scaffold; (c-d) SEM morphology of MMT@ Ag powders; (e) EDS spectra of spots 1 and 2 in (d).

around 518 and 464 cm^{-1}, indicating the presence of MMT. Combining the results of XRD and FTIR, the existence of MMT@ Ag in the scaffold was verified. The morphology of MMT@ Ag was characterized by SEM, as shown in Fig. 3-16(c)-Fig. 3-16(d). It could be seen that there were some white particles distributing on MMT particles [Fig. 3-16(c)-Fig. 3-16(d)]. According to the results of EDS analysis [Fig. 3-16(e)], they were just the synthesized Ag.

The Ag$^+$ release behaviors of the PGA-MMT@ Ag scaffolds were investigated by immersing in deionized water for different time with selecting PGA-7.5% MMT@ Ag as a representative sample [Fig. 3-17(a)-Fig. 3-17(b)]. It could be seen that the release rate of Ag$^+$ gradually decreased with immersion time increasing, based on analyzing the slope of the curves. The release behavior of Ag$^+$ showed two stages: a fast release of about 3 days and a following slow and sustained release for 28 days. The first stage was associated with the diffusion of Ag$^+$ from the scaffold/water interface with a low resistance. The second stage was attributed to the dual barrier effects of impermeable MMT. On one hand, the layered structure of MMT barriered the attack of water on Ag in the

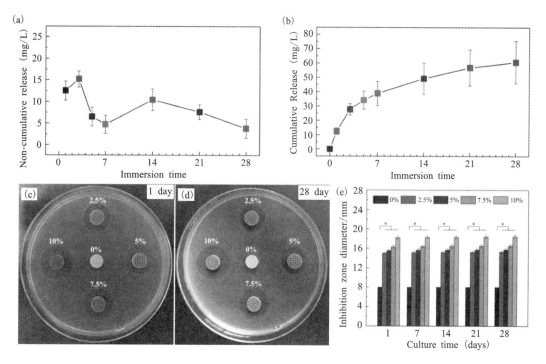

Fig. 3-17　(a) The non-cumulative release and (b) cumulative release of Ag$^+$ from PGA-7.5% MMT@ Ag scaffolds after immersion in deionized water for different time; Ag$^+$ showed a slow and sustained release for 28 days except an initial fast release of about 3 days; (c-d) the photographs of inhibition zones formed around the PGA-MMT@ Ag scaffolds (diameter 8 mm) after culture for (c) 1 and (d) 28 days; there was transparent inhibition zone forming around all of the MMT@ Ag contained scaffolds and there was no significant difference in the size of the inhibition zone around the same scaffold on 1st and 28th day; (e) the inhibition zone diameters calculated from the photographs; the inhibition zone diameters almost remained unchanged with the culture time prolonging, indicating the scaffolds had long-lasting antibacterial properties.

interlayer space. On the other hand, the layered structure hindered the diffusion of Ag$^+$ in the interlayer space. The initial fast release was beneficial for quickly and effectively killing initial bacteria, while the followed slow and sustained release was beneficial for long-lasting antibacterial activities. The long-term antibacterial properties of the PGA-MMT@ Ag scaffolds were assessed by inhibition zone test, as shown in Fig. 3-17 (c)-Fig. 3-17 (d). It was evident that there existed transparent inhibition zones around all of the MMT@ Ag contained scaffolds after 1 day of culture [Fig. 3-17(c)], and their diameters increased with MMT@ Ag content increasing (15.0, 15.5, 16.3 and 18.4 mm for the scaffolds containing 2.5%, 5%, 7.5% and 10% MMT@ Ag, respectively). It was worth noting that there was no significant difference in the diameters of the inhibition zones around the same scaffold after 1 and 28 days of culture [Fig. 3-17(c) and Fig. 3-17 (d), respectively]. In fact, the inhibition zone diameters almost remained unchanged during 28 days of culture, indicating the scaffolds had long-lasting antibacterial properties.

The bacterial inhibition rate of the scaffolds was tested using turbidimetry method, as shown in Fig. 3-18(a-b). Compared with the blank group (incubating without scaffolds) and control group (incubating with PGA scaffolds), all the bacterial suspensions incubating with MMT@ Ag contained scaffolds became transparent after 24 h immersion. According to the results from absorbance measurement [Fig. 3-18(b)], the antibacterial rate of the scaffolds gradually increased with MMT

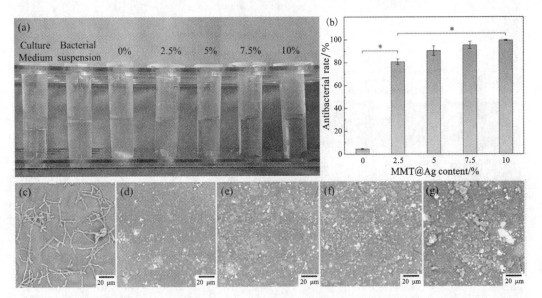

Fig. 3-18 (a) The photograph showing the E. coil suspensions after incubating with the PGA-MMT@ Ag scaffolds for 24 h; the suspensions immersed with MMT@ Ag contained scaffolds became transparent, indicating the amount of E. coil decreased; (b) the antibacterial rate calculated from the results of the absorbance measurement of the suspensions; it increased with MMT@ Ag content increasing; (c-g) the adhesion conditions of E. coil on the scaffolds containing (c) 0, (d) 2.5, (e) 5, (f) 7.5 and (g) 10% of MMT@ Ag; large amounts of bacteria adhered on the PGA scaffold without MMT@ Ag while there were hardly any bacteria on the MMT@ Ag contained scaffolds.

@ Ag content increasing, which were 80.7%, 90.4%, 95.3% and 99.5% for 2.5%, 5%, 7. 5% and 10% of MMT@ Ag, respectively. The adhesion conditions of the bacteria after culture on the scaffolds for 24 h were observed by SEM, as shown in Fig. 3-18 (c)-Fig. 3-18 (g). It was evident that large amounts of bacteria adhered on the PGA scaffold without MMT@ Ag. In contrast, there were hardly any bacteria on the MMT@ Ag contained scaffolds. It indicated MMT@ Ag imparted high antibacterial activities to the scaffolds through releasing Ag^+, which was generated via the oxidization of Ag by water and oxygen. It was noteworthy that Ag^+ could interact with many components in bacterial cells, damaging many significant structure and physiological functions. It could damage the membrane structure, causing loss of intracellular substances; binded to sulfhydryl groups in proteins and enzymes, impairing respiration and substance metabolism; and even interacted with nucleic acids in DNA, preventing the reproduction of bacterial cells.

3.2.4　Conclusions

In this study, MMT with unique interlayer space was incorporated to PGA scaffolds prepared via additive manufacturing to increase the mechanical properties, decreasing the degradable rate, and imparting sustained release and antibacterial properties. The results indicated MMT played the role in rigid reinforcements dispersing well in the PGA matrix, effectively transferring and absorbing the stresses in the matrix, which significantly increased the compressive properties and hardness of the scaffolds. Moreover, MMT acted as impermeable barriers, hindering the diffusion of water and its attack on the PGA matrix, which inhibited the hydrolysis and hence significantly lowered the degradable rate of the scaffolds. More importantly, Ag^+ was loaded into the interlayer space of MMT via ion exchange, which was further chemically reduced to metallic Ag with higher stability. The impermeable layered structure of MMT barriered the attack of water and the diffusion of Ag^+, contributing a slow and sustained Ag^+ release of the scaffolds. Hence, the scaffolds showed not only a high bacterial inhibition rate but also a long-lasting antibacterial activity.

3.3　Lanthanum-Containing Magnesium Alloy with Antitumor Function Based on Increased Reactive Oxygen Species

3.3.1　Introduction

Currently, surgical resection is a popular treatment method for tumor-induced bone defects. Nevertheless, the surgical resection cannot eliminate bone tumor cells completely. The residual bone tumor cells may lead to the relapse of the bone tumor. Therefore, it is important to develop antitumor implants to repair bone defects and prevent bone tumor relapse. Ma et al. had reported that a bifunctional graphene oxide-modified β-tricalcium phosphate implant showed excellent photothermal effects in killing bone-tumor cells, which could be used for therapy of tumor-related bone defects. Li et al. also reported that zoledronic acid-loaded magnesium-strontium alloys could inhibit giant bone cell tumors, which could be a potential implant in repairing the bone defects after removal of tumor.

Compared to normal cells, hydrogen peroxide levels are greatly increased in many types of cancer cells. It helps cancer cells to infiltrate and metastasize to other tissues, and hydrogen peroxide is also an important signal molecule regulating the entire process of tumor cell survival, proliferation, and apoptosis. As tumor cells have elevated reactive oxygen species levels and are under increased intrinsic oxidative stress, this provides an opportunity to kill the tumor cells based on their vulnerability to reactive oxygen species insults.

Lanthanum (La), a rare earth element, has received increasing attention due to its antitumor property. The radius and valence of the La ion are 1.061 Å and trivalent, respectively. The La ion possesses a large ratio of the electric charge to ion radius, enabling a high ability to bind to the divalent metal binding sites on mitochondria. This binding leads to irreversible alteration of its structure and loss of biological activity, which results in disruption of tumor cell function and death. Heffeter et al. reported that lanthanum compounds could selectively inhibit or kill tumor cells even in drug-resistant tumor cells. Chen et al. reported that lanthanum chloride could inhibit proliferation and induce the cervical tumor cells. Considering the antitumor property of La, it is reasonable to speculate that La could be used as an antitumor agent to proude implants the ability to kill bone tumor cells.

As promising bone implant materials, magnesium (Mg) and its alloys possess degradability, good biocompatibility, and desirable mechanical properties. They can gradually degrade in the human body, thereby avoiding the second surgery for implant removal and decreasing the pain for patients. Mg as a necessary element in the human body can promote new bone formation, which is beneficial to bone defects repairing. Furthermore, Mg alloys possess similar elastic modulus and density to those of natural human bones, thus mitigating the stress shielding effect induced by serious mismatch in modulus between implants and natural bones. To our knowledge, there are very few reports about the antitumor property of Mg alloy containing La.

In this study, La was alloyed to Mg-6Zn-0.5Zr (mass fraction, ZK60) through a selective laser melting technique to endow it with antitumor properties. Meanwhile, alloying is an effective approach to enhance the Mg degradation resistance by tailoring the phase morphology, distribution, potential, and size of the matrix. The antitumor property of ZK60 – La was evaluated and the potential mechanisms were discussed. Furthermore, the degradation properties were investigated.

3.3.2　Experimental Methods

3.3.2.1　Preparation of ZK60 – La Samples

The spherical Mg-6Zn-0.5Zr (ZK60) powder (mean particle size 50 μm) [Fig. 3-19(a)] and polyangular La powder (mean particle size 8 μm) [Fig. 3-19(b)] were used as raw materials. These two powders were blended homogeneously using ball milling at a rate of 100 r/min for 10 h under argon gas protection to obtain mixed powders with different La contents (0.5%, 1.0%, 1.5% and 2.0%).

The selective laser melting system [Fig. 3-19(c)] was composed of a fiber laser, an optical focus system, an automatic powder dispensing apparatus, an argon gas protection device, and a

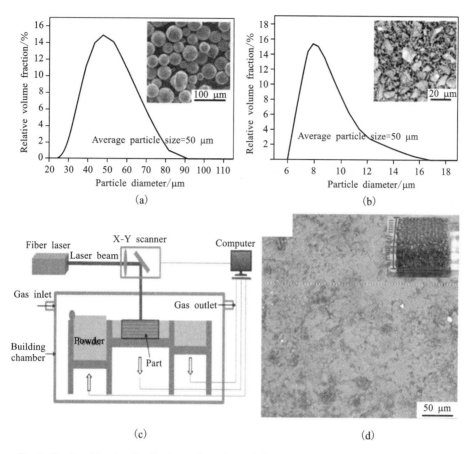

Fig. 3-19　Particle size distributions of powders: (a) ZK60 and (b) La; (c) schematic of selective laser melting system; (d) the surface of the selective laser melted sample.

computer-based control setup system. Selective laser melting was carried out in the following parameters: Laser beam diameter 100 μm, laser power 70 W, scanning speed 600 mm/min, and scan line spacing 50 μm. The building chamber was filled with argon gas to prevent oxidation. Then, ZK60 and ZK60 − xLa (x = 0.5%, 1.0%, 1.5% and 2.0%) samples (10 mm × 10 mm × 5 mm) were prepared. The surface of as-built samples was completely dense with no obvious pores or cracks [Fig. 3-19(d)].

3.3.2.2　Microstructure Characterization and Mechanical Properties Tests

The samples were polished on abrasive papers and finally etched with the picral solution for 10 s. Subsequently their metallurgical structure was observed by optical microscopy. The composition distribution was studied using a scanning electron microscopy (SEM) equipped with an energy dispersive spectroscopy (EDS) detector. The phase compositions were analyzed through X-ray diffraction. The hardness was carried out using a HXD-1000TM/LCD device (load of 2.942 N). The compressive strength test was operated at a constant crosshead speed (0.2 mm/min) using an Instron machine.

3.3.2.3 Degradation Properties Assays

The potentiodynamic polarization curves were performed using an electrochemical workstation (Gamry 2000 +) with a standard three-electrode configuration. To obtain a stable open circuit potential, the samples were immersed in the simulated body fluid (SBF) solution for 5 min. Then, the measurement was conducted in a potential ranging from −300 mV to 300 mV compared to the open circuit potential. The potentiodynamic scanning rate for the test was 1 mV/s. The corrosion current density (i_{corr}) and corrosion potential (E_{corr}) were obtained through Tafel extrapolation method.

Immersion tests were carried out in SBF solution at (37 ± 0.5) ℃. The ratio of the exposed area to the volume of SBF solution was 1.25 cm^2/mL. Each specimen was immersed in SBF solution for 14 d, then removed from the solution and subsequently washed with distilled water 3 times. The morphology and the composition of the degradation product film on sample surface were assessed by SEM and EDS. After immersion for 3, 7, and 14 d, each specimen was removed from the solution. The degradation products were removed by immersing the samples in chromic acid solution for 20 min for the weight loss test. The weight loss rate $\Delta W [mg/(cm^2 \cdot d^{-1})]$ was calculated by the formula given in Reference. The degradation rate (P_w, mm/a) was calculated based on the weight loss rate by the equation: $P_w = 2.10\Delta W$, as in Reference.

3.3.2.4 Antitumor Property and Cytocompatibility

The extracts for the antitumor tests were conducted as follow. ZK60 and ZK60 − La samples were sterilized using ultraviolet radiation for 1 h. Then the samples were immersed in Dulbecco's modified Eagle's medium (DMEM) for 5 d, and the extraction medium ratio (the specimen surface area/medium volume) was kept at 1.25 cm^2/mL. All the extracts were subsequently centrifuged at 3000 r/min for 5 min, collected supernates, and added 10% fetal bovine serum (FBS). The pH values of the extracts were characterized by a pH meter. The ion concentrations of the extracts were analyzed by an inductively coupled plasma-atomic emission spectroscopy.

The human osteosarcoma cells (U2OS cells) were purchased from the Type Culture Collection of the Chinese Academy of Sciences. Cells were maintained in DMEM supplemented with 10% FBS in a humidified atmosphere with 5% CO_2 at 37℃. The medium was changed every two or three days. Human embryonic kidney 293 cells (HEK 293 cells) were purchased from Chinese Infrastructure of Cell Line Resources. The cells were cultured at 37℃ in a humidified atmosphere of 5% CO_2. The cell culture medium was DMEM supplemented with 10% FBS.

The U2OS cells were adopted to evaluate the antitumor property. DMEM with 10% fetal bovine serum was used as blank control. U2OS cells (2×10^4 cells/mL) were seeded in 96 − well plates and cultured with DMEM supplemented with 10% FBS for 24 h. The incubated medium was then substituted by 200 μL of ZK60 or ZK60 − La extracts. At 1st, 3th, and 5th d, the incubated medium was then removed and 200 μL medium containing 10 μL cell counting kit-8 (CCK-8) solution (Dojindo Laboratories, Tokyo, Japan) was introduced, followed by continuous incubation for another 2 h. Optical density (OD) values at 570 nm were obtained through a microplate reader. The relative growth rate (RGR) of cells was calculated according to the equation: RGR = (OD of the sample/OD of blank control group) × 100%. Human embryonic kidney 293 cells (HEK 293 cells) were used to assess the cytocompatibility. The cells (1 × 10^5 cells/mL) were incubated in a 96 – well plate for 24 h. Then, 100 μL of extracts were added to each well to replace the medium. Then, 10 μL CCK-8 solution was added to each well after incubating for 1 d, 3 d, and 5 d, and subsequently incubated for another 2 h. OD values at 570 nm were obtained using a microplate reader.

For live/dead staining studies, tumor cells (1 × 10^5 cells/mL) were seeded in 24 – well plates cultured in an incubator for 24 h to allow attachment, and then, 200 μL extracts were added to each well to replace the medium. Subsequently, the medium was removed and the live/dead staining was performed with 0.2 mL of combination dye (Live/Dead Cell Viability Assay, Invitrogen). Briefly, 1 μmol/L calcien AM and 2 μmol/L ethidium homodimer-1 solutions were prepared in PBS. After the removal of the extracts medium, the cells were washed with PBS solution for 3 times, followed by addition of 100 μL of 1 μmol/L calcein AM and 2 μmol/L ethidium homodimer-1 solution. The fluorescent images of cells were then taken by a fluorescence microscope (BX60, Olympus, Japan). The viable cells combined with calcein-AM were stained green, whereas the dead cells combined with ethidium homodimer-1 were stained red. For live/dead staining studies, HEK 293 cells (1 × 10^5 cells/mL) were seeded in 24 – well plates for 24 h, and then, 200 μL extracts were added to each well to replace the medium. Subsequently, the medium was removed and the live/dead staining was performed.

The potential of mitochondrial membrane was detected by the mitochondrial permeability JC-1 fluorescent dye. Briefly, cells (5 × 10^3 cells/mL) were seeded into a 96 – well plate in 200 μL medium for 24 h. Then, 400 μL of extracts were added to each well to replace the medium and the cells were cultured for further 24 h. Then, the medium was then replaced by 10 μL of 5 mmol/L JC-1 staining solution, and the plate was incubated for 15 min at (37 ± 0.5)℃. The plate was centrifuged for 5 min and the supernatant was removed, and then, 200 μL of PBS solution was added. Cells were resuspended in 1 mL PBS, and instantly assessed with flow cytometry.

The reactive oxygen species (ROS) level was detected using a 6 – corboxy-2′7′-dichlorodihydro fluorescein diacetate (DCFH-DA) fluorescent probe. Cells were cultured in 6 – well plates and allowed to attach. Cells were washed with PBS solution after culturing with extract for 24 h. Subsequently, they were incubated with DCFH-DA solution (10 μmol/L in DMEM) for 20 min at (37 ±0.5)℃. Afterward, cells were washed twice with PBS solution to remove the excess staining solution and instantly assessed with flow cytometry. Differential expression was expressed as the ratio of the fluorescence intensities of experimental samples and the control sample.

3.3.2.5 Statistical Analysis

Data were expressed as mean ± standard deviation of three independent experiments. The statistical differences were analyzed between different groups to determine the p values by student's t test, which were considered significant when a p value < 0.05.

3.3.3 Results and Discussion

3.3.3.1 Antitumor Property

The fluorescence images of the U2OS cells after culturing in the different extracts for 5 d were shown in Fig. 3-20(a)-Fig. 3-20(f). No dead cells were observed in the control group [Fig. 3-20 (a)]. Few dead cells were observed in the ZK60 extract [Fig. 3-20(b)]. Significantly, dead cells gradually increased and live cells decreased in ZK60 – La extracts with La content increasing. In addition, the cells cultured in the ZK60 – La extracts exhibited an unhealthy shrinkage shape. These results indicated that ZK60 – La exhibited antitumor property, and higher La content exhibited

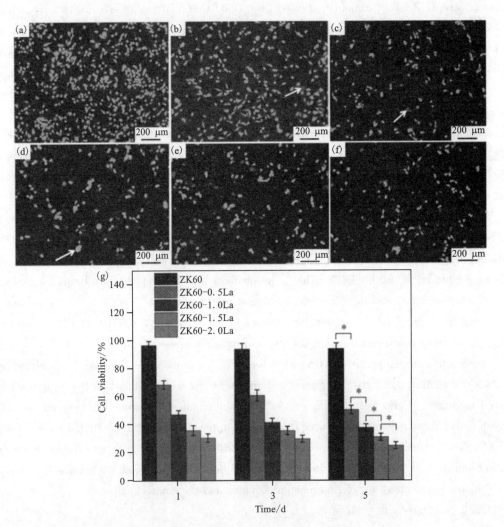

Fig. 3-20 U2OS cells after culturing in extracts for 5 d and stained with live/dead assay; red represented the dead cells and green represented the live cells: (a) Control (b) ZK60, (c) ZK60 – 0.5La, (d) ZK60 – 1.0La, (e) ZK60 – 1.5La, (f) ZK60 – 2.0La; (g) cell viability of U2OS cells in different extracts after culturing for 1, 3, and 5 d.

higher antitumor efficiency.

The cell viability of the U2OS cells was studied by CCK8 assay, with results shown in Fig. 3-20 (g). The cell viability of the U2OS cells after culturing in ZK60 extract for 5 d was 94.2%. As a comparison, the cell viability of the U2OS cells cultured in ZK60 − 0.5La, ZK60 − 1.0La, ZK60 − 1.5La, and ZK60 − 2.0La extracts were 50.8%, 38.1%, 31.4%, and 25.2%, respectively. It indicated that the alloying of La inhibited the growth of U2OS cells, and the cell inhibition rate gradually increased with La content increasing. Among these, ZK60 − 1.0La extract exhibited a cell inhibition rate of 61.9%. These results were in accordance with the fluorescence staining test.

The fluorescence images of the HEK 293 cells after culturing in the different extracts for 5 d were exhibited in Fig. 3-21(a)-Fig. 3-21(f). From the results of live/dead staining, almost no dead

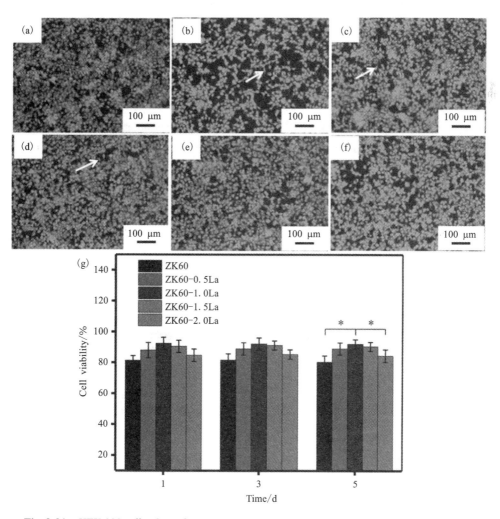

Fig. 3-21　HEK 293 cells after culturing in extracts for 5 d and stained with live/dead assay; red represented the dead cells and green represented the live cells: (a) Control (b) ZK60, (c) ZK60 − 0.5La, (d) ZK60 − 1.0La, (e) ZK60 − 1.5La, (f) ZK60 − 2.0La; (g) cell viability of HEK 293 cells in different extracts after culturing for 1, 3 and 5 d.

cells were observed. The morphology of the cells was in spindle-like shape after culturing in different extracts, which indicated that the ZK60 – La exhibited compatibility to normal cells. The CCK8 assay was used to assess the cytocompatibility for HEK 293 cells, with results shown in Fig. 3-21 (g). The cell viability of HEK 293 cells after culturing in extract of ZK60, ZK60 – 0.5La, ZK60 – 1.0La, ZK60 – 1.5La, and ZK60 – 2.0La for 5 d was 80.3%, 88.9%, 91.9%, 90.3%, and 84.4%, respectively. The viability of the cells cultured in ZK60 – La extract was higher than 80% (grade 1, according to the Standard), indicating that ZK60 – La showed no toxicity to HEK 293 cells.

Compared to normal cells, tumor cells had a high ROS level, and were more vulnerable to oxidative insults under increased intrinsic oxidative stress. It was well known that the mitochondria were the main ROS factory in the cells. Thus, the level of mitochondrial membrane potential (MMP) and that of ROS in U2OS cells were measured. As shown in Fig. 3-22(a), the level of MMP after incubating in ZK60 extract was 95.2%, and the level of MMP decreased in the U2OS cells with the La content increasing. Specifically, the obtained MMP in the extract of ZK60 – La was reduced to 88.6% for ZK60 – 0.5La, 80.2% for ZK60 – 1.0La, 76.7% for ZK60 – 1.5La, and 73.2% for ZK60 – 2.0La, respectively. Meanwhile, the ROS levels in U2OS cells after incubating in the different extracts were shown in Fig. 3-22(b). The ROS level after incubating in ZK60 extract was 109.2%, and the ROS level increased in the U2OS cells with the La content increasing. Specifically, the obtained ROS level in the extract of ZK60 – La was increased to 122.3% for ZK60 – 0.5La, 138.5% for ZK60 – 1.0La, 145.8% for ZK60 – 1.5La, and 152.1% for ZK60 – 2.0La, respectively.

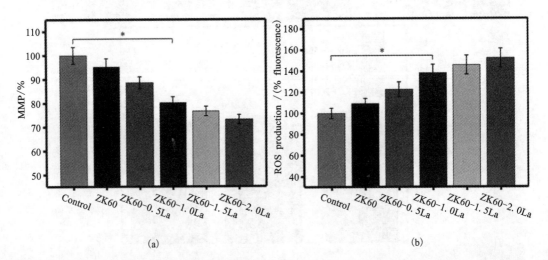

(a)　　　　　　　　　　　　　(b)

Fig. 3-22 (a) The mitochondrial membrane potential (MMP) and (b) reactive oxygen species (ROS) in U2OS cells after incubating in the different extracts.

The degradation of Mg metals led to metal ions release accompanying by high alkalinity, which might be key factors causing cell death. The pH values of the ZK60 and ZK60 – La extracts after immersing for 5 d were shown in Fig. 3-23(a). The pH value of the ZK60 extract was 8.8. The pH values of ZK60 – La extracts were lower than that of the ZK60 extract, and pH value of ZK60 – 1. 0La extract was 8.2, which was the lowest among them. It could be inferred that ZK60 – 1.0La had the slowest degradation rate and the least OH⁻ release, providing a more favorable environment for cell growth. Thus, HEK 293 cells exhibited the highest cell viability in ZK60 – 1.0La extract. The ion concentrations of the extracts were illustrated in Fig. 3-23(b). The La ion concentrations in ZK60 – La extracts were (0.5 ± 0.1) μg/mL for ZK60 – 0.5La alloy, (1.2 ± 0.2) μg/mL for ZK60 – 1.0La alloy, (1.9 ± 0.1) μg/mL for ZK60 – 1.5La alloy, and (3.5 ± 0.1) μg/mL for ZK60 – 2.0La alloy. The concentration of La ion increased with the La content increasing in ZK60 – La. Although higher concentrations of La ions were more conducive to killing tumor cells, they also impaired the biocompatibility of ZK60 – La.

The mechanism of ZK60 – La inducing tumor cell death was illustrated in Fig. 3-23(c). The

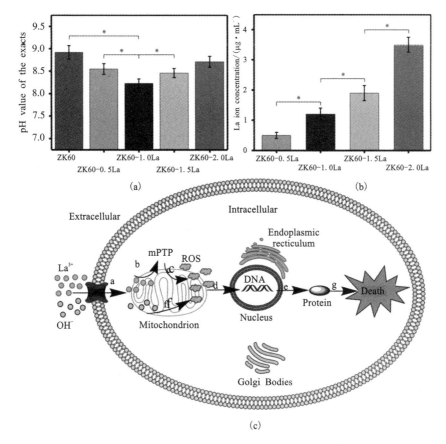

(a)   (b)   (c)

Fig. 3-23   Characterization of the extracts: (A) pH value; (B) La³⁺ concentration; (C) Mechanism of ZK60 – La inducing tumor cell death: (a) La³⁺ and OH⁻ transported into cell; (b) the mitochondrial permeability transition pore (mPTP) opening; (c) ROS accumulated in mitochondrion; (d) regulated the gene expression; (e) regulated the expression levels of protein; (f) ROS accumulation caused by OH⁻; and (g) regulation of protein expression led cell death.

ZK60 – La released a mass of La^{3+} when they were degraded. The La^{3+} was transported into the tumor cell through the ion channels on the cell membrane. The radius of the La^{3+} (1.061 Å) were close to that of calcium ion (Ca^{2+}) (0.99 Å). However, the La^{3+} possessed the greater ratio of the electric charge to radius (3/1.061 Å = 2.83) than that of the Ca^{2+} (2/0.99 Å = 2.02), which made it possess a stronger bonding force with divalent binding sites than the Ca^{2+}[137]. Thus, the La^{3+} could replace the Ca^{2+} binding to the binding sites on the mitochondrial permeability transition pore (mPTP). The opening of mPTP could result in ionic balance disorders between the mitochondrial matrix and cytoplasm. The redistribution of ions on both sides of the membrane led to the decrease of mitochondrial membrane potential. As a result, the electron transport chain was blocked, which resulted in the reactive oxygen species generation. In addition, the ability to scavenge free radicals for cells could also be weakened in a high alkaline environment by suppressed activity of related enzymes in cells, leading to the reactive oxygen species accumulation. The ROS accumulated in the tumor cells could result in oxidative stress, regulating the expression of related proteins, finally causing tumor cell apoptosis. The apoptosis was a typically form of programmed cell death regulated by genes, which played a role in the cell death. A local burst of ROS also could induce oxidation of nucleotides in DNA. Irreparable DNA damage prevented proper protein synthesis, which led to cell death.

3.3.3.2 Degradation Properties

The polarization curves of ZK60 and ZK60 – La immersed in SBF were presented in Fig. 3-24 (a). The E_{corr} and I_{corr} estimated using Tafel extrapolation were shown in Tab. 3-4. The E_{corr} and I_{corr} of ZK60 were 1.61 V and 50.2 $\mu A/cm^2$. It should be noted that ZK60 – 1.0La had the highest E_{corr} (– 1.41 V) and the lowest I_{corr} (26.3 $\mu A/cm^2$), which suggested that it had the best degradation resistance.

The degradation rate of ZK60 and ZK60 – La calculated from the weight loss were exhibited in Fig. 3-24 (b). The degradation rate increased with the immersion time increasing from 3 d to 7 d, while it decreased with the immersion time increasing from 7 d to 14 d. It could be attributed to the reduction of surface area for the samples in the degradation process. When the samples immersed in the solution, the surface of the sample was exposed to the solution causing several thermopositive reactions, thus increasing the degradation rate. While, protective films would form on the samples with prolonged immersion in SBF, which prohibited the contact between the samples and corrosive medium, thus decreasing the degradation rate. The degradation rate of ZK60 was 2.13 mm/a after exposure to SBF for 14 d. When the content of La increased to 1.0%, the degradation rate decreased to 1.23 mm/a. Clearly, various La content exerted an effect on the pH of extract, as shown in Fig. 3-23(a). With La content increasing to 1.0%, the degradation rate was reduced. Thus, the released OH^- was decreased. With La content further increased, the degradation was accelerated, and the pH value was consequently increased.

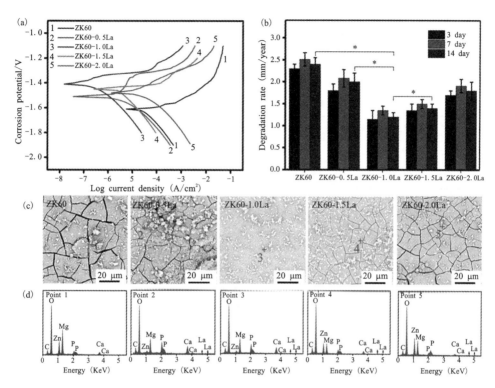

Fig. 3-24   (a) Polarization curves of ZK60 and ZK60 – La immersed in SBF solution; (b) Degradation rates of ZK60 and ZK60 – La calculated from the weight loss; (c) Morphologies of the ZK60 and ZK60 – La after immersing in SBF solution for 14 d; (d) Energy dispersive spectroscopy (EDS) spectra of the degradation products indicated by the red point in (c).

Tab. 3-4   **The corrosion potential and current density of ZK60 and ZK60 – La estimated using Tafel extrapolation.**

	E_{corr}/V	$I_{corr}/(\mu A \cdot cm^{-2})$
ZK60	-1.61 ± 0.01	50.2 ± 7
ZK60 – 0.5La	-1.51 ± 0.01	39.4 ± 5
ZK60 – 1.0La	-1.41 ± 0.01	26.3 ± 3
ZK60 – 1.5La	-1.45 ± 0.01	35.1 ± 5
ZK60 – 2.0La	-1.48 ± 0.01	43.7 ± 5

Tab. 3-5　EDS results of the degradation products indicated by the red point in Fig. 3-24(c).

Point	Mg	Zn	La	C	O	Ca	P
	at%	at%	at%	at%	at%	at%	at%
1	14.72	4.62	–	17.90	58.37	2.51	1.88
2	7.15	0.89	0.30	18.72	61.34	6.61	4.99
3	8.07	1.12	0.45	17.32	62.69	5.79	4.56
4	6.50	3.79	0.21	21.42	21.42	2.90	2.25
5	10.05	6.25	0.84	21.49	58.20	1.61	1.56

The morphologies of ZK60 and ZK60 – La after immersing in SBF solution for 14 d were shown in Fig. 3-24(c). They were all covered with degradation product layer. Many cracks were observed for ZK60, while the surface film of ZK60 – 1.0La maintained integrity. The EDS spectra of the degradation products were shown in Fig. 3-24(c). It was shown that the degradation products were primarily constituted of O, C, and Mg. The La and Zn, along with Ca, P, were also detected in the degradation products. The atomic ratio of Ca to P was about 1.34, which was between the ones of octacalcium phosphate and hydroxyapatite.

3.3.3.3　Microstructure

The metallurgical structures of ZK60 and ZK60 – La obtained by optical microscopy were shown in Fig. 3-25. Both ZK60 and ZK60 – La consisted of dendrite grains and intermetallics. The average grain size was 13.1 μm for ZK60, 10.2 μm for ZK60 – 0.5La, 7.6 μm for ZK60 – 1.0La, 6.3 μm for ZK60 – 1.5La, and 5.1 μm for ZK60 – 2.0La, respectively. The results showed that alloying La to the ZK60 contributed to grain refinement. The related refinement mechanism was as follows: during solidification, the solute La atoms possessed strong segregation ability and formed constitutional undercooling in a diffusion layer. The constitutional undercooling could reduce the diffusion rate of solute atoms, which restricted grain growth and promoted the primary Mg matrix nucleation. Moreover, the La-containing intermetallic could form at grain boundary, which could further prevent the grain growth.

The distribution of the intermetallic phase was analyzed by SEM and EDS. The ZK60 constituted of the α-Mg phase and intermetallic phase. The intermetallic phase in ZK60 was sparsely distributed along grain boundary with an island-like structure. Some intermetallic phase with short-bar shape appeared after alloying 0.5% or 1.0% La and increased with the La content increasing. The intermetallic phase with short-bar shape was widened and gradually connected to form a semi-continuous network as La content reached 1.5% or 2.0%. The EDS results revealed that the phase with the island-like shape [point A in Fig. 3-25(a)] was constituted of Mg (89.41%) and Zn (10.59%) [Fig. 3-25(f)], and the phase with short-bar shape [point B in Fig. 3-25(c)] was constituted of Mg (91.27%), Zn (7.60%) and La (1.13%) [Fig. 3-25(g)]. The phase with semi-continuous network shape [point C in Fig. 3-25(e)] was constituted of Mg (88.53%), Zn

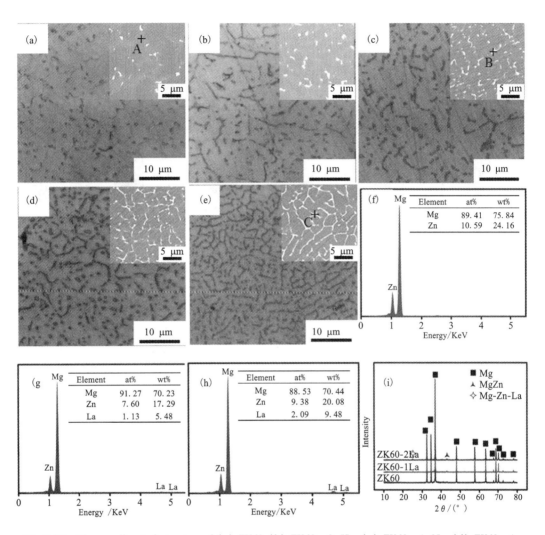

Fig. 3-25   The metallurgical structure of (a) ZK60 (b) ZK60 – 0.5La (c) ZK60 – 1.0La (d) ZK60 – 1. 5La (d) ZK60 – 2.0La; EDS results of the secondary phase indicated by the points (f) point A in Fig. 3-25 (a); (g) point B in Fig. 3-25(c); (h) point C in Fig. 3-25(e); (i) XRD spectra of the samples.

(9.38%) and La (2.09%) [Fig. 3-25(h)]. The XRD spectra of the samples were presented in Fig. 3-25(i). Combined with the EDS results, the phase with island-like shape was suggested to be MgZn, the phase with short-bar shape and phase with semi-continuous network shape was suggested to be the MgZnLa phase.

3.3.3.4   Mechanical Properties

The mechanical properties of the samples were shown in Fig. 3-26. The compressive strengths of ZK60, ZK60 – 0.5La, ZK60 – 1.0La, ZK60 – 1.5La, and ZK60 – 2.0La were (134.5 ± 4.5) MPa, (151.2 ± 4.3) MPa, (169.4 ± 5.1) MPa, (163.7 ± 4.5) MPa, and (158.8 ± 5.0) MPa, respectively. The compressive strength increased as the La content increased, and ZK60 – 1.0La possessed the highest compressive strength. The enhanced compression strength was partly ascribed

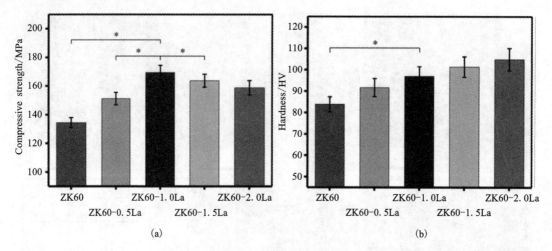

Fig. 3-26 The mechanical properties of ZK60 and ZK60 − La: (a) Compressive strength, (b) Hardness.

to the strengthening effect of grain refinement and uniformly dispersed MgZnLa phase with short-bar shape. When the La content increased further, the compressive strength decreased. It was ascribed to the fact that continuity of the Mg matrix was destroyed by the semi-continuous network MgZnLa phase along the grain boundary, and stress accumulation could form at the interfaces between the MgZnLa phase and matrix during plastic deformation. In addition, with the increase of La content, the hardness of the samples increased from (83.9 ± 3.5) HV for ZK60 to (104.9 ± 5.2) HV for the ZK60 − 2.0La. It was attributed to the strengthening effect of grain refinement and precipitation strengthening of the high hardness MgZnLa phase.

3.3.4　Conclusions

In this chapter, ZK60 − La was successfully prepared by selective laser melting technology. ZK60 − 1.0La revealed a high cell inhibition rate of 61.9% for bone tumor cells and high cell viability of 91.9% for normal kidney cells, indicating its good anti-tumor property. It further revealed that the MMP of U2OS cells after incubating in ZK60 − La extracts was reduced as the La content increased. Meanwhile, the ROS levels in U2OS cells after incubating in the ZK60 − La extracts increased with the La content increasing. In addition, its degradation rate of 1.23 mm/a was lower than that of ZK60 alloy with 2.13 mm/a, which was mainly attributed to the grain refinement.

Chapter 4

Promotion of Osteogenic Ability

Fe_3O_4 nanoparticle is a kind of superparamagnetic material with strong magnetism and good biocompatibility, which can produce stable magnetic field in the surrounding space after magnetization. The magnetic field can directly affect the osteoblasts, promote the proliferation and differentiation of osteoblasts, accelerate the apoptosis of osteoclasts, inhibit bone resorption and increase bone formation. It can also stimulate the mineralization process of bone repair by regulating the metabolism of bone growth factor to effectively promote bone growth. In addition, the magnetic field also generates local biological current, which affects local metabolism and cartilage calcification. In this chapter, Fe_3O_4 nanoparticle was introduced into bone implants to promote the osteogenic ability.

4.1   Physical Stimulations and Their Osteogenesis-inducing Mechanisms

4.1.1   Introduction

Millions of people around the world are suffering from bone defects caused by bone diseases, traumas, infections, natural disasters, etc.. In USA alone, there are about seven million patients suffering bone defects. In recent years, bone graft is widely used to treat bone defects, including autologous, allograft and artificial bone graft. Artificial bone graft consists of seeding osteogenic cells onto 3D porous scaffolds which can be fabricated via 3D printing technology to induce osteogenesis. While there still exists delayed union or nonunion resulting from the loss of cell activity or cell death during bone defect repair. Chemical stimulations such as growth factors, osteogenic chemical inducers and hormones were utilized to improve the activity of bone cells. Nonetheless, they displayed some disadvantages. For example, growth factors (such as bone morphogenetic proteins, transforming growth factors, etc.) display short half-life, and their activities lost rapidly. Physical stimulations such as magnetic, electric and mechanical stimulation can constantly act on bone defect sites to enhance and maintain cell activity via activating signal pathways, modulating ion channels, regulating bone-related gene expressions, etc.. More importantly, physical stimulations have been proved to be safe and can control the bone growth direction depending on the direction of stimulations, thereby accelerating bone formation and regeneration.

Magnetic stimulation is a safe and non-invasive method to treat bone defect, which is produced by magnetic fields and electromagnetic fields, mainly including static magnetic field and pulse electromagnetic field stimulation. Electric stimulation is a widely recognized approach for stimulating bone growth, which is preformed by various currents mainly including direct current, biphasic electric current and alternating electric current stimulation. Mechanical stimulation is conducive to bone regeneration and healing, which is produced by ultrasound and other mechanical methods, mainly including ultrasonic, compressive stress, tensile stress and fluid shear stress stimulation. Some summaries about the physical stimulations toward bone repair applications, including classifiation and producing methods as well as advantages and disadvantages, were presented in Tab. 4-1. These physical stimulations can enhance cell activity and promote bone regeneration, which have been described as functional adaptation primarily owing to their osteogenesis-inducing ability. Detailedly, Hall effect produced by magnetic stimulations, inverse piezoelectric effect induced by electrical stimulations, and mechanotransduction effect caused by mechanical stimulations, can change local microenvironment of bone defect sites, alter cell membrane functions, activate signaling pathways, and regulate bone-related gene expressions, etc., thereby enhancing cell activity and promoting bone regeneration. These mechanisms are responsible for accelerating bone formation and bone repair.

Tab. 4-1　Physical stimulations for bone repair.

Physical stimulations	Classify	Producingmethods	Advantages	Disadvantages	References
Magnetic Stimulation	→Static magnetic field	Magnets Passing direct current through coils	Safe non-invasive No infection No side effects Ease of use	Need for additional equipment Less well defined stimulation site	[16,23,24]
	Pulse electromagnetic field	Passing pulse current through Helmholtz coils			
Electric Stimulation	Biphasic current	Biphasic current stimulator deliver biphasic stimulation currents	Ease of operation Stable strength Reproducible	The insufficient biocompatibility of electrodes can cause local infection	[25 – 28]
	Direct current	Passing direct electric current through electrodes			
	Alternating current	A generator produce alternating current			

Continued to Tab. 4-1

Physical stimulations	Classify	Producingmethods	Advantages	Disadvantages	References
Mechanical Stimulation	Ultrasonic	Ultrasound	Safe non-invasive No infection Less complication	Difficult to apply on freely moving animals Difficult to precisely measure stimulus intensity	[29 – 32]
	Compressive stress	Compressive apparatus			
	Tensile stress	Tension apparatus			
	Fluid shear stress	Flow chamber			

In this paper, the different osteogenesis-inducing mechanisms of physical stimulations in bone repair process were systematically combed. The bioeffects of physical stimulations on cell behavior and bone formation which were investigated by numerous of studies in vitro and in vivo were summarized. Meanwhile, the synergetic effects of physical stimulations and bone scaffolds, especially the 3D printed bone scaffolds, on cells were presented. Besides, the equipments of physical stimulation systems were discussed, and the application prospects of these stimulations in bone repair were also analyzed.

4.1.2 The Osteogenesis-inducing Mechanisms of Physical Stimulations

Bone is a constantly updated tissue composed of metabolically active cells. Cell behaviors such as migration, proliferation, differentiation and apoptosis play a significant role in bone repair process. Physical stimulations can accelerate the proliferation and differentiation of osteoblasts and inhibit the formation of osteoclasts. In order to better understand the bioeffects of physical stimulations on cell activity and bone growth, the osteogenesis-inducing mechanisms of them were systematically combed according to relevant researches.

4.1.2.1 Magnetic Stimulation

The osteogenesis-inducing mechanisms of magnetic stimulation were explained as follows: (1) Producing Hall effect: The moving charged ions between bone matrix and osteocyte membrane would encounter a Lorentz force in magnetic field, and then formd Hall voltage to induce the further migration of ions and improved permeability of cell membrane, thereby contributing the extracellular ions to pass through cell membrane to enhance cell activity. (2) Improving cell membrane permeability: Phospholipid molecules on cell membrane possess diamagnetic anisotropy, they could be suffered magnetic field force, then rotated and orientated along the direction of the magnetic fields which caused the expansion of ion channels on cell membrane. Therefore, numerous ions could pass through the cell membrane, thus increasing conductivity and inducing much powerful current which produced a series of bioeffects to promote bone formation. (3) Regulating calcium ions concentration: calcium ions were the basic substance of all cells, which could affect the activity of intracellular enzymes, participate in cell signal transduction, regulate cell metabolism and cell activity, etc.. Magnetic fields could activate calcium ion-dependent protein kinase by altering calcium ions level, further regulate nuclear factors including cyclin which played a regulatory role in osteoblasts. (4) Activating the cyclic adenosine monophosphate system: Magnetic stimulation could activate the cyclic adenosine monophosphate system, and then activated various enzyme systems which could induce bone cells to produce special physiological functions, thereby accelerating bone growth.

4.1.2.2　Electric Stimulation

The osteogenesis-inducing mechanisms of electric stimulation were explained as follows: (1) Inducing inverse piezoelectric effect: When an electric field was applied to bone defect sites, the stress and strain could generat between the anode and cathode of the defect sites which could produce electric signals, thereby regulating bone cell behaviors. (2) Up-regulating calcium level: Electric field could facilitate the calcium salt to move to the cathode, and elevate intracellular calcium level by promoting extracellular calcium ion influx into cells, thereby accelerating proliferation of cell and calcification and mineralization of bone tissue. (3) Regulating growth factors: Electrical stimulation could regulate the expression of growth factors, such as insulin-like growth factors Ⅰ and Ⅱ, transforming growth factors, fibroblast growth factors, bone morphogenetic proteins, etc., thereby promoting bone formation. (4) Changing local microenvironment: Electrical stimulation could improve local blood circulation and cause biochemical changes in the microcirculation around the bones and chondrocytes, such as elevated pH, thereby promoting ossification.

4.1.2.3　Mechanical Stimulation

The osteogenesis-inducing mechanisms of mechanical stimulation were explained as follows: (1) Mechanical stimulation could activate various signaling pathways when the stimulation acted on bone cells, and transduce the extracellular mechanical signals into the corresponding biochemical signals, such as calcium ion channel, G proteins, insulin-like growth factor, integrins, transforming growth factor-β and/or bone morphogenetic protein, extracellular matrix, Wnt, etc. (Fig. 4-1), thereby inducing a series of gene expression to promote proliferation, differentiation, apoptosis of bone cell. (2) Mechanical stimulation could activate the calcium ion channel on cell membrane which induced the extracellular calcium ion flow into the cell to increase the intracellular calcium concentration, thereby conducing to bone healing. (3) The pressure wave produced by the ultrasound could enhance the fluid flow in the fracture area to increase the supply of nutrients and the removal of metabolites, and thus contributing to the proliferation and differentiation of osteoblasts and fibroblasts. (4) Bone tissues possess of abundant interconnected microchannels, mechanical stress could produce strain gradients and cause ionic current flow along the microchannels, which played an important role in the process of mechanotransduction.

4.1.3　The Effects of Physical Stimulations on Bone Cells

The effectiveness of physical stimulations in bone repair has been investigated in vitro and in vivo. It was proved that physical stimulations could promote bone mesenchymal stem cells differentiate to osteoblasts, accelerate osteoblasts proliferation and differentiation, and inhibit osteoclasts formation, thereby contributing to bone repair and regeneration.

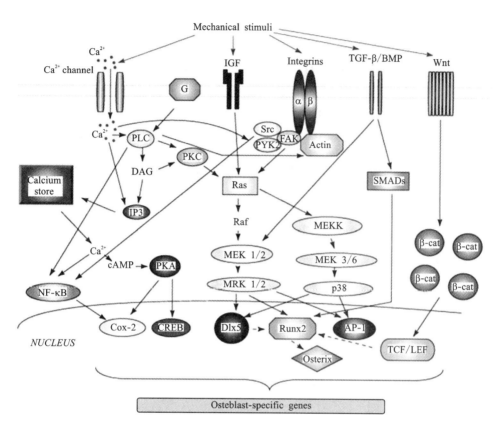

Fig. 4-1　Schematic of interactions of various signaling pathways under mechanical stimulation. Ca^{2+} channels, Gproteins (G), insulin-like growth factor (IGF), transforming growth factor-β (TGF-β) and/ or BMP, integrins and Wnt receptors were stimulated by mechanical stimulation, thereby inducing a series of transcription factors to regulate proliferation and differentiation of osteoblast.

4.1.3.1　Magnetic Stimulation on Bone Cells

The studies of magnetic stimulation used to stimulate bone cells were mainly focused on the static magnetic field and pulse electromagnetic field. In general, static magnetic field could promote proliferation and differentiation of osteoblasts as well as inhibited formation of osteoclasts, thereby promoting the process of bone repair. Moreover, the strong static magnetic field (> 1 T) could regulate the orientation of bone cells and matrix proteins. Yamamoto et al. investigated the effects of 0.16 T static magnetic field continuously exposing 20 days on the rat calvaria cell and found that static magnetic field significantly increased activity of alkaline phosphatase and osteocalcin content. Zhang et al. investigated the bioeffects of 16 T static magnetic field on osteoblasts and osteoclasts. They found that static magnetic field enhanced osteoblast differentiation determined by the formed nodules area and the calcium deposition, and inhibited osteoclast formation evaluated by tartrate-resistant acid phosphatase, integrin β_3, matrix metalloproteinase 9, receptor activator of nuclear factor kB ligand, etc. Di et al. also found that 16 T static magnetic field inhibited osteoclasts formation and differentiation due to the decreases of tartrate-resistant acid phosphatase activity, and resulted in osteoclasts apoptosis and necrosis. Kotani et al. found that 8 T static magnetic field stimulated the osteoblast transformed to rod-like shapes, cells differentiation and matrix synthesis. Moreover, static magnetic field regulated the orientation of cells and bone formation parallel to the static magnetic field direction [Fig. 4-2(b) and 4-2(c)]. Some studies have shown that magnetic nanoparticles in 3D printed scaffolds could also produce magnetic stimulation on bone cells. Huang et al. investigated the effects of magnetic stimulation which produced by incorporation of Fe_3O_4 magnetic nanoparticle in polylactic-co-glycolic acid/collagen/hydroxyapatite composite scaffolds on bone mesenchymal stem cells. They found that the magnetic nanocomposite scaffolds obviously enhanced the proliferation and differentiation of bone mesenchymal stem cells.

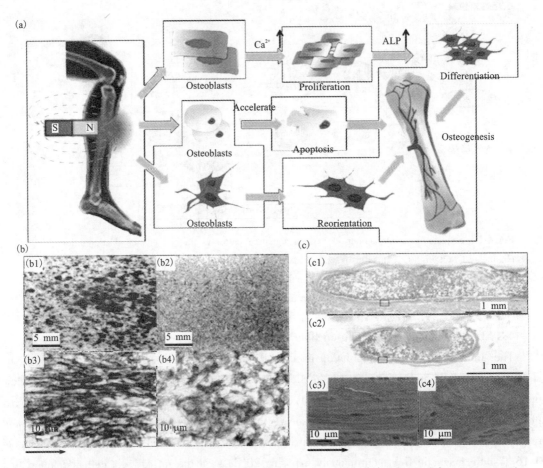

Fig. 4-2 (a) Schematic of static magnetic field promoted osteogenesis. (b) Effects of the static magnetic field on the cell differentiation: the alkaline phosphatase activity increased in exposed groups (b1, b3) compared with control groups (b2, b4). The orientation of cells maintained parallel to the direction of static magnetic field. (c) Effects of the static magnetic field on the bone formation: the bone formation in exposed groups (c1) significantly increased compared with control groups (c2). The orientation of bone formation was parallel to the direction of static magnetic field. The squares in (c1) and (c2) represent the areas in (c3) and (c4), respectively. The arrow indicated the direction of static magnetic field.

Pulse electromagnetic field could induce bone formation as well as inhibit bone resorption by regulating the formation, proliferation and differentiation of osteoblasts and osteoclasts. The effectiveness of regulation depended on the magnetic field intensity. It was owing to the nonlinear intensity window effect of pulse electromagnetic field in the process of cell behaviors regulating. Zhou et al. investigated the bioeffects of 50 Hz sinusoidal electromagnetic fields at different intensities (0.9, 1.2, 1.5, 1.8, 2.1, 2.4, 2.7 and 3.0 mT) on the differentiation of osteoblasts and the expression of Collagen-I mRNA and bone morphogenetic protein-2. The results showed that the electromagnetic fields at 1.5 – 2.4 mT groups significantly increased the differentiation of osteoblasts and the expression of Collagen-I mRNA and bone morphogenetic protein-2. Moreover, the calcium content and calcified nodules of the 1.8 mT group were higher than other groups. Kamolmatyakul et al. reported that pulse electromagnetic field (50 Hz, 1.5 mV/cm) significantly increased the proliferation rate of osteoblast-like cells. Diniz et al. proposed that pulse electromagnetic field (15 Hz, 7 mT) could promote osteoblasts differentiation in the proliferation and differentiation stage, and they pointed out that the promotion was not associated with the increased number of cells. Wang et al. investigated the effects of 15 Hz pulse electromagnetic field with various intensities of 0, 0.5, 1, 2 and 3 mT on osteoclast. The results showed that 0.5 mT pulse electromagnetic field significantly inhibited the formation and maturation of osteoclast. Chang et al. examined the effects of pulse electromagnetic field (7.5Hz, 4.8 μV/cm) on osteoclasts, and they found that the pulse electromagnetic field obviously inhibited the osteoclastogenesis.

4.1.3.2   Electric Stimulation on Bone Cells

The main sources of electric stimulation on bone cells are biphasic electric current, direct current and alternating electric current. The action modes and intensity of electric current have significant influences on cell behaviors. Kim et al. investigated the effect of biphasic electric current (1.5 μA/cm^2, 3000 Hz) on the proliferation, differentiation and synthesized cytokines of osteoblasts in the interrupted and continuous modes. The results showed that the proliferation of osteoblasts increased 31% after continuous stimulating 2 days, whereas unchanged in the interrupted mode, indicating that the continuous stimulation was more effective than the interrupted stimulation. The bone mesenchymal stem cells possess the capability to osteogenic differentiation which effectively accelerate bone healing and bone remodeling, so the migration of bone mesenchymal stem cells play an important role in bone repair. Electric field could promote the migration of bone mesenchymal stem cells, and the migration rate of the bone mesenchymal stem cells was controlled by the electric field intensity. Banks et al. were also verified this viewpoint, and found that the bone mesenchymal stem cells became significantly elongated and were perpendicular to the electric field vector. Creecy et al. exposed bone mesenchymal stem cells to alternating electric current of either 10 mA or 40 mA for 6 h/day, and they found that the stimulations significantly increased the gene expressions of osteopontin, osteocalcin and runt-related transcription factor 2, thereby promoting the differentiation of bone mesenchymal stem cells to osteoblasts. Wang et al. reported that direct current electric stimulation promoted bone mesenchymal stem cells migration. The optimal intensity and duration were 200 mV/mm and 4 h, respectively, and they up-regulated the osteocalcin, alkaline phosphatase and runt-related transcription factor 2 expressions which benefited to bone mesenchymal stem cells proliferation and differentiation. In addition, some scholars investigated the cell responses to electrical stimulation combining with 3D printed bone scaffolds. Grunert et al. studied the effects of electric stimulation on osteoblasts which cultured on 3D printed calcium phosphate/collagen composite scaffolds. The results indicated that the stimulation promoted the proliferation and differentiation of osteoblasts.

4.1.3.3 Mechanical Stimulation on Bone Cells

The mechanical stimulation is mainly including the ultrasonic stimulation and mechanical stress stimulation. The ultrasound is a high frequency mechanical wave which can be transmitted into biological tissues to produce biochemical reactions. Mechanical stresses are mainly divided into compressive stress, tensile stress and fluid shear stress. The effects of mechanical stimulation on bone cells mainly depend on loading mode, intensity, frequency and duration. The low intensity pulsed ultrasound (< 100 mW/cm^2) could modulate the proliferation and differentiation of osteoblasts and osteoclast through regulating bone-related gene expressions, and the regulatory effects were related with intensity. Yang et al. examined the effect of ultrasonic stimulation with different intensities (62.5 mW/cm^2, 125 mW/cm^2 and 250 mW/cm^2) on the osteoblasts differentiation and osteoclastogenesis. The results indicated that the ultrasound at 125 mW/cm^2 obviously enhanced the mineralization, collagen synthesis and alkaline phosphatase activity of osteoblasts. Moreover, low intensity pulsed ultrasound at 62.5 mW/cm^2 and 125 mW/cm^2 significantly inhibited the formation and differentiation of osteoclasts. Sun et al. reported that low intensity pulsed ultrasound (1 MHz, 68 mW/cm^2) obviously increased the osteoblast cell counts and alkaline phosphatase level after ultrasonic stimulation for 7 days, and significantly reduced the osteoclast cell counts. Korstjens et al. found that low intensity pulsed ultrasound (1.5 MHz, 30 mW/cm^2) treating at 20 min/day for 3 days or 6 days significantly increased the bone collar volume and calcified cartilage. It was worth noting that ultrasound stimulation displayed pronounced biological effects on cells which cultured on 3D printed bone scaffolds. Zhou et al. investigated the effects of low intensity pulsed ultrasound on human bone marrow mesenchymal stem cells seeded on hydroxyapatite scaffolds, and they found that the ultrasound stimulation combining with scaffolds significantly improved the alkaline phosphatase activity and calcium deposition.

The mechanical stresses with amplitude, frequency and duration of various peak stress had different influences on cell behaviors. Bone cells could distinguish different stress magnitude and adjust the bio-chemical response accordingly. Tang et al. investigated the bioeffects of cyclic stretching (500 $\mu\varepsilon$, 1000 $\mu\varepsilon$ and 1500 $\mu\varepsilon$) on osteoblasts. The results indicated that the stretching at 500 $\mu\varepsilon$ increased osteoblast collagen synthesis, while the stretching at 1000 $\mu\varepsilon$ and 1500 $\mu\varepsilon$ inhibited collagen production, indicating that the response of osteoblasts was dependent on the stretching magnitude. Jagodzinski et al. proved the mechanical strain with an elongation of 2% and 8% increased the alkaline phosphatase levels and osteocalcin secretion of mesenchymal stem cells after loading 4 days, and the increase rate of 8% stretching group was higher than 2% stretching group. Kearney et al. found that the 2.5%, 0.17 Hz cyclic tensile mechanical strain obviously reduced mesenchymal stem cells proliferation after 2 and 3 days, and increased the expression of transcription factor Cbfa1, osteocalcin, collagen type I and bone morphogenetic protein-2 which was related to osteogenic differentiation [Fig. 4-3(a)]. Sanchez et al. reported the cyclic compression stress (1 MPa at 1 Hz) significantly increased the genes expression of cyclooxygenase 2, interleukin-6, receptor activator of nuclear factor κB ligand, etc. which involved in bone remodeling and bone formation. Li et al. investigated the bioeffects of different oscillating frequencies, peak shear stress amplitudes, and total flow durations on osteocyte activity. The results indicated that the three dynamic fluid flow parameters could regulate the osteocyte activity, faster oscillating frequencies, higher peak shear stress amplitudes and longer loading durations, beneficial to bone formation. Liu et al. proved that fluid shear stress at 1.6 Pa and 1.9 Pa significantly induced the cell elongation and reorientation parallel to the direction of fluid flow, indicating that the fluid shear stress could influence the cell growth direction. Li et al. found that the fluid shear stress at 12 dyn/cm^2 could reorganize the cytoskeleton in MC3T3 – E1 pre-osteoblasts which was critical for mechanosensation and intracellular signal transduction. And the actin filaments rapidly reorganized

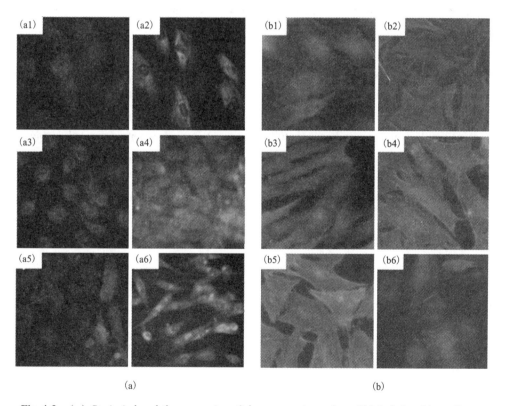

Fig. 4-3　(a) Strain induced the expression of the osteogenic markers Cbfα1 (a1, a2), collagen type I (a3, a4), and osteocalcin (a5, a6). mesenchymal stem cells in static culture for 6 days (a1, a3, a5), mesenchymal stem cells exposed to mechanical strain (2.5%) after 6 days (a2, a4, a6). (b) The fluid shear stress at 12 dyn/cm^2 induced stress fibre formation in different time spans. The cells were loaded for 0, 5, 15, 45, 90 and 120 min, respectively) (b1-b6).

into thick parallel bundles of fibres, and the fibre formation was induced by shear stress loading 0 – 90 min whereas the cytoskeleton was disrupted over loading 90 min [Fig. 4-3(b)]. Besides, fluid shear stress could produce bioeffects to cells which seeded on 3D printed bone scaffolds. Stiehler et al. studied the effect of fluid shear stress on human mesenchymal stem cells cultured on porous poly(D, L-lactide-co-glycolide) scaffolds, and the results showed that the fluid shear stress markedly enhanced alkaline phosphatase activity, increased Ca^{2+} content and promoted cells growth.

4.1.3.4　Physical Stimulations on Artificial Bone

In terms of bone defects repair, bone scaffolds need to possess interconnected internal porous structure that provide channels for the adhesion and migration of bone cells, the transmission of nutrients, and the growth of bone tissue. Meanwhile, bone scaffolds also need to possess customized external geometries that can exactly match bone defects, which is beneficial for the structural and functional remodeling of bone. The customized porous scaffolds present a great challenge for manufacturing process. 3D printing is one of the advanced manufacturing technologies which fabricate objects directly from the given computer-aided design model via layer by layer printing. It can fabricate the interconnected internal porous structure and the customized external shape of bone scaffolds. Moreover, bone scaffolds require excellent biocompatibility to encourage cell adhesion and migration. Bioceramics (such as hydroxyapatite, bioactive glass, etc.) and biopolymers (such as polycaprolactone, polylactide, etc.) are suitable materials for the fabrication of bone scaffolds owing to their good biological properties. Magnetic materials (such as Fe_3O_4, γ-Fe_2O_3, etc.) and conductive materials (such as carbon nanotube, graphene, etc.) are incorporated in bioceramics and/or biopolymers to enhance the biological and physical properties of scaffolds. Zhang et al. incorporated Fe_3O_4 nanoparticles into polycaprolactone and mesoporous bioactive glass composites, and found that the 3D printed composite scaffold significantly stimulated cells proliferation and differentiation. Therefore, the bone scaffold fabricated via 3D printing technology with physical stimulations (such as magnetic or conductive materials) is a promising and efficient candidate for bone formation and healing.

The physical stimulations combining with bone scaffolds have great potential in bone repair because they can fully reflect the synergetic effects of bone scaffolds and physical fields in bone repair process. Yun et al. found that static magnetic field synergized with magnetic bone scaffolds promoted the osteoblastic differentiation including enhanced alkaline phosphatase activity and up-regulated gene expressions of osterix and runt-related transcription factor 2. Feng et al. investigated the bioeffects of 4000 G static magnetic field on the osteoblasts cultured on poly-L-lactide substrates surface and found that alkaline phosphatase activity was significantly increased, indicating that static magnetic field combining with scaffolds could promote cell differentiation. Arjmand et al. proved that the extremely low frequency pulse electromagnetic field combining with polycaprolactone (PCL) nanofibrous scaffold significantly enhanced the proliferation and osteogenic differentiation of mesenchymal stem cells by analyzing alizarin red staining, alkaline phosphatase activity, calcium content, related genes expressions such as collagen type I, runt-related gene 2, osteonectin and osteocalcin. Some studies have shown that scaffold materials have a significant impact on bone repair. Jin et al. investigated the effects of electric stimulation combining with three-dimensional porous scaffolds (PCL, PCL/carbon nanotubes (CNT) and PCL/ β-tricalcium phosphate (β-TCP) scaffold) on the osteoblasts. They found that the electric stimulation enhanced the alkaline phosphatase activity and calcium mineralization of osteoblasts in all scaffolds, and the enhancement of bone mineralization in PCL/β-TCP scaffold was the highest [Fig. 4-4(a)]. The results indicated that the electric stimulation and scaffold materials both played a significant role in bone repair. Sun et al. reported that the electric stimulation induced the reorientation of fibroblasts in three-dimensional collagen scaffold and along the direction of the electric stimulation. Chen et al. investigated synergistic action of fluid shear stress and three-dimensional porous scaffolds (collagen/ hydroxyapatite, Col/HA) on the biological behaviors of mesenchymal stem cells. The results showed that the viability of mesenchymal stem cells in the all scaffolds significantly increased under oscillatory shear stress cultured for 3 weeks compared with control group. Moreover, the oscillatory shear stress significantly enhanced the osteogenic differentiation of mesenchymal stem cells in the scaffolds [Fig. 4-4(b)].

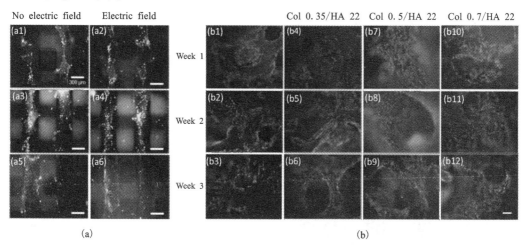

Fig. 4-4 (a) Live/dead assay of MG63 cells seeded on PCL (a1, a2), PCL/CNT (a3, a4), and PCL/β-TCP scaffolds (a5, a6) with and without electric stimulation after 14 days. (b) Live/dead assay of mesenchymal stem cells seeded on the midline section of different scaffolds for 1, 2, and 3 weeks under oscillatory perfusion. (b1 – b3) Static culture mesenchymal stem cells. The scale bar indicates 50 μm. Living cells (green) and dead cells (red).

4.1.4　In vivo Studies of Physical Stimulation

In vivo studies mainly include animal experiments and clinical trials. Animal experiments can provide theoretical supports for clinical trials. Many animal experiments and clinical trials have been carried out to determine the effects of magnetic, electric and mechanical stimulation on bone repair.

4.1.4.1　In vivo Studies of Magnetic Stimulation

The magnetic stimulation produced by magnetic fields and electromagnetic fields could conduce to accelerate bone repair due to that they could promote bone formation and inhibit bone resorption. Taniguchi et al. investigated the effects of 30 mT static magnetic field on the bone mineral density of ovariectomized rat model under whole body exposure. The results indicated that bone mineral density significantly increased after 12 weeks because static magnetic field increased the level of locomotor activity in rats model. Besides, the bone mass was also higher than control group. Puricelli et al. assessed the effect of the magnetized metal device on the repair of femur cavity of rats. The results showed that the 4.1 mT magnetic field accelerated the bone formation compared with control group on 15th, 45th, 60th days after the implantation, thereby enhancing the bone healing. Leesungbok et al. compared the bone formation ability of titanium implant with or without magnets in a rabbit tibia. The results showed that the titanium implants with magnet enhanced early implant bone formation compared with there without magnet implants. It was worth noting that static magnetic field, combining with magnetic nanocomposite scaffolds which consisted of polymer and magnetic nanoparticles, could own the advantages of them in bone repair. Yun et al. investigated the effects of static magnetic field synergized with magnetic scaffolds on osteoblastic functions of mouse calvarium. The results showed that static magnetic field combining with magnetic scaffolds

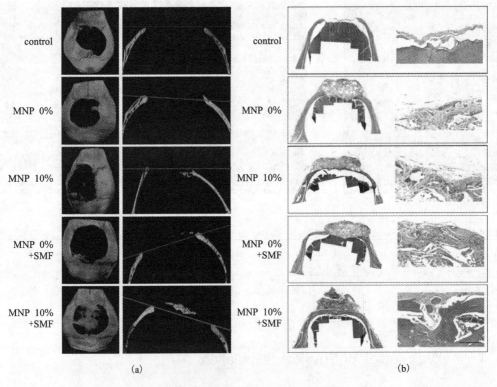

(a)　　　　　　　　　　　　　　　　(b)

Fig. 4-5 Effects of static magnetic field and PCL/MNP (magnetic nanoparticle) scaffolds on bone regeneration of calvarial defect in mouse after 6 weeks of implantation. (a) μCT images constructed for the calcified tissues in the defects (left: top view; right: lateral cross-section view). (b) H&E-stained images (left: gross cross-section view, right: magnified image of newly formed tissues).

significantly enhanced the new bone formation after exposure of 6 weeks (Fig. 4-5). Inoue et al. investigated the effects of pulse electromagnetic field on late bone healing phase of canine mid-tibia osteotomy model. The results revealed that the stimulation of 1 h/day for 8 weeks significantly increased the new bone formation and mechanical strength. Zaki et al. researched the effectiveness of pulse electromagnetic field on the fractures healing of patients at different treatment stages. The results showed that pulse electromagnetic field significantly accelerated the bone healing of patients at 12th week who were continued subjecting to pulse electromagnetic field treatment compared with control group which was only treated with plaster cast, and the late treatment group which received pulse electromagnetic field treatment with the cast removed also increased the osteocalcin level, indicating that the pulse electromagnetic field could enhance the fracture healing.

4.1.4.2   In vivo Studies of Electric Stimulation

Bone tissue would respond to electrical stimulation signals which produced by various electric currents, thereby generating a series of biochemical reactions which were conducive to bone repair. El-Hakim et al. investigated the effects of direct current of 10 μA on mandibular distraction osteogenesis of adult goats in different distraction periods. The results showed that direct current played a positive role on mandibular distraction osteogenesis when it was applied to the distraction areas during activation and consolidation periods. Fredericks et al. reported that the direct current stimulation could promote bone formation of rabbit posterolateral fusion model. Park et al. investigated the effects of electric stimulation of 1 h/day for 4 weeks on 3 mm gapped osteotomies in mid-tibial of rabbit models, and the two electrodes were placed on the above patellar tendon and lateral thigh, respectively. The results showed that the callus area and mineral content were 27% and 31% higher than control osteotomies, respectively, and the biomechanical properties were significantly higher than control group. It indicated that the electric stimulation could increase the mineralization and callus development of the bone healing regions, thereby enhancing the biomechanical properties. Chen et al. evaluated the changes in bone mineral density of fifteen males with spinal cord injury after the intervention of functional electric stimulation for 6 months. The results showed that the bone mineral density increased significantly, whereas the effect would disappear when the stimulation was removed.

4.1.4.3   In vivo Studies of Mechanical Stimulation

Mechanical stimulation can accelerate the bone repair process and induce healing of nonunions, which depends on the intensity, frequency and duration of loading. Azuma et al. investigated the effects of ultrasonic stimulation (30 mW/cm^2, 20min/day) on fracture healing in the different duration (1 – 8, 9 – 16, 17 – 24 and 1 – 24 days). The radiography and histological results demonstrated that the low intensity pulsed ultrasound could accelerate fracture healing at each treatment period, and the 1 – 24 days group was more effective than other treated groups (Fig. 4-6). Moreover, the mechanical torsion properties of treated femurs were significantly higher than nontreated femurs, and the properties in the 1 – 24 days group were the highest. Takikawa et al. established nonunion model of tibia fracture in rat, and utilized low intensity pulsed ultrasound (30 mW/cm^2) to treat the fracture sites. They found that the healing rates of tibia samples were 30.8%

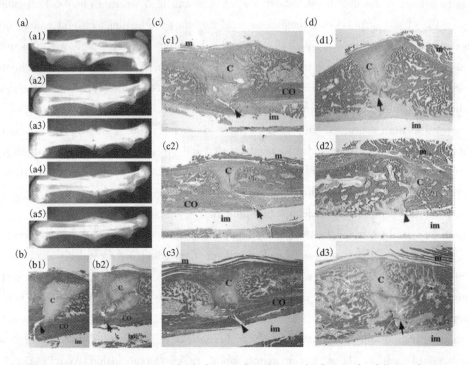

Fig. 4-6 Effects of low intensity pulsed ultrasound on fracture healing in the different duration. (a) Radiography of treated femur (a2 – a5, treatment duration at 1 – 8, 9 – 16, 17 – 24 and 1 – 24 days, respectively) and nontreated femur (a1) at 25th day after fracture. The treated groups had better bone healing than control group. (b-d) Histological analyses of low intensity pulsed ultrasound treatment on fracture healing at different duration. At 9th day, early endochondral ossification in treated femur (b2) was greater than in the control (b1). At 17th day, endochondral ossification and remodeling in the control femur (c1) were less than treated femur for 16 days (days 1 – 16, c2) and 8 days (days 9 – 16, c3). At 25th day, bone bridging in the control femur (d1) was less than treated for 24 days (days 1 – 24, d2) and 8 days (days 17 – 24, d3).

and 50% after treated for 4 weeks and 6 weeks, respectively, while the samples in control group were not healing. Nolte et al. studied the bioeffect of low intensity pulsed ultrasound (20 min/day) on the fracture nonunion sites of 29 patients. The results showed that 86% of patients obtained complete healing after 22 weeks. Fritton et al. investigated the skeletal responsed to compressive loads by applying controlled cyclic axial load on mouse tibia and analyzed the bone mineral content of loaded and unloaded limbs. The results showed that the average trabecular thickness, bone mineral content and bone volume fraction increased 12%, 14% and 15%, respectively. Lambers et al. studied the effects of cyclically load of 8 N on the bone formation and resorption of mouse tail vertebrae. The results showed that the 8 N group significantly increased trabecular bone volume fraction and cortical area fraction. Moreover, the bone strength increased due to the increasing of bone formation area and the decreasing of bone resorption area (Fig. 4-7). Peptan et al. investigated the effects of cyclic tensile or compressive forces (1 N, 8 Hz) on remodeling and growth of intramembranous bone and cranial sutures of rabbit models. The results showed that the high-frequency cyclic tensile and compressive forces both induced the modeling and growth of cranial sutures.

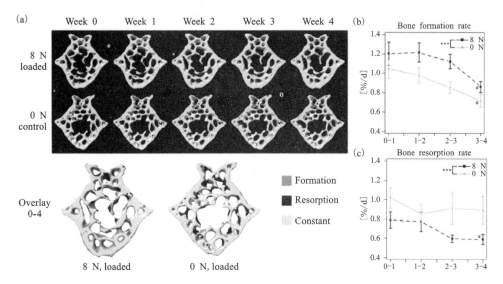

Fig. 4-7 Bone microstructure of mice in the 8 N and 0 N group in vivo micro-CT scans (a). The trabecular structure of the 8 N group thickened with increasing stimulation time and there was little change in 0 N group. Curves of dynamic bone formation rate (b) and bone resorption rate (c) over time. The bone formation rate of 8 N group was obviously higher than 0 N group and the bone resorption rate showed the opposite result.

4.1.5 The Equipments of Physical Stimulation Systems

In vitro and in vivo studies have shown that different physical stimulations had different effects on bone cells. As the source of physical stimulations, the physical stimulation systems played an important role in bone repair. To date, there were no unified stimulation systems for each kind of physical stimulation, and the representative physical stimulation systems were shown in Fig. 4-8.

4.1.5.1 The Magnetic Stimulation Systems

The static magnetic field and pulse electromagnetic field were widely used in the treatment of various bone-related diseases such as fracture, osteoporosis, bone delayed union or nonunion, etc., owing to their non-invasive, no infection, no side effects and ease of use. In vivo studies, many researchers implanted magnet rods, magnetic plates and magnetic washers into bone defect sites to construct static magnetic field. Some researchers constructed static magnetic field stimulation equipments composed of magnetic plates which were fixed on outside of cage [Fig. 4-8 (a)] or utilized signal generator to produce direct current transferring to a pair of Helmholtz coils to expose animals. In vitro studies, the static magnetic field exposure systems which were used to expose bone cells had various modes, such as magnets, a magnetic shield box, parallel arranged magnetic plates, etc.. The construction of pulse electromagnetic field usually adopted the tunable pulse

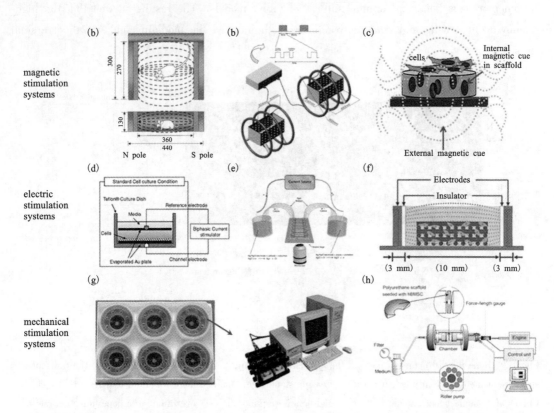

Fig. 4-8 The schematic of the physical stimulation systems. (a) static magnetic field exposure system. (b) pulse electromagnetic field exposure system. (c) Magnetic stimulation on artificial bone. (d) Biphasic electric current stimulation system. (e) Direct current electric stimulation system. (f) Electric stimulation consisted of a parallel electrode used to stimulate cells seeded on scaffold. (g) Flexercell compression plus system was used to compress osteoblasts membrane. (h) Mechanical stimulation bioreactor system was used to perfuse scaffolds seeded with cells.

generator to produce pulse current with specific frequency, waveform and peak. Jing D. et al. designed a pulse electromagnetic field generator consisting of three identical Helmholtz coils [Fig. 4-8(b)] and it could output different waveforms and parameters.

4.1.5.2   The Electric Stimulation Systems

In vivo studies, the modes of electrical stimulations mainly included invasive, semi-invasive and non-invasive way in bone repair. The invasive way meant embedding cathode and anode in the injury sites, and the semi-invasive way meant embedding the cathode into the injury sites and placing the anode in a cephalad paraspinous locus. The non-invasive way referred to place the injury sites in an electric field or place the electrodes on the surface of the treatment sites. It had been widely accepted by patients owing to the small trauma. In vitro studies, some researchers placed electrodes on top and bottom surfaces of each well and then connected the electric field device to stimulate cells. Many researchers used sinusoidal alternating electric field which consisted of function generator and parallel electrodes to expose bone cells. Kim et al. designed a biphasic electric current system to stimulate osteoblasts which consisted of Teflon© culture dish, two evaporated Au plates, media and biphasic current stimulator. The anodes and cathodes of each well were connected to form an electrical shunt configuration and all electrodes were connected to the biphasic electric current stimulator chip [Fig. 4-8(d)]. Banks et al. customized an ibidi© device to create an electric field stimulation system which allowed to simultaneously stimulate six cell migration chambers, and 6 pairs of agar bridges in physiologic buffered saline connected cell migration channels to reservoirs of physiologic buffered saline, in which Ag-AgCl electrodes were immersed [Fig. 4-8(e)].

4.1.5.3   The Mechanical Stimulation Systems

Low intensity pulsed ultrasound treatment had received widespread attention in treatment bone fracture due to the advantages of safety, non-invasive, no infection and less complication. The ultrasonic stimulation used by most researchers was usually generated by the Sonic Accelerated Fracture Healing System, which could produce different frequencies and intensities. Different devices were used to carry out different mechanical stimulations for bone cells and tissues. The BiopressTM system was used by many researchers to apply compressive loads. It could control load magnitude to compress osteoblasts membrane to investigate the effects of compression stress on osteoblasts. Zhong et al. designed a cellular cyclic tension and compression apparatus to investigate the biological response of osteoblasts under stretching or compressing. The apparatus could control the carrier rod to precisely shift up and down. Many researchers used a parallel-plate flow chamber to induce fluid flow over the cells to construct fluid shear stress. You L. et al. established a flow system which was driven by an electromagnetic actuator.

4.1.6   The Opportunities and Challenges of Physical Stimulations

Physical stimulations have been demonstrated to be effective in promoting bone repair. It is urgently require further systematic investigations to find the underlying mechanisms, thereby getting better understanding of the bioeffects and providing adequate theoretical supports for the application in bone repair. Bone is a dynamic tissue composed of several cell types such as osteocytes, osteoblasts, osteoclasts and bone mesenchymal stem cells. The cells play an important role in maintaining normal bone homeostasis. Current researches mainly focused on the bone formation by osteoblasts. Therefore, future researches should comprehensively evaluate the bioeffects of physical stimulations on various cells, and the mutual regulation between cells under physical stimulations should also be considered.

4.2　Disperse magnetic Sources Constructed with Functionalized Fe_3O_4 Nanoparticles in Poly-l-lactic Acid Scaffolds

4.2.1　Introduction

Fe_3O_4 nanoparticles have been extensively applied in biomedicine due to the excellent magnetism, good biocompatibility and nontoxicity. Particularly, the Fe_3O_4 nanoparticles were incorporated into scaffolds made of biopolymers or bioceramics, aiming to utilize the nanoparticles as magnetic sources to induce a series of cell behaviors, thereby promoting bone regeneration. Bock et al integrated Fe_3O_4 nanoparticles into scaffolds made of hydroxyapatite and collagen by dip-coating. Results demonstrated the ability of the magnetic scaffolds to promote cell adhesion and proliferation. Santis et al developed a magnetic scaffold by incorporating Fe_3O_4 nanoparticles into poly (e-caprolactone) via three dimensional fiber-deposition technique, and found that the presence of Fe_3O_4 nanoparticles promoted cells adhesion and spreading. It was worth noting that Fe_3O_4 nanoparticles tended to aggregate in scaffolds as a result of high surface energy and anisotropic dipolar attractions. In this case, their specific properties related to single magnetic domain and magnetic nanostructures would be compromised, thus limiting their enhancement effect in bone regeneration.

Functionalization is considered to be an effective method to improve the dispersion of nanoparticles. Shrestha et al. functionalized multi-wall carbon nanotubes by carboxylation and found that the functionalized carbon nanotubes could uniformly disperse in nanotopographical polyurethane bioactive scaffolds. Anwar et al synthesized nanohydroxyapatites which were functionalized using vinylphosphonic acid and methacrylic acid, respectively. Results revealed that the functionalized nanohydroxyapatites could disperse in a liquid phase. Zhang et al functionalized nanodiamond with phospholipids and proved that the functionalized nanodiamond could disperse in a poly (lactic-co-glycolic acid) matrix.

Oleic acidic monofunctional fatty acid possesses a carboxylic acid group and a hydrocarbon chain. The carboxylic acid groups of oleic acid may interact with hydroxyl groups of Fe_3O_4 nanoparticles in case of aqueous medium. And hydrocarbon chains of oleic acid are consequently toward the outside of nanoparticles and mutually exclusive. Therefore, oleic acid may functionalize the nanoparticles and thus improve the dispersion of nanoparticles in the scaffolds. In addition, oleic acid is one of the major component of membrane phospholipids that express high affinity to cell membrane. From this point of view, oleic acid could directly or indirectly interact with cell membrane, thus promoting the cell adhesion.

Herein, oleic acid functionalized Fe_3O_4 nanoparticles were incorporated into PLLA scaffolds fabricated by selective laser sintering (SLS) technique. The magnetic, thermal and mechanical properties of the scaffolds were evaluated. The cytocompatibility such as viability, adhesion, proliferation and differentiation of cells cultured on the scaffolds were also assessed.

4.2.2   Materials and Methods

4.2.2.1   Materials

PLLA powders (M_w: 150 kDa, purity: >99%, density: 1.25 g/cm^3) were provided by Shenzhen Polymtek Biomaterial Co., Ltd. (Shenzhen, China). Fe$_3$O$_4$ nanoparticles (average particle size: 20 nm, purity: >99%, density: 5.18 g/cm^3) were purchased from Nanjing Emperor Nano Material Co., Ltd. (Nanjing, China). Oleic acid was received from Tianjin Chemical Co., Ltd. (Tianjin, China). Sodium pyruvate, fetal bovine serum and phosphate buffered saline were purchased from Gibco Co., Ltd. (Grand Island, USA). Penicillin and streptomycin were purchased from Hyclone Co., Ltd. (Logan, USA). Cell counting kit-8 (CCK-8) solution was obtained from Selleck Chemicals (Houston, USA). MG63 cells were provided by Chinese Academy of Sciences (Shanghai, China). The other chemicals and solvents were acquired from Sinopharm Chemical Reagent Co., Ltd (Shanghai, China).

4.2.2.2   Synthesis of Oleic Acid Functionalized Fe$_3$O$_4$ Nanoparticles

The synthesis process of oleic acid functionalized Fe$_3$O$_4$ nanoparticles was shown in Fig.4-9(a). Concretely, Fe$_3$O$_4$ nanoparticles were dispersed in a mixture of distilled water (50 mL) and ethanol

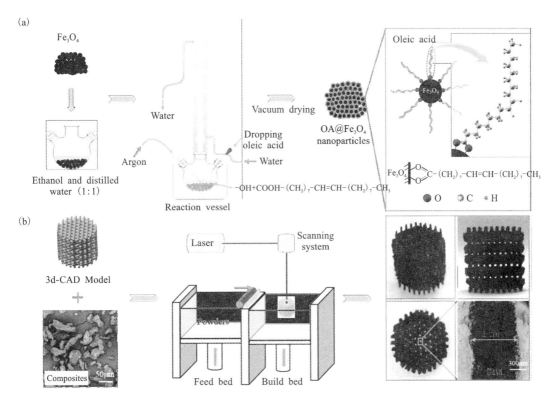

Fig.4-9   Principle diagram of the synthesis of oleic acid functionalized Fe$_3$O$_4$ (OA@ Fe$_3$O$_4$) nanoparticles (a) and scaffold preparation (b).

(50 mL) in a 250 mL three neck flask. Afterwards, the mixture solution was introduced to a reaction vessel and then was vigorous magnetic stirring under argon. Oleic acid (6 mL) was added dropwise to the vigorously stirred solution after the solution temperature reached 75 ℃. And the reaction proceeded for another hour. After that, the mixture was cooled to room temperature. And then the oleic acid functionalized Fe_3O_4 ($OA@Fe_3O_4$) nanoparticles were collected magnetically and washed several times with ethanol and distilled water. Finally, the nanoparticles were dried under vacuum at 50℃ for 10 hours.

4.2.2.3 Composite Powders and Scaffolds Preparation

Composite powders with different contents of $OA@Fe_3O_4$ nanoparticles (0, 4%, 8%, 12% and 16%) were prepared. Briefly, PLLA powders were added into ethanol solution at 10% w/v and then were dispersed for 20 minutes by water bath ultrasound at 40 kHz frequency. Subsequently, the well dispersed $OA@Fe_3O_4$ nanoparticles in ethanol solution were added dropwise to the PLLA solution. The concentrations of $OA@Fe_3O_4$ nanoparticles in PLLA solution were determined as 0, 4%, 8%, 12% and 16%. The resulting mixtures were ultrasonic dispersed for another hour to obtain uniformly dispersed solutions. After that, the solutions were purified by centrifugation and dried using dry box to obtain composite powders.

Independently developed SLS system was utilized to prepare magnetic scaffolds. According to the contents of $OA@Fe_3O_4$ nanoparticles (0%, 4%, 8%, 12% and 16%), the obtained scaffolds were named as 0FNPs, 4FNPs, 8FNPs, 12FNPs and 16FNPs scaffolds, respectively. The preparation illustration of the magnetic scaffold was shown in Fig. 4-1 (b). The designed three-dimensional (3D) scaffold model was imported into the SLS system and sliced. Then the composite powders were sintered selectively according to the slice file. After preparation, the excess powders were removed. Finally, the magnetic scaffolds with 3D porous structure were obtained.

4.2.2.4 Characterization of $OA@Fe_3O_4$ Nanoparticles and Magnetic Scaffolds

The surface functional groups of oleic acid, Fe_3O_4 and $OA@Fe_3O_4$ nanoparticles were detected with Fourier transform infrared (FTIR, Nicolet 6700, Thermo Electron Scientific Instruments, USA) spectrometer over the range from 4000 cm^{-1} to 400 cm^{-1}. The crystal structures of Fe_3O_4, $OA@Fe_3O_4$ nanoparticles and the phase identification of the magnetic scaffolds were analyzed by X-ray diffraction (XRD, DMAX 2500, Japan Science Corporation, Japan) in the 2θ scanning range from 20° to 70° employing a scanning rate of 8°/min. Microstructure of the magnetic scaffolds was observed using scanning electron microscopy (SEM, Phenom ProX, Phenom-World BV, Netherlands). The pore sizes of the magnetic scaffolds were measured by calibration of the scale baron micrographs via the ImageJ software. Ten repeated measurements were performed for different pores in each scaffold. Dispersion capability of Fe_3O_4, $OA@Fe_3O_4$ nanoparticles in PLLA matrix was characterized using SEM. And the distribution of Fe elements in the matrix were detected using energy dispersive spectroscopy (EDS) integrated in the SEM.

Magnetic properties of Fe_3O_4 nanoparticles, $OA@Fe_3O_4$ nanoparticles and the scaffolds (0FNPs, 4FNPs, 8FNPs, 12FNPs and 16FNPs scaffolds) were detected by a vibration sample magnetometer (VSM, MPMS3, Quantum Design China, China) at room temperature. Compressive strength and modulus of scaffolds were tested by universal testing machine at a speed of 0.5 mm/min. Five samples in each group were repeated in the experiments for the averages. The decomposition process of scaffolds was assessed via thermogravimetric analysis and differential scanning calorimetry using a thermogravimetric analyzer (Nanjing Dazhan Electromechanical Technology Institute, Nanjing, China) following the same thermal conditions (range from 30℃ to 500℃ at a heating rate of 20 ℃/min) under nitrogen atmosphere.

4.2.2.5　Cytocompatibility

MG63 cells were incubated in Dulbecco's Modified Eagle Medium supplemented with 10% fetal bovine serum and 1% (volume fraction) streptomycin/penicillin at 37 ℃ in a humidified 5% CO_2 atmosphere. And the incubate medium was updated every 2 days. Magnetic scaffold samples (8 mm ×8 mm ×2 mm) were sterilized under exposure to ultraviolet light for 2 hours before cell seeding, and then transferred to 24 – well culture plates as well as secured using Viton O-rings. After cell counting, MG63 cells were seeded on each scaffold at a density of 10^5 cells per well. And the incubate medium was refreshed every day. After MG63 cells seeding on scaffolds for 1, 4 and 7 days, the cell-scaffold samples were rinsed three times using phosphate buffered saline. Then, calcein acetoxymethyl ester was added to stain cells for 40 min at 37℃. The stained cell-scaffold samples were washed by phosphate buffered saline and then analyzed using a fluorescence microscope. At different culture times, the adhesion and spreading morphologies of cells on the samples were visualized by SEM.

The proliferation capability of MG63 cells cultured on the scaffolds was assessed using CCK-8 assay. The cells were cultured on the scaffold samples at a density of 10^5 cells per well for 1, 4 and 7 days. At each evaluation period, 40 μL of CCK-8 solution and 400 μL of culture medium were added to each well and incubated for another 4 hours at 37℃. Then, 100 μL solution from each well was transferred to a 24 well plate. Subsequently, the light absorbance of the solutions was measured at 450 nm using a spectrophotometric microplate reader. The early differentiation of the cells, after being cultured on the scaffold samples for 7 days and 14 days, was measured by alkaline phosphatase (ALP) activity. At the predetermined time point, the ALP activity of the cells was analyzed by measuring the light absorbance at 450 nm using microplate reader. All the experiments were carried out in triplicate.

4.2.2.6　Statistical Analysis

All data in the present study were collected from at least three separate experiments, which were analyzed by one-way analysis of variance. And they expressed as means ± standard deviation. In all statistical analyses, probability values of less than 0.05 and 0.01 were considered to be significant, which were represented as ' * ' and ' * * ', respectively.

4.2.3　Results and Discussion

4.2.3.1　Characterization of OA@ Fe_3O_4 Nanoparticles

The FTIR spectra of oleic acid, Fe_3O_4 and OA@ Fe_3O_4 nanoparticles were shown in Fig. 4-10 (a). Clearly, peaks at 2925, 2854, 1710 and 1415 cm^{-1} corresponding to methyl symmetric, methylene asymmetric stretching vibration, carbonyl stretching band and carboxyl symmetric stretching band were detected in oleic acid. And peak at 582 cm^{-1} corresponding to Fe—O appeared in Fe$_3$O$_4$ nanoparticles. As for OA@ Fe$_3$O$_4$ nanoparticles, peaks at 2921, 2850 and 1405 cm^{-1} indicated that the existence of oleic acid on the Fe$_3$O$_4$ nanoparticles surfaces. It should be noted that the peak at 1710 cm^{-1} assigned to carbonyl stretch bond of oleic acid disappeared, indicating that there was no free oleic acid on the surface of the nanoparticles. Besides, peak corresponding to Fe—O shifted from 582 cm^{-1} to 568 cm^{-1}, which could be attributed to the interaction between Fe—O of Fe$_3$O$_4$ and carboxylate of oleic acid. All the results above suggested that Fe$_3$O$_4$ nanoparticles were functionalized by oleic acid.

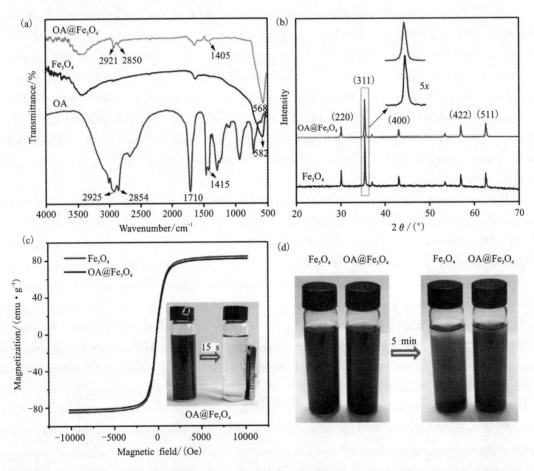

Fig. 4-10 Characterization of OA@ Fe$_3$O$_4$ nanoparticles. (a) FTIR of oleic acid, Fe$_3$O$_4$ nanoparticles and OA@ Fe$_3$O$_4$ nanoparticles. (b) XRD patterns of OA@ Fe$_3$O$_4$ and Fe$_3$O$_4$ nanoparticles. (c) Magnetic hysteresis loops of OA@ Fe$_3$O$_4$ and Fe$_3$O$_4$ nanoparticles. The inset is an image of OA@ Fe$_3$O$_4$ nanoparticles dispersed in mixture of distilled water and ethanol (1 : 1) and attracted by a magnet. (d) Dispersion capability of the OA@ Fe$_3$O$_4$ and Fe$_3$O$_4$ nanoparticles in mixture of distilled water and ethanol (1:1).

The XRD patterns of Fe_3O_4 and OA@ Fe_3O_4 nanoparticles were shown in Fig. 4-10(b). Basing on standard patterns of Fe_3O_4 (JCPDS #19 – 629), the diffraction peaks of OA@ Fe_3O_4 nanoparticles exhibited on obvious deviation from those of Fe_3O_4 nanoparticles, indicating that the functionalization resulted in no change on the crystal structure of nanoparticles. Interestingly, the peaks of OA@ Fe_3O_4 nanoparticles became broad and intensity consequently decreased, compared with Fe_3O_4 nanoparticles. The broadened peaks might be closely related to the decrease of particle size, which could be calculated by Scherrer's equation:

$$D = K\lambda / (\beta cos\theta)$$

Where K, λ, β and θ were the shape factor, X-ray wavelength, full width at half maximum and diffraction angle, respectively. As calculated from the strongest peak (311), the average particle sizes for Fe_3O_4 and OA@ Fe_3O_4 nanoparticles were (19.5 ± 0.03) nm and (15.2 ± 0.02) nm, respectively. On the other hand, the broadened peaks for OA@ Fe_3O_4 nanoparticles could also be ascribed to the amorphous oleic acid on the surface of crystalline Fe_3O_4 induced microstrain.

The hysteresis loops of the Fe_3O_4 and OA@ Fe_3O_4 nanoparticles were shown in Fig. 4-10(c). It could be seen that their remanences were both close to zero. And their saturation magnetizations were 84.5 emu/g and 82.2 emu/g, respectively. It indicated that the functionalization had little effect on the superparamagnetic property and magnetic saturation strength of Fe_3O_4 nanoparticles. As shown in the inset, the OA@ Fe_3O_4 nanoparticles dispersing in the mixture of distilled water and ethanol exhibited a markedly magnetic response to a magnet, indicating the excellent magnetic properties. In order to investigate the dispersion capability of the Fe_3O_4 and OA@ Fe_3O_4 nanoparticles, they dispersed in the mixture of distilled water and ethanol, as shown in Fig. 4-10 (d). It was observed that the OA@ Fe_3O_4 nanoparticles dispersed more efficiently in the mixture solution as compared to the Fe_3O_4 nanoparticles. It indicated that the functionalized nanoparticles presented significantly improved dispersion capability, so that it was expected to be uniformly dispersed in PLLA matrix.

4.2.3.2　Characterization of Magnetic Scaffolds

In this paper, magnetic scaffolds prepared via SLS possessed interconnected pore structures, as shown in Fig. 4-9(b). Obviously, the pores of the magnetic scaffolds were presented clearly. The pore sizes of the scaffolds, measured by ImageJ software, were (650 ± 30) μm ($n = 10$). Respect to microstructure, the pore sizes were greater than 100 μm and connectivity were generally considered to be the minimum requirement for cell migration and proliferation. Whereas increas of pore sizes would result in a reduction of mechanical properties of scaffolds, which would affect the biomechanical support requirements for the scaffolds in bone repairing. Therefore, aiming to maintain a balance between the cell behaviors and mechanical properties, the scaffolds with preferred pore size ranging from 100 μm to 1000 μm not only permited in growth of cells and new bone tissues, but also ensured the mechanical properties of scaffolds. From the point of views above, the scaffolds prepared in the presented investigation were almost ideal.

The dispersion states of Fe_3O_4 and OA@ Fe_3O_4 nanoparticles in PLLA matrix were shown in Fig. 4-11. Obviously, Fe_3O_4 nanoparticles dispersed well in PLLA matrix when the content was no more than 8% [Figs. 4-11(a) and 4-11(b)]. However, they aggregated significantly ['red zone' showed in Figures 4-11(c) and 4-11(d)] once the content reached 12% and 16%, owing to the high surface energy and anisotropic dipolar attraction of Fe_3O_4 nanoparticles. It should be noted that the OA@ Fe_3O_4 nanoparticles uniformly dispersed in matrix when the content increased from 4% to 12% [Figures 4-11(e)-4-11(g)]. And only exhibited slight agglomeration ('red zone') even though their content reached as high as 16% [Fig. 4-11(h)]. Furthermore, the dispersion states of OA@ Fe_3O_4 nanoparticles in PLLA matrix were further evidenced by the dispersion of Fe element, as shown in the EDS maps [Fig. 4-11(e1) − 4-11(h1)]. It could be seen that Fe element uniformly dispersed in PLLA matrix when the content was no more than 12% [Fig. 4-11(e1) − 4-11(g1)]. Conclusively, OA @ Fe_3O_4 nanoparticles exhibited better dispersion capability than Fe_3O_4 nanoparticles in PLLA matrix. It was attributed to a layer of oleic acid adsorbed on the surface of Fe_3O_4 nanoparticles by interaction of carboxylic acid groups and hydroxyl groups. Meanwhile, the mutually exclusive hydrocarbon chains were oriented toward the PLLA matrix, thereby facilitating the dispersion of the nanoparticles in PLLA scaffolds.

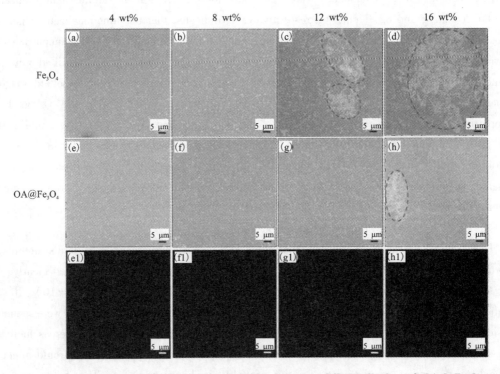

Fig. 4-11 Morphological analyses of the scaffolds containing different Fe_3O_4 and OA @ Fe_3O_4 nanoparticle contents (4%, 8%, 12% and 16%) using SEM and EDS mapping. (a-d) Surface morphology of the scaffolds containing different Fe_3O_4 nanoparticles contents. (e-h) Surface morphology of the scaffolds containing different OA@ Fe_3O_4 nanoparticles contents. (e1 − h1) EDS maps of Fe element in the scaffolds.

Mechanical properties of magnetic scaffolds including compressive strength and compressive modulus were evaluated (Fig. 4-12). It was seen that the compressive strength of 4FNPs, 8FNPs, 12FNPs and 16FNPs scaffolds were relatively higher than that of 0FNPs scaffold ($p < 0.05$), demonstrating a positive effect of the nanoparticles on the mechanical properties of scaffolds. In particular, the compressive strength of the 12FNPs scaffolds was 40.5 MPa, which was significantly higher than that of 0FNPs scaffolds with a compressive strength of 20.8 MPa (increased by 95%). And the compressive modulus of the 12FNPs scaffolds was 3.5 GPa, which increased by 68% than that of 0FNPs scaffolds (1.9 GPa). While the compressive strength and modulus of 16FNPs scaffolds were 36.5 MPa and 3.2 GPa, which decreased by 10% and 8%, respectively, compared to that of 12FNPs scaffolds. It is well known that the good dispersion of rigid nanoparticles in matrix is an important factor for improved mechanical properties. In the presented study, the mechanical properties of the scaffolds were closely related to the contents and the dispersion states of nanoparticles in scaffolds. In fact, at uniform dispersion state, more rigid $OA@Fe_3O_4$ nanoparticles could provide more effective resistance against the plastic deformation of polymer chains, thus contributing to an improved mechanical strength. However, excessive nanoparticles would lead to aggregation, which acted as impurities rather than a strengthening role, thus in turn deteriorating the mechanical properties.

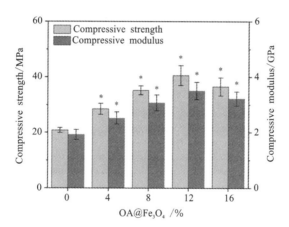

Fig. 4-12   Compressive strength and compressive modulus of scaffolds (0FNPs, 4FNPs, 8FNPs, 12FNPs and 16FNPs scaffolds, $n = 5$, $^*p < 0.05$).

The magnetic hysteresis loops, magnetization saturation and hysteresis loop areas of the scaffolds were characterized by VSM at 300 K (Fig. 4-13). Clearly, the three parameters increased significantly as the $OA@Fe_3O_4$ nanoparticles content gradually increased to 16%. Concretely, the magnetization saturation of the 0FNPs, 4FNPs, 8FNPs, 12FNPs and 16FNPs scaffolds were 0, 2.1, 4.4, 8.1 and 10.7 emu $\cdot$ g^{-1} [Fig. 4-13(a) and 4-13(b)], respectively. Besides, the hysteresis loop area, as another important parameter reflect the magnetization saturation, was calculated from the magnetic hysteresis loops, with results shown in Fig. 4-13(c). Similarly, the area values increased gradually with the increase of OA@ Fe_3O_4 nanoparticles content. In particularly, the area values reached at 16.3×10^3 erg/g with 12% OA@ Fe_3O_4 nanoparticles.

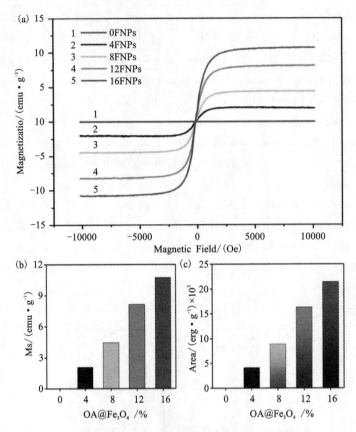

Fig. 4-13 Magnetization properties of the magnetic scaffolds (0FNPs, 4FNPs, 8FNPs, 12FNPs and 16FNPs scaffolds). (a) Magnetic hysteresis loops measured at 300 K. (b) Magnetization saturation, M_s. (c) Integrated loop area, calculated from the magnetic hysteresis loops.

The phase composition of the scaffolds was characterized by XRD, as shown in Fig. 4-13(a). It could be observed that the 0FNPs scaffolds exhibited strong characteristic peaks of PLLA. Meanwhile, diffraction peaks corresponding to Fe_3O_4 were also observed in 4FNPs, 8FNPs, 12FNPs and 16FNPs scaffolds. And the diffraction intensities were positively related to the OA@ Fe_3O_4 content. Furthermore, no additional peaks and obvious peaks shift was observed in the XRD patterns, indicating that the structures of Fe_3O_4 nanoparticles remained unchanged. The thermal behaviors of the scaffolds were assessed by thermogravimetric analysis [Fig. 4-13(b)], which provided quantitative information of Fe_3O_4 nanoparticles presenting in the scaffold samples. It could be seen that all the samples exhibited similar thermal behaviors. Obvious weight loss of the samples occurred in the range of 300 – 400 ℃, which was due to the decomposition caused by the breakage of PLLA macromolecules chains. Notably, the residues for 0FNPs, 4FNPs, 8FNPs, 12FNPs and

16FNPs scaffold samples were 0%, 3.6%, 7.7%, 11.3% and 15.4%, respectively, which were well-matched to the OA@ Fe_3O_4 nanoparticles contents initially incorporated in the PLLA matrix.

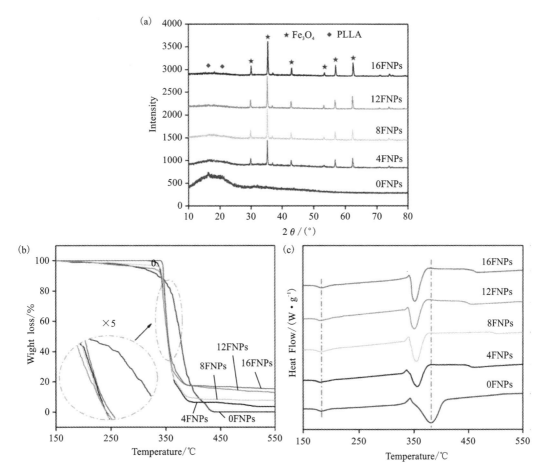

Fig. 4-14   (a) XRD patterns of the magnetic scaffolds. (b) Thermogravimetric analysis and (c) differential scanning calorimetry analysis of the magnetic scaffolds during thermal treatment.

Differential scanning calorimetry analysis curve provided information on the melting and decomposition temperature of scaffolds [Fig. 4-14 (c)]. It was seen that the OA @ Fe_3O_4 nanoparticles had no effect on the melting temperatures of PLLA (about 180 ℃). It should be noted that the decomposition temperatures of the 4FNPs, 8FNPs, 12FNPs and 16FNPs scaffolds shifted to lower temperatures as compared to 0FNPs scaffolds, similarly to the magnification in thermogravimetric analysis curves [Fig. 4-14(b)]. Tab. 4-2 summarized the quantitative results for the decomposition temperatures of scaffolds when they decomposed to 20%, 50% and 90%. It was revealed that the decomposition temperatures of the scaffolds decreased at each decomposition point as the nanoparticles content gradually increased to 12%. It was believed that the OA @ Fe_3O_4 nanoparticles in the scaffolds catalyzed the decomposition of the PLLA molecules chains. However, the decomposition temperatures increased slightly when the nanoparticles content further increased to

16%. The analysis showed that the high loading of nanoparticles tended to aggregate during heating, which reduced effective surface area and thereby reduced their catalytic effectiveness for the decomposition of PLLA molecules chains.

Tab. 4-2 **Thermal decomposition data of composite scaffolds**

Scaffolds	$T_{20\%}$	$T_{50\%}$	$T_{90\%}$
0FNPs	358.9	381.8	407.9
4FNPs	344.8	356.2	377.7
8FNPs	343.6	354.6	373.8
12FNPs	342.4	350.5	371.2
16FNPs	344.9	351.6	372.8

4.2.3.3 Investigation of Cytocompatibility of Magnetic Scaffolds

It is well accepted that the cytocompatibility of scaffolds is essential for bone regeneration. The 12FNPs scaffolds with excellent comprehensive properties were selected for further cytocompatibility studies, with 0FNPs scaffold as control. Cell viability and adhesion of MG63 cells cultured on the 12FNPs scaffold and 0FNPs scaffold were assessed using staining and morphology assay (Fig. 4-15). Obviously, the numbers of green fluorescent cell on the 12FNPs and 0FNPs scaffolds were positively related to the culture time. There was little difference in the number of cells on the 12FNPs and 0FNPs scaffolds after 1 day of culture. Significantly, more cells presented on 12FNPs scaffold than that on 0FNPs scaffold at 4th day and 7th day of the cultivation period [Fig. 4-15 (a)]. It indicated that the OA@ Fe_3O_4 nanoparticlesin scaffolds were beneficial to cell growth.

The cell adhesion is of great importance for subsequent cell expansion, proliferation, and differentiation. Thus, the adhesion morphologies of MG63 cells cultured for 4 days and 7 days on the 12FNPs and 0FNPs scaffolds were characterized by SEM [Fig. 4-15(b)]. It was seen that the cells cultured on 12FNPs and 0FNPs scaffolds both spread with the increase of culture time. Concretely, cells were attached to the surface of 12FNPs and 0FNPs scaffolds and presented similar elongated morphology after 1 day of culture. The cells cultured on 12FNPs scaffolds for 4 days presented some filopodia which facilitated cell adhesion to the scaffolds, whereas the cells on 0FNPs scaffolds displayed fusiform shape. After culture of 7 days, cells on the 12FNPs scaffolds extensively spread. And more cells covered most part of the surface. As control, cells on the 0FNPs scaffolds displayed some filopodia. It indicated that the OA@ Fe_3O_4 nanoparticles in scaffolds were beneficial to improve cell viability and adhesion. The effectiveness of magnetic nanoparticles in improving cell adhesion has also been confirmed by other studies. Guo et al. applied colloidal assembly of magnetic nanoparticles on agarose hydrogel to form magnetichydrogel substrate, and they found that the magnetichydrogel substrate could promote cells adhesion and growth. Hu et al fabricated magnetic polyacrylamide hydrogel by incorporating magnetic nanoparticles assemblies into hydrogel matrix, and proved that the nanoparticles effectively improved cell-adhesive properties.

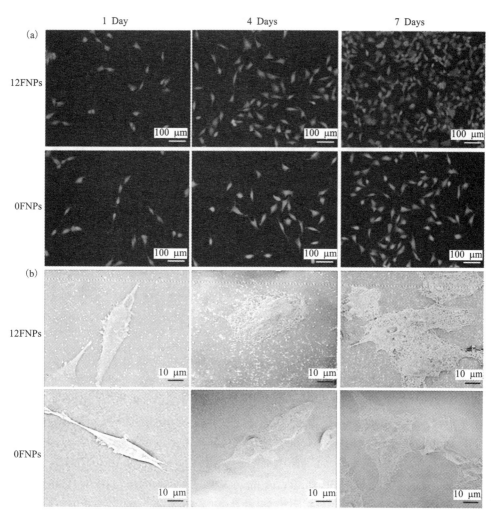

Fig. 4-15　(a) Confocal fluorescence micrographs and (b) morphologies analysis of MG63 cells cultured on the 12FNPs and 0FNPs scaffolds for 4 days and 7 days.

The proliferation levels of MG63 cells cultured on 12FNPs and 0FNPs scaffolds were measured by CCK-8 assays [Fig. 4-16(a)]. With culture time increasing from 1 day to 7 days, the cell proliferation level on 12FNPs and 0FNPs scaffolds gradually increased. And the proliferation level of the 12FNPs scaffolds was significantly higher than that of the 0FNPs scaffolds at each evaluation time point ($p < 0.01$), indicating that the 12FNPs scaffolds as guiding and stimulating matrix were more conducive to cell proliferation. The differentiation levels of MG63 cells cultured on 12FNPs and 0FNPs scaffolds were studied by ALP activity tests (Fig. 4-16(b)). The cell differentiation levels on 12FNPs and 0FNPs scaffolds increased with the culture time (7 days and 14 days). Furthermore, the ALP activity of the 12FNPs scaffolds was significantly higher than that of the 0FNPs scaffolds on 7th day and 14th day ($p < 0.01$), suggesting that the 12FNPs scaffolds exhibited better cell differentiation ability than 0FNPs scaffolds.

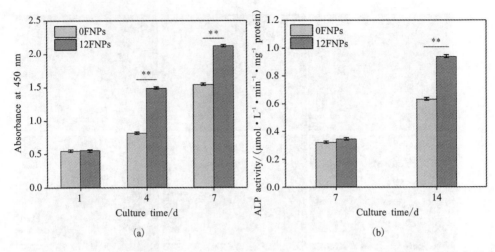

Fig. 4-16 (a) Proliferation capabilities of MG63 cells cultured on the 12FNPs and 0FNPs scaffolds for 1 day, 4 days and 7 days ($n = 3$, $**p < 0.01$). (b) Differentiation capabilities of MG63 cells cultured on the 12FNPs and 0FNPs scaffolds for 7 days and 14 days ($n = 3$, $**p < 0.01$).

The viability, adhesion, proliferation and differentiation of the MG63 cells on the 12FNPs scaffolds were significantly better than those on the 0FNPs scaffolds, indicating that $OA@Fe_3O_4$ nanoparticles in the 12FNPs scaffolds stimulated these capabilities of cells. The mechanisms of stimulation were shown in Fig. 4-17. Each $OA@Fe_3O_4$ nanoparticle could be considered as a single magnetic domain that produced a nanoscale magnetic field. Therefore, numerous nanoscale magnetic fields were contained within the scaffolds. On one hand, the magnetic fields could create micro magnetic driving force inducing cells close proximity to the nanoparticles in the scaffolds, which was conducive to cell adhesion. On the other hand, the magnetic fields could induce membrane

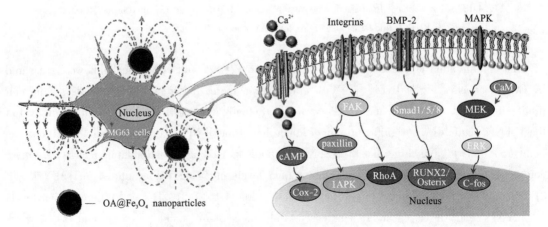

Fig. 4-17 Stimulation mechanisms of $OA@Fe_3O_4$ nanoparticles to the adhesion, proliferation and differentiation of MG63 cells on scaffolds.

phospholipids rearrangement and trigger physical sensing system of cells, such as activated the calcium ion (Ca^{2+}) channels on cell membrane and stimulated various signaling pathways including integrin, BMP-2 and mitogen-activated protein kinase (MAPK) pathways, which were essential for osteoblastic differentiation. Therefore, the creation of micro magnetic driving force, activation of Ca^{2+} channels and stimulation of various signaling pathways induced by OA@Fe_3O_4 nanoparticles were considered extremely important in the magnetic scaffold-induced cell adhesion, proliferation and differentiation. Besides, the OA@Fe_3O_4 nanoparticles in scaffolds could increase the roughness and surface area, which also promoted the initial cell adhesion and spreading.

4.2.4　Conclusions

Oleic acid was selected in present study to functionalize the Fe_3O_4 nanoparticles in order to improve their dispersion in PLLA scaffolds. With a biocompatible oleic acid surface layer, the OA@Fe_3O_4 nanoparticles exhibited better dispersion capability in scaffolds than non-functionalized Fe_3O_4 nanoparticles. The magnetic scaffolds with uniformly dispersed OA@Fe_3O_4 nanoparticles (12%) presented compressive strength and modulus increasing, which was 40.5 MPa and 3.5 GPa, respectively. Furthermore, the magnetic scaffolds effectively enhanced cell viability, adhesion, proliferation and differentiation. In conclusion, the magnetic scaffolds with uniformly dispersed OA@Fe_3O_4 nanoparticles possessed good mechanical and biological properties, which was conductive toits application in bone regeneration.

References ━━━━━━━━━━━━━━━━━━━━━━━━━━━━━━━━━━━━

［1］ Feyerabend F, Fischer J, Holtz J, et al. Evaluation of short-term effects of rare earth and other elements used in magnesium alloys on primary cells and cell lines［J］. Acta biomaterialia, 2010, 6(5): 1834-1842.

［2］ Tian P, Liu X. Surface modification of biodegradable magnesium and its alloys for biomedical applications ［J］. Regenerative biomaterials, 2015, 2(2): 135-151.

［3］ Erinc M, Sillekens W H, Mannens R, et al. Applicability of existing magnesium alloys as biomedical implant materials［J］. 2009.

［4］ Tan L, Yu X, Wan P, et al. Biodegradable materials for bone repairs: a review［J］. Journal of Materials Science & Technology, 2013, 29(6): 503-513.

［5］ Levy G, Aghion E. Effect of diffusion coating of Nd on the corrosion resistance of biodegradable Mg implants in simulated physiological electrolyte［J］. Acta biomaterialia, 2013, 9(10): 8624-8630.

［6］ Liang X, Qi Y, Pan Z, et al. Design and preparation of quasi-spherical salt particles as water-soluble porogens to fabricate hydrophobic porous scaffolds for tissue engineering and tissue regeneration［J］. Materials Chemistry Frontiers, 2018, 2(8): 1539-1553.

［7］ El-Rahman S S A. Neuropathology of aluminum toxicity in rats (glutamate and GABA impairment)［J］. Pharmacological Research, 2003, 47(3): 189-194.

［8］ Nakamura Y, Tsumura Y, Tonogai Y, et al. Differences in the Toxicological Behavior among the Chlorides of Seven Rare Earth Elements Administered Intravenously to Rats (PROCEEDINGS OF 24TH SYMPOSIUM ON TOXICOLOGY AND ENVIRONMENTAL HEALTH)［J］. Journal of Health Science, 1999, 45(1): P15-15.

［9］ Xu Q, Hashimoto M, Dang T T, et al. Preparation of monodisperse biodegradable polymer microparticles using a microfluidic flow-focusing device for controlled drug delivery［J］. Small, 2009, 5(13): 1575-1581.

［10］ Zare E N, Lakouraj M M, Mohseni M. Biodegradable polypyrrole/dextrin conductive nanocomposite: synthesis, characterization, antioxidant and antibacterial activity［J］. Synthetic Metals, 2014, 187: 9-16.

［11］ Chaya A, Yoshizawa S, Verdelis K, et al. In vivo study of magnesium plate and screw degradation and bone fracture healing［J］. Acta biomaterialia, 2015, 18: 262-269.

［12］ Gao C, Feng P, Peng S, et al. Carbon nanotube, graphene and boron nitride nanotube reinforced bioactive ceramics for bone repair［J］. Acta biomaterialia, 2017, 61: 1-20.

［13］ Yin G Z, Yang X M, Zhou Z, et al. A green pathway to adjust the mechanical properties and degradation rate of PCL by blending bio-sourced poly (glycerol-succinate) oligoesters［J］. Materials Chemistry Frontiers, 2018, 2(3): 544-553.

[14] Oriňák A, Oriňáková R, Králová Z O, et al. Sintered metallic foams for biodegradable bone replacement materials[J]. Journal of Porous Materials, 2014, 21(2): 131-140.

[15] Serre C M, Papillard M, Chavassieux P, et al. Influence of magnesium substitution on a collagen-apatite biomaterial on the production of a calcifying matrix by human osteoblasts[J]. Journal of Biomedical Materials Research: An Official Journal of The Society for Biomaterials, The Japanese Society for Biomaterials, and the Australian Society for Biomaterials, 1998, 42(4): 626-633.

[16] Saris N E L, Mervaala E, Karppanen H, et al. Magnesium: an update on physiological, clinical and analytical aspects[J]. Clinica chimica acta, 2000, 294(1-2): 1-26.

[17] Seal C K, Vince K, Hodgson M A. Biodegradable surgical implants based on magnesium alloys-A review of current research[C]//IOP conference series: materials science and engineering. IOP Publishing, 2009, 4(1): 012011.

[18] Zheng Y F, Gu X N, Witte F. Biodegradable metals[J]. Materials Science and Engineering: R: Reports, 2014, 77: 1-34.

[19] Zhang E, Chen H, Shen F. Biocorrosion properties and blood and cell compatibility of pure iron as a biodegradable biomaterial [J]. Journal of Materials Science: Materials in Medicine, 2010, 21 (7): 2151-2163.

[20] Liu X, Sun J, Zhou F, et al. Micro-alloying with Mn in Zn-Mg alloy for future biodegradable metals application[J]. Materials & Design, 2016, 94: 95-104.

[21] Tie D, Guan R, Liu H, et al. An in vivo study on the metabolism and osteogenic activity of bioabsorbable Mg-1Sr alloy[J]. Acta biomaterialia, 2016, 29: 455-467.

[22] Witte F, Kaese V, Haferkamp H, et al. In vivo corrosion of four magnesium alloys and the associated bone response[J]. Biomaterials, 2005, 26(17): 3557-3563.

[23] Li Z, Gu X, Lou S, et al. The development of binary Mg-Ca alloys for use as biodegradable materials within bone[J]. Biomaterials, 2008, 29(10): 1329-1344.

[24] Gu X N, Zheng W, Cheng Y, et al. A study on alkaline heat treated Mg-Ca alloy for the control of the biocorrosion rate[J]. Acta Biomaterialia, 2009, 5(7): 2790-2799.

[25] Rink L, Rink L. Zinc in human health. [J]. Zinc in Human Health, 2011, 11(2-3):63-87.

[26] Zomorodian A, Garcia M P, e Silva T M, et al. Corrosion resistance of a composite polymeric coating applied on biodegradable AZ31 magnesium alloy[J]. Acta biomaterialia, 2013, 9(10): 8660-8670.

[27] Yang L, Zhang E. Biocorrosion behavior of magnesium alloy in different simulated fluids for biomedical application[J]. Materials science and engineering: C, 2009, 29(5): 1691-1696.

[28] M. A. Ze-Qun, F. U. Guang-Yan, et al. The Effect of Ball Milling Time on Corrosion Resistance of Mechanical Alloying Mg-2Mn Alloy [J]. Journal of Shengyang University of Chemical Technology, 2017,02: 167-170.

[29] Liu C, Fu X, Pan H, et al. Biodegradable Mg-Cu alloys with enhanced osteogenesis, angiogenesis, and long-lasting antibacterial effects[J]. Scientific reports, 2016, 6: 27374.

[30] Tie D, Feyerabend F, Mueller W D, et al. Antibacterial biodegradable Mg-Ag alloys[J]. European cells & materials, 2013, 25: 284-98; discussion 298.

[31] Zhang E, Yang L, Xu J, et al. Microstructure, mechanical properties and bio-corrosion properties of Mg-Si (-Ca, Zn) alloy for biomedical application[J]. Acta biomaterialia, 2010, 6(5): 1756-1762.

[32] Seyedraoufi Z S, Mirdamadi S. Synthesis, microstructure and mechanical properties of porous Mg⊹Zn scaffolds[J]. J Mech Behav Biomed Mater, 2013, 21(3):1-8.

［33］ Zhang S, Zhang X, Zhao C, et al. Research on an Mg-Zn alloy as a degradable biomaterial［J］. Acta biomaterialia, 2010, 6(2): 626-640.

［34］ Cheng J, Zheng Y F. In vitro study on newly designed biodegradable Fe-X composites (X = W, CNT) prepared by spark plasma sintering［J］. Journal of Biomedical Materials Research Part B: Applied Biomaterials, 2013, 101(4): 485-497.

［35］ Liu B, Zheng Y F. Effects of alloying elements (Mn, Co, Al, W, Sn, B, C and S) on biodegradability and in vitro biocompatibility of pure iron［J］. Acta biomaterialia, 2011, 7(3): 1407-1420.

［36］ Čapek J, Stehlíková K, Michalcová A, et al. Microstructure, mechanical and corrosion properties of biodegradable powder metallurgical Fe-2 wt% X (X = Pd, Ag and C) alloys［J］. Materials Chemistry and Physics, 2016, 181: 501-511.

［37］ Hänzi A C, Gunde P, Schinhammer M, et al. On the biodegradation performance of an Mg-Y-RE alloy with various surface conditions in simulated body fluid［J］. Acta biomaterialia, 2009, 5(1): 162-171.

［38］ Schinhammer M, Hänzi A C, Läffler J F, et al. Design strategy for biodegradable Fe-based alloys for medical applications［J］. Acta biomaterialia, 2010, 6(5): 1705-1713.

［39］ Liu B, Zheng Y F, Ruan L. In vitro investigation of Fe30Mn6Si shape memory alloy as potential biodegradable metallic material［J］. Materials Letters, 2011, 65(3): 540-543.

［40］ Li H F, Xie X H, Zheng Y F, et al. Development of biodegradable Zn-1X binary alloys with nutrient alloying elements Mg, Ca and Sr［J］. Scientific reports, 2015, 5: 10719.

［41］ Niu J, Tang Z, Huang H, et al. Research on a Zn-Cu alloy as a biodegradable material for potential vascular stents application［J］. Materials Science and Engineering: C, 2016, 69: 407-413.

［42］ Yue R, Huang H, Ke G, et al. Microstructure, mechanical properties and in vitro degradation behavior of novel Zn-Cu-Fe alloys［J］. Materials Characterization, 2017, 134: 114-122.

［43］ Liu Y, Wang L, Cao L, et al. Understanding and suppressing side reactions in Li-air batteries［J］. Materials Chemistry Frontiers, 2017, 1(12): 2495-2510.

［44］ Berglund I S, Brar H S, Dolgova N, et al. Synthesis and characterization of Mg-Ca-Sr alloys for biodegradable orthopedic implant applications［J］. Journal of Biomedical Materials Research Part B: Applied Biomaterials, 2012, 100(6): 1524-1534.

［45］ Shen C, Liu X, Fan B, et al. Mechanical properties, in vitro degradation behavior, hemocompatibility and cytotoxicity evaluation of Zn-1.2 Mg alloy for biodegradable implants［J］. RSC Advances, 2016, 6(89): 86410-86419.

［46］ Bowen P K, Drelich J, Goldman J. Zinc exhibits ideal physiological corrosion behavior for bioabsorbable stents ［J］. Advanced materials, 2013, 25(18): 2577-2582.

［47］ Strukturne M I N C, Lastnosti N E. Structural, mechanical and cytotoxicity characterization of as-cast biodegradable Zn-xMg (x = 0.8-8.3%) alloys［J］. Materiali in tehnologije, 2014, 48(5): 623-629.

［48］ Wang X, Xu S, Zhou S, et al. Topological design and additive manufacturing of porous metals for bone scaffolds and orthopaedic implants: A review［J］. Biomaterials, 2016, 83: 127-141.

［49］ Zhen Z, Xi T, Zheng Y. A review on in vitro corrosion performance test of biodegradable metallic materials ［J］. Transactions of Nonferrous Metals Society of China, 2013, 23(8): 2283-2293.

［50］ Pogorielov M, Husak E, Solodivnik A, et al. Magnesium-based biodegradable alloys: Degradation, application, and alloying elements［J］. Interventional Medicine and Applied Science, 2017, 9(1): 27-38.

［51］ Xu W, YANG K. Study on properties of a novel biodegradable Fe-30Mn-1C alloy［J］. Acta Metall Sin, 2011, 47(10): 1342-1347.

[52] Zheng Y, WU Y. Revolutionizing metallic biomaterials[J]. Acta Metall Sin, 2017, 53(3): 257-297.

[53] Agarwal S, Curtin J, Duffy B, et al. Biodegradable magnesium alloys for orthopaedic applications: A review on corrosion, biocompatibility and surface modifications[J]. Materials Science and Engineering: C, 2016, 68: 948-963.

[54] Bajger P, Ashbourn J M A, Manhas V, et al. Mathematical modelling of the degradation behaviour of biodegradable metals[J]. Biomechanics and modeling in mechanobiology, 2017, 16(1): 227-238.

[55] Zheng Y, Li Y, Chen J, et al. Surface characteristics and corrosion resistance of biodegradable magnesium alloy ZK60 modified by Fe ion implantation and deposition[J]. Progress in Natural Science: Materials International, 2014, 24(5): 547-553.

[56] Hong D, Chou D T, Velikokhatnyi O I, et al. Binder-jetting 3D printing and alloy development of new biodegradable Fe-Mn-Ca/Mg alloys[J]. Acta biomaterialia, 2016, 45: 375-386.

[57] Gu X N, Xie X H, Li N, et al. In vitro and in vivo studies on a Mg-Sr binary alloy system developed as a new kind of biodegradable metal[J]. Acta biomaterialia, 2012, 8(6): 2360-2374.

[58] Hong D, Saha P, Chou D T, et al. In vitro degradation and cytotoxicity response of Mg-4% Zn-0.5% Zr (ZK40) alloy as a potential biodegradable material[J]. Acta biomaterialia, 2013, 9(10): 8534-8547.

[59] Mueller W D, Fernandez Lorenzo de Mele M, Nascimento M L, et al. Degradation of magnesium and its alloys: Dependence on the composition of the synthetic biological media[J]. Journal of Biomedical Materials Research Part A: An Official Journal of The Society for Biomaterials, The Japanese Society for Biomaterials, and The Australian Society for Biomaterials and the Korean Society for Biomaterials, 2009, 90(2): 487-495.

[60] Chen Y, Xu Z, Smith C, et al. Recent advances on the development of magnesium alloys for biodegradable implants[J]. Acta biomaterialia, 2014, 10(11): 4561-4573.

[61] Chou D T, Hong D, Saha P, et al. In vitro and in vivo corrosion, cytocompatibility and mechanical properties of biodegradable Mg-Y-Ca-Zr alloys as implant materials[J]. Acta biomaterialia, 2013, 9(10): 8518-8533.

[62] Mouzou E, Paternoster C, Tolouei R, et al. CO-rich atmosphere strongly affects the degradation of Fe-21Mn-1C for biodegradable metallic implants[J]. Materials Letters, 2016, 181: 362-366.

[63] Hofstetter J, Martinelli E, Pogatscher S, et al. Influence of trace impurities on the in vitro and in vivo degradation of biodegradable Mg-5Zn-0.3 Ca alloys[J]. Acta biomaterialia, 2015, 23: 347-353.

[64] Zhang J, Xu C, Jing Y, et al. New horizon for high performance Mg-based biomaterial with uniform degradation behavior: Formation of stacking faults[J]. Scientific reports, 2015, 5: 13933.

[65] Witte F, Fischer J, Nellesen J, et al. In vivo corrosion and corrosion protection of magnesium alloy LAE442 [J]. Acta biomaterialia, 2010, 6(5): 1792-1799.

[66] Niinomi M, Nakai M, Hieda J. Development of new metallic alloys for biomedical applications[J]. Acta biomaterialia, 2012, 8(11): 3888-3903.

[67] Jamesh M, Wu G, Zhao Y, et al. Effects of silicon plasma ion implantation on electrochemical corrosion behavior of biodegradable Mg-Y-RE alloy[J]. Corrosion Science, 2013, 69: 158-163.

[68] Yeung K W K, Wong K H M. Biodegradable metallic materials for orthopaedic implantations: A review[J]. Technology and Health Care, 2012, 20(5): 345-362.

[69] Cho S Y, Chae S W, Choi K W, et al. Biocompatibility and strength retention of biodegradable Mg-Ca-Zn alloy bone implants[J]. Journal of Biomedical Materials Research Part B: Applied Biomaterials, 2013, 101 (2): 201-212.

[70] Čapek J, Kubásek J, Vojtěch D, et al. Microstructural, mechanical, corrosion and cytotoxicity characterization of the hot forged FeMn30 (wt.%) alloy[J]. Materials Science and Engineering: C, 2016,

58: 900-908.

[71] Song G, Song S. A possible biodegradable magnesium implant material[J]. Advanced Engineering Materials, 2007, 9(4): 298-302.

[72] Csaderova L, Martines E, Seunarine K, et al. A Biodegradable and Biocompatible Regular Nanopattern for Large-Scale Selective Cell Growth[J]. Small, 2010, 6(23): 2755-2761.

[73] Hänzi A C, Gerber I, Schinhammer M, et al. On the in vitro and in vivo degradation performance and biological response of new biodegradable Mg-Y-Zn alloys[J]. Acta Biomaterialia, 2010, 6(5): 1824-1833.

[74] Liu X, Sun J, Qiu K, et al. Effects of alloying elements (Ca and Sr) on microstructure, mechanical property and invitro corrosion behavior of biodegradable Zn-1.5Mg alloy[J]. Journal of Alloys & Compounds, 2016, 664:444-452.

[75] Zhao L, Zhang Z, Song Y, et al. Mechanical properties and in vitro biodegradation of newly developed porous Zn scaffolds for biomedical applications[J]. Materials & Design, 2016, 108: 136-144.

[76] Nagels J, Stokdijk M, Rozing P M. Stress shielding and bone resorption in shoulder arthroplasty[J]. Journal of shoulder and elbow surgery, 2003, 12(1): 35-39.

[77] Hung F Y, Lui T S, Chen L H, et al. Vibration behavior of light metals: Al-Zn alloy and Mg-Al-Zn alloy [J]. Journal of materials science, 2007, 42(13): 5020-5028.

[78] Brar H S, Platt M O, Sarntinoranont M, et al. Magnesium as a biodegradable and bioabsorbable material for medical implants[J]. Jom, 2009, 61(9): 31-34.

[79] Jiang J, Zhang F, Ma A, et al. Biodegradable behaviors of ultrafine-grained ze41a magnesium alloy in dmem solution[J]. Metals, 2016, 6(1): 3.

[80] Torroni A, Xiang C, Witek L, et al. Biocompatibility and degradation properties of WE43 Mg alloys with and without heat treatment: In vivo evaluation and comparison in a cranial bone sheep model [J]. Journal of Cranio-Maxillofacial Surgery, 2017, 45(12): 2075-2083.

[81] Torroni A, Xiang C, Witek L, et al. Histo-morphologic characteristics of intra-osseous implants of WE43 Mg alloys with and without heat treatment in an in vivo cranial bone sheep model [J]. Journal of Cranio-Maxillofacial Surgery, 2018, 46(3): 473-478.

[82] Duygulu O, Kaya R A, Oktay G, et al. Investigation on the potential of magnesium alloy AZ31 as a bone implant[C]//Materials Science Forum. Trans Tech Publications, 2007, 546: 421-424.

[83] Tan L, Wang Q, Lin X, et al. Loss of mechanical properties in vivo and bone-implant interface strength of AZ31B magnesium alloy screws with Si-containing coating [J]. Acta biomaterialia, 2014, 10 (5): 2333-2340.

[84] Ulum M F, Nasution A K, Yusop A H, et al. Evidences of in vivo bioactivity of Fe-bioceramic composites for temporary bone implants[J]. Journal of Biomedical Materials Research Part B: Applied Biomaterials, 2015, 103(7): 1354-1365.

[85] Sӑndulache F, Stanciu S, Cimpoşu N, et al. Preliminary Results on the Surface of a New Fe-Based Metallic Material after "In Vivo" Maintaining[C]//IOP Conference Series: Materials Science and Engineering. IOP Publishing, 2017, 209(1): 012049.

[86] Xiao C, Wang L, Ren Y, et al. Indirectly extruded biodegradable Zn-0.05 wt% Mg alloy with improved strength and ductility: In vitro and in vivo studies[J]. Journal of materials science & technology, 2018, 34 (9): 1618-1627.

[87] Vojtěch D, Kubásek J, Šerák J, et al. Mechanical and corrosion properties of newly developed biodegradable Zn-based alloys for bone fixation[J]. Acta Biomaterialia, 2011, 7(9): 3515-3522.

［88］ Li X, Chu C, Chu P K. Effects of external stress on biodegradable orthopedic materials: a review［J］. Bioactive materials, 2016, 1(1): 77-84.

［89］ Kirkland N T, Birbilis N, Staiger M P. Assessing the corrosion of biodegradable magnesium implants: a critical review of current methodologies and their limitations［J］. Acta biomaterialia, 2012, 8(3): 925-936.

［90］ Gu X N, Zheng Y F. A review on magnesium alloys as biodegradable materials［J］. Frontiers of Materials Science in China, 2010, 4(2): 111-115.

［91］ Yu L, Wenjiang D. Current State and Protection Technique of Magnesium Alloys［J］. Materials Review, 2005, 11.

［92］ Qizhou W X Q G C, Bokang W. The Effect of Rare Earth on Corrosion of AZ91 Magnesium Alloy in NaCl Solution［J］. Development and Application of Materials, 2002, 5.

［93］ Tekumalla S, Seetharaman S, Almajid A, et al. Mechanical properties of magnesium-rare earth alloy systems: A review［J］. Metals, 2015, 5(1): 1-39.

［94］ Liu C, Xin Y, Tang G, et al. Influence of heat treatment on degradation behavior of bio-degradable die-cast AZ63 magnesium alloy in simulated body fluid［J］. Materials Science and Engineering: A, 2007, 456(1-2): 350-357.

［95］ Kuwahara H, Mazaki N, Mabuchi M, et al. Behavior of magnesium in Hank's solution aimed to trabecular pattern of natural bone［C］//Materials Science Forum. Trans Tech Publications, 2003, 419(Ⅱ): 1007-1012.

［96］ Zhang X P, Zhao Z P, Wu F M, et al. Corrosion and wear resistance of AZ91D magnesium alloy with and without microarc oxidation coating in Hanks solution［J］. Journal of Materials Science, 2007, 42(20): 8523-8528.

［97］ Wang H X, Guan S K, Wang X, et al. In vitro degradation and mechanical integrity of Mg-Zn-Ca alloy coated with Ca-deficient hydroxyapatite by the pulse electrodeposition process［J］. Acta Biomaterialia, 2010, 6(5): 1743-1748.

［98］ Hiromoto S, Inoue M, Taguchi T, et al. In vitro and in vivo biocompatibility and corrosion behaviour of a bioabsorbable magnesium alloy coated with octacalcium phosphate and hydroxyapatite［J］. Acta biomaterialia, 2015, 11: 520-530.

［99］ Xu L, Pan F, Yu G, et al. In vitro and in vivo evaluation of the surface bioactivity of a calcium phosphate coated magnesium alloy［J］. Biomaterials, 2009, 30(8): 1512-1523.

［100］ Yan T, Tan L, Zhang B, et al. Fluoride conversion coating on biodegradable AZ31B magnesium alloy［J］. Journal of Materials Science & Technology, 2014, 30(7): 666-674.

［101］ Pereda M D, Alonso C, Burgos-Asperilla L, et al. Corrosion inhibition of powder metallurgy Mg by fluoride treatments［J］. Acta Biomaterialia, 2010, 6(5): 1772-1782.

［102］ Wang H, Estrin Y, Zúberová Z. Bio-corrosion of a magnesium alloy with different processing histories［J］. Materials letters, 2008, 62(16): 2476-2479.

［103］ Song Y, Zhang S, Li J, et al. Electrodeposition of Ca-P coatings on biodegradable Mg alloy: in vitro biomineralization behavior［J］. Acta Biomaterialia, 2010, 6(5): 1736-1742.

［104］ Obayi C S, Tolouei R, Paternoster C, et al. Influence of cross-rolling on the micro-texture and biodegradation of pure iron as biodegradable material for medical implants［J］. Acta biomaterialia, 2015, 17: 68-77.

［105］ WANG W, LU S, QI M. Powder-metallurgical preparation and biodegradation property of Fe-Zn alloy［J］. Journal of Functional Materials, 2013 (4): 2.

［106］ Huang T, Cheng J, Bian D, et al. Fe-Au and Fe-Ag composites as candidates for biodegradable stent materials［J］. Journal of Biomedical Materials Research Part B: Applied Biomaterials, 2016, 104 (2):

225-240.

[107] Moravej M, Prima F, Fiset M, et al. Electroformed iron as new biomaterial for degradable stents: Development process and structure-properties relationship[J]. Acta biomaterialia, 2010, 6(5): 1726-1735.

[108] Moravej M, Purnama A, Fiset M, et al. Electroformed pure iron as a new biomaterial for degradable stents: In vitro degradation and preliminary cell viability studies[J]. Acta Biomaterialia, 2010, 6(5): 1843-1851.

[109] Lin G, Hu R, Law W C, et al. Biodegradable Nanocapsules as siRNA Carriers for Mutant K-Ras Gene Silencing of Human Pancreatic Carcinoma Cells[J]. Small, 2013, 9(16): 2757-2763.

[110] Gong H, Wang K, Strich R, et al. In vitro biodegradation behavior, mechanical properties, and cytotoxicity of biodegradable Zn-Mg alloy[J]. Journal of Biomedical Materials Research Part B: Applied Biomaterials, 2015, 103(8): 1632-1640.

[111] Witte F, Fischer J, Nellesen J, et al. In vitro and in vivo corrosion measurements of magnesium alloys[J]. Biomaterials, 2006, 27(7): 1013-1018.

[112] Liu X, Yue Z, Romeo T, et al. Biofunctionalized anti-corrosive silane coatings for magnesium alloys[J]. Acta biomaterialia, 2013, 9(10): 8671-8677.

[113] Staiger M P, Pietak A M, Huadmai J, et al. Magnesium and its alloys as orthopedic biomaterials: a review [J]. Biomaterials, 2006, 27(9): 1728-1734.

[114] Gui Z, Kang Z, Li Y. Mechanical and corrosion properties of Mg-Gd-Zn-Zr-Mn biodegradable alloy by hot extrusion[J]. Journal of Alloys and Compounds, 2016, 685: 222-230.

[115] Yang J, Koons G L, Cheng G, et al. A review on the exploitation of biodegradable magnesium-based composites for medical applications[J]. Biomedical Materials, 2018, 13(2): 022001.

[116] Liu L, Chen X, Pan F, et al. Effect of Y and Ce additions on microstructure and mechanical properties of Mg-Zn-Zr alloys[J]. Materials Science and Engineering: A, 2015, 644: 247-253.

[117] Brar H S, Wong J, Manuel M V. Investigation of the mechanical and degradation properties of Mg-Sr and Mg-Zn-Sr alloys for use as potential biodegradable implant materials[J]. Journal of the mechanical behavior of biomedical materials, 2012, 7: 87-95.

[118] Li Y, Zhang K, LI X, et al. Influence of extrusion on microstructures and mechanical properties of Mg-5.0 Y-7.0 Gd-1.3 Nd-0.5 Zr magnesium alloy [J]. The Chinese Journal of Nonferrous Metals, 2010, 9: 1692-1697.

[119] Drynda A, Hassel T, Bach F W, et al. In vitro and in vivo corrosion properties of new iron-manganese alloys designed for cardiovascular applications [J]. Journal of Biomedical Materials Research Part B: Applied Biomaterials, 2015, 103(3): 649-660.

[120] Hermawan H, Purnama A, Dube D, et al. Fe-Mn alloys for metallic biodegradable stents: degradation and cell viability studies[J]. Acta biomaterialia, 2010, 6(5): 1852-1860.

[121] Hermawan H, Dubé D, Mantovani D. Degradable metallic biomaterials: design and development of Fe-Mn alloys for stents[J]. Journal of Biomedical Materials Research Part A: An Official Journal of The Society for Biomaterials, The Japanese Society for Biomaterials, and The Australian Society for Biomaterials and the Korean Society for Biomaterials, 2010, 93(1): 1-11.

[122] Hermawan H, Dubé D, Mantovani D. Development of degradable Fe-35Mn alloy for biomedical application [C]//Advanced Materials Research. Trans Tech Publications, 2007, 15: 107-112.

[123] Li H, Zheng Y, Qin L. Progress of biodegradable metals [J]. Progress in Natural Science: Materials International, 2014, 24(5): 414-422.

[124] Demir A G, Monguzzi L, Previtali B. Selective laser melting of pure Zn with high density for biodegradable

implant manufacturing[J]. Additive Manufacturing, 2017, 15: 20-28.

[125] Liu Z, Wang F, Qiu D, et al. The effect of solute elements on the grain refinement of cast Zn[J]. Metallurgical and Materials Transactions A, 2013, 44(9): 4025-4030.

[126] Liu Z, Qiu D, Wang F, et al. The grain refining mechanism of cast zinc through silver inoculation[J]. Acta Materialia, 2014, 79: 315-326.

[127] Sikora-Jasinska M, Mostaed E, Mostaed A, et al. Fabrication, mechanical properties and in vitro degradation behavior of newly developed ZnAg alloys for degradable implant applications[J]. Materials Science and Engineering: C, 2017, 77: 1170-1181.

[128] Wang L, Ji B, Hu Y, et al. A review on in situ phytoremediation of mine tailings[J]. Chemosphere, 2017, 184: 594-600.

[129] Cheng J, Liu B, Wu Y H, et al. Comparative in vitro study on pure metals (Fe, Mn, Mg, Zn and W) as biodegradable metals[J]. Journal of Materials Science & Technology, 2013, 29(7): 619-627.

[130] Li H, Peng Q, Li X, et al. Microstructures, mechanical and cytocompatility of degradable Mg-Zn based orthopedic biomaterials[J]. Materials & Design, 2014, 58: 43-51.

[131] Windhagen H, Radtke K, Weizbauer A, et al. Biodegradable magnesium-based screw clinically equivalent to titanium screw in hallux valgus surgery: short term results of the first prospective, randomized, controlled clinical pilot study[J]. Biomedical engineering online, 2013, 12(1): 62.

[132] Hänzi A C, Dalla Torre F H, Sologubenko A S, et al. Design strategy for microalloyed ultra-ductile magnesium alloys[J]. Philosophical Magazine Letters, 2009, 89(6): 377-390.

[133] Zheng Y, Liu B, GU X. Research Progress in Biodegradable Metallic Materials for Medical Application[J]. Materials Review, 2009, 1.

[134] Vojtech D, Kubasek J, Capek J, et al. Comparative mechanical and corrosion studies on magnesium, zinc and iron alloys as biodegradable metals[J]. Mater. Technol, 2015, 49: 877-882.

[135] Wegener B, Sievers B, Utzschneider S, et al. Microstructure, cytotoxicity and corrosion of powder-metallurgical iron alloys for biodegradable bone replacement materials[J]. Materials Science and Engineering: B, 2011, 176(20): 1789-1796.

[136] Li H, Yang H, Zheng Y, et al. Design and characterizations of novel biodegradable ternary Zn-based alloys with IIA nutrient alloying elements Mg, Ca and Sr[J]. Materials & Design, 2015, 83: 95-102

[137] Bobe K, Willbold E, Morgenthal I, et al. In vitro and in vivo evaluation of biodegradable, open-porous scaffolds made of sintered magnesium W4 short fibres[J]. Acta Biomaterialia, 2013, 9(10): 8611-8623.

[138] Loher S, Schneider O D, Maienfisch T, et al. Micro-organism-triggered release of silver nanoparticles from biodegradable oxide carriers allows preparation of self-sterilizing polymer surfaces[J]. Small, 2008, 4(6): 824-832.

[139] You J, Shao R, Wei X, et al. Near-infrared light triggers release of paclitaxel from biodegradable microspheres: photothermal effect and enhanced antitumor activity[J]. Small, 2010, 6(9): 1022-1031.

[140] Dziuba D, Meyer-Lindenberg A, Seitz J M, et al. Long-term in vivo degradation behaviour and biocompatibility of the magnesium alloy ZEK100 for use as a biodegradable bone implant[J]. Acta biomaterialia, 2013, 9(10): 8548-8560.

[141] Drynda A, Deinet N, Braun N, et al. Rare earth metals used in biodegradable magnesium-based stents do not interfere with proliferation of smooth muscle cells but do induce the upregulation of inflammatory genes[J]. Journal of Biomedical Materials Research Part A: An Official Journal of The Society for Biomaterials, The Japanese Society for Biomaterials, and The Australian Society for Biomaterials and the Korean Society for

Biomaterials, 2009, 91(2): 360-369.

[142] Gu X, Zheng Y, Cheng Y, et al. In vitro corrosion and biocompatibility of binary magnesium alloys[J]. Biomaterials, 2009, 30(4): 484-498.

[143] Li L, Gao J, Wang Y. Evaluation of cyto-toxicity and corrosion behavior of alkali-heat-treated magnesium in simulated body fluid[J]. Surface and Coatings Technology, 2004, 185(1): 92-98.

[144] Ulum M F, Paramitha D, Estuningsih S, et al. Metal ion level and polymorphonuclear leukocyte cells number as determination factors for early in vivo rejection of biodegradable metals[J]. European Cells and Materials, 2013, 26(5): 59.

[145] Yun Y H, Dong Z, Yang D, et al. Biodegradable Mg corrosion and osteoblast cell culture studies[J]. Materials Science and Engineering: C, 2009, 29(6): 1814-1821.

[146] Hermawan H, Alamdari H, Mantovani D, et al. Iron-manganese: new class of metallic degradable biomaterials prepared by powder metallurgy[J]. Powder Metallurgy, 2008, 51(1): 38-45.

[147] Wang S, Xu Y, Zhou J, et al. In vitro degradation and surface bioactivity of iron-matrix composites containing silicate-based bioceramic[J]. Bioactive materials, 2017, 2(1): 10-18.

[148] Kubásek J, Vojtěch D, Jablonská E, et al. Structure, mechanical characteristics and in vitro degradation, cytotoxicity, genotoxicity and mutagenicity of novel biodegradable Zn-Mg alloys[J]. Materials Science and Engineering: C, 2016, 58: 24-35.

[149] Jin G, Qin H, Cao H, et al. Synergistic effects of dual Zn/Ag ion implantation in osteogenic activity and antibacterial ability of titanium[J]. Biomaterials, 2014, 35(27): 7699-7713.

[150] Murni N S, Dambatta M S, Yeap S K, et al. Cytotoxicity evaluation of biodegradable Zn-3Mg alloy toward normal human osteoblast cells[J]. Materials Science and Engineering: C, 2015, 49: 560-566.

[151] Witte F, Hort N, Vogt C, et al. Degradable biomaterials based on magnesium corrosion[J]. Current opinion in solid state and materials science, 2008, 12(5-6): 63-72.

[152] GAO J, HU D, SONG C. Medical magnesium alloy degradation and its impact on human physiology [J]. Journal of Functional Materials, 2012, 19.

[153] Yamamoto A, Honma R, Sumita M. Cytotoxicity evaluation of 43 metal salts using murine fibroblasts and osteoblastic cells [J]. Journal of Biomedical Materials Research: An Official Journal of The Society for Biomaterials, The Japanese Society for Biomaterials, and the Australian Society for Biomaterials, 1998, 39(2): 331-340.

[154] Di Nicola M, Carlo-Stella C, Magni M, et al. Human bone marrow stromal cells suppress T-lymphocyte proliferation induced by cellular or nonspecific mitogenic stimuli[J]. Blood, 2002, 99(10): 3838-3843.

[155] Molly L, Vandromme H, Quirynen M, et al. Bone formation following implantation of bone biomaterials into extraction sites[J]. Journal of periodontology, 2008, 79(6): 1108-1115.

[156] Witte F, Reifenrath J, Müller P P, et al. Cartilage repair on magnesium scaffolds used as a subchondral bone replacement[J]. Materialwissenschaft und Werkstofftechnik: Entwicklung, Fertigung, Prüfung, Eigenschaften und Anwendungen technischer Werkstoffe, 2006, 37(6): 504-508.

[157] Castellani C, Lindtner R A, Hausbrandt P, et al. Bone-implant interface strength and osseointegration: Biodegradable magnesium alloy versus standard titanium control [J]. Acta biomaterialia, 2011, 7(1): 432-440.

[158] Peng Q, Huang Y, Zhou L, et al. Preparation and properties of high purity Mg-Y biomaterials [J]. Biomaterials, 2010, 31(3): 398-403.

[159] Zhang S, Li J, Song Y, et al. In vitro degradation, hemolysis and MC3T3-E1 cell adhesion of biodegradable

Mg-Zn alloy[J]. Materials Science and Engineering: C, 2009, 29(6): 1907-1912.

[160] Ostrowski N, Lee B, Enick N, et al. Corrosion protection and improved cytocompatibility of biodegradable polymeric layer-by-layer coatings on AZ31 magnesium alloys [J]. Acta Biomaterialia, 2013, 9 (10): 8704-8713.

[161] Yang Y, Yuan F, Gao C, et al. A combined strategy to enhance the properties of Zn by laser rapid solidification and laser alloying[J]. Journal of the Mechanical Behavior of Biomedical Materials, 2018, 82: 51-60.

[162] Gao C, Peng S, Feng P, et al. Bone biomaterials and interactions with stem cells[J]. Bone Research, 2017, 5(4): 17059.

[163] Shuai C, Li S, Peng S, et al. Biodegradable metallic bone implants [J]. Materials Chemistry Frontiers, 2019.

[164] Rink L. Zinc in human health[M]. Ios Press, 2011.

[165] Prasad A S. Zinc in Human Health: Effect of Zinc on Immune Cells[J]. Molecular Medicine, 2008, 14(5-6): 353-357.

[166] Aggett P J, Comerford J G. Zinc and human health[J]. Nutrition Reviews, 1995, 53(9 Pt 2): S16.

[167] Brown K H, Wuehler S E, Peerson J M. The importance of zinc in human nutrition and estimation of the global prevalence of zinc deficiency[J]. Food and Nutrition Bulletin, 2001, 22(2): 113-125.

[168] Tapiero H, Tew K D. Trace elements in human physiology and pathology: zinc and metallothioneins[J]. Biomedicine & Pharmacotherapy, 2003, 57(9): 386-398.

[169] Xiang Wang, Hongmei Lu, Xinlin Li, et al. Effect of cooling rate and composition on microstructures and properties of Zn-Mg alloys[J]. Transactions of Nonferrous Metals Society of China, 2007, 17(s1): 122-125.

[170] Bakhsheshi-rad H R, Hamzah E, Low H T, et al. Fabrication of biodegradable Zn-Al-Mg alloy: Mechanical properties, corrosion behavior, cytotoxicity and antibacterial activities[J]. Materials Science & Engineering C Materials for Biological Applications, 2017, 73: 215.

[171] Bowen P K, Ii R J G, SHEARIER E R, et al. Metallic Zinc Exhibits Optimal Biocompatibility for Bioabsorbable Endovascular Stents[J]. Materials Science & Engineering C, 2015, 56: 467-472.

[172] Arrens A, Liu M, Abidin N I Z, et al. 3-Corrosion of magnesium (Mg) alloys and metallurgical influence [J]. Corrosion of Magnesium Alloys, 2011: 117-165.

[173] Sayir A, Farmer S C. The effect of the microstructure on mechanical properties of directionally solidified $Al_2O_3/ZrO_2(Y_2O_3)$ eutectic[J]. Acta Materialia, 2000, 48(18-19): 4691-4697.

[174] Stein F, Palm M, Sauthoff G. Mechanical properties and oxidation behaviour of two-phase iron aluminium alloys with $Zr(Fe,Al)_2$ Laves phase or $Zr(Fe,Al)$ 12 τ 1 phase[J]. Intermetallics, 2005, 13 (12): 1275-1285.

[175] Nikanorov S P, Volkov M P, Gurin V N, et al. Structural and mechanical properties of Al-Si alloys obtained by fast cooling of a levitated melt[J]. Materials Science & Engineering A, 2005, 390(1): 63-69.

[176] Jin M P, Sohn S W, Kim T E, et al. Nanostructure-dendrite composites in the Fe-Zr binary alloy system exhibiting high strength and plasticity[J]. Scripta Materialia, 2007, 57(12): 1153-1156.

[177] Barbier, Huang, M. X, et al. A novel eutectic Fe-15 wt % Ti alloy with an ultrafine lamellar; structure for high temperature applications[J]. Intermetallics, 2013, 35(3): 41-44.

[178] Lliê N, Rein R, Göken M, et al. Properties of eutectic Ru-Al alloy produced by ingot metallurgy [J]. Materials Science and Engineering: A, 2002, 329: 38-44.

[179] Bei H, George E. Microstructures and mechanical properties of a directionally solidified NiAl-Mo eutectic

alloy[J]. Acta Materialia, 2005, 53(1): 69-77.

[180] Shuai C, Wang B, Yang Y, et al. 3D honeycomb nanostructure-encapsulated magnesium alloys with superior corrosion resistance and mechanical properties[J]. Composites Part B: Engineering, 2019, 162: 611-620.

[181] Shuai C, Li Y, Wang G, et al. Surface modification of nanodiamond: Toward the dispersion of reinforced phase in poly-l-lactic acid scaffolds[J]. International journal of biological macromolecules, 2019, 126: 1116-1124.

[182] Croker M N, Fidler R S, Smith R W. The Characterization of Eutectic Structures[J]. Proceedings of the Royal Society of London, 1973, 335(1600): 15-37.

[183] Schlieter A, Kühn U, Eckert J, et al. Anisotropic mechanical behavior of ultrafine eutectic TiFe cast under non-equilibrium conditions[J]. Intermetallics, 2011, 19(3): 327-335.

[184] Okamoto H, Kacprzak L, Subramanian P. Binary alloy phase diagrams[M]. ASM international, 1996.

[185] Ku C-H, Pioletti D P, Browne M, et al. Effect of different Ti-6Al-4V surface treatments on osteoblasts behaviour[J]. Biomaterials, 2002, 23(6): 1447-1454.

[186] Burnatowskahledin M A, Mayor G H, Lau K. Renal handling of aluminum in the rat: clearance and micropuncture studies[J]. American Journal of Physiology, 1985, 249(2 Pt 2): F192.

[187] Wang, H. T, Yang, et al. In Vitro Evaluation of the Feasibility of Commercial Zn Alloys as Biodegradable Metals[J]. Journal of Materials Science & Technology, 2016, 32(9): 909-918.

[188] Ebrahimi S H S, Emamy M, Pourkia N, et al. The microstructure, hardness and tensile properties of a new super high strength aluminum alloy with Zr addition[J]. Materials & Design, 2010, 31(9): 4450-4456.

[189] Büyük U, Engin S, Maraşl N. Directional solidification of Zn-Al-Cu eutectic alloy by the vertical Bridgman method[J]. Journal of Mining and Metallurgy, Section B: Metallurgy, 2015, 51(1): 67-72.

[190] Yang Y, Guo X, He C, et al. Regulating Degradation Behavior by Incorporating Mesoporous Silica for Mg Bone Implants[J]. ACS Biomaterials Science & Engineering, 2018, 4(3): 1046-1054.

[191] Astm G. Standard test method for conducting potentiodynamic polarization resistance measurements[J]. Annual Book of ASTM Standards, 2009, 3: 237-239.

[192] Internasional A. Astm G31-72: Standart Practice for Laboratory Immersion Corrosion Testing of Metals[J]. United State, 2004.

[193] ISO I. 8407: 2009 (E). Corrosion of Metals and Alloys-Removal of Corrosion Products from Corrosion Test Specimens[J]. International Standards Organization: Geneva, Switzerland, 2009.

[194] Li H, Li Z, Liu Y, et al. Effect of zirconium on the microstructure and mechanical properties of Zn-4% Al hypoeutectic alloy[J]. Journal of Alloys & Compounds, 2014, 592(14): 127-134.

[195] Liu C, He P, Wan P, et al. The in vitro biocompatibility and macrophage phagocytosis of Mg17 Al12 phase in Mg-Al-Zn alloys[J]. Journal of Biomedical Materials Research Part A, 2015, 103(7): 2405-2415.

[196] Pei F, Ping W, Gao C, et al. A Multimaterial Scaffold With Tunable Properties: Toward Bone Tissue Repair [J]. Advanced Science, 2018, 5(6): 1700817.

[197] Mostaed E, Sikorajasinska M, Mostaed A, et al. Novel Zn-based alloys for biodegradable stent applications: Design, development and in vitro degradation[J]. Journal of the Mechanical Behavior of Biomedical Materials, 2016, 60: 581-602.

[198] Bagha P S, Khaleghpanah S, Sheibani S, et al. Characterization of nanostructured biodegradable Zn-Mn alloy synthesized by mechanical alloying[J]. Journal of Alloys & Compounds, 2017.

[199] Yang H, Qu X, Lin W, et al. In vitro and in vivo studies on zinc-hydroxyapatite composites as novel biodegradable metal matrix composite for orthopedic applications[J]. Acta Biomaterialia, 2018.

[200] Miao Y, George C, Cao Y, et al. Microstructure, corrosion, and mechanical properties of compression-molded zinc-nanodiamond composites[J]. Journal of Materials Science, 2014, 49(10): 3629-3641.

[201] Liu X, Sun J, Yang Y, et al. Microstructure, mechanical properties, in vitro degradation behavior and hemocompatibility of novel Zn-Mg-Sr alloys as biodegradable metals[J]. Materials Letters, 2016, 162: 242-245.

[202] Haynes W M. CRC Handbook of Chemistry and Physics[M]. 2011.

[203] 10993-5 I. Biological evaluation of medical devices-Part 5: Tests for in vitro cytotoxicity: International Organization for Standardization Geneve, Switzerland, 2009.

[204] Hu Y, Gu X, Yang Y, et al. Facile fabrication of poly (l-lactic acid)-grafted hydroxyapatite/poly (lactic-co-glycolic acid) scaffolds by pickering high internal phase emulsion templates[J]. ACS applied materials & interfaces, 2014, 6(19): 17166-17175.

[205] Sprott M R, Gallego-Ferrer G, Dalby M J, et al. Functionalization of PLLA with Polymer Brushes to Trigger the Assembly of Fibronectin into Nanonetworks[J]. Advanced healthcare materials, 2019, 8(3): 1801469.

[206] Lizundia E, Fortunati E, Dominici F, et al. PLLA-grafted cellulose nanocrystals: Role of the CNC content and grafting on the PLA bionanocomposite film properties[J]. Carbohydrate polymers, 2016, 142: 105-113.

[207] Fitzgerald R, Vleggaar D. Using poly-L-lactic acid (PLLA) to mimic volume in multiple tissue layers[J]. Journal of drugs in dermatology: JDD, 2009, 8(10 Suppl): s5-14.

[208] Rajzer I, Kurowska A, Jabłoński A, et al. Layered gelatin/PLLA scaffolds fabricated by electrospinning and 3D printing-for nasal cartilages and subchondral bone reconstruction[J]. Materials & Design, 2018, 155: 297-306.

[209] Chen J P, Su C H. Surface modification of electrospun PLLA nanofibers by plasma treatment and cationized gelatin immobilization for cartilage tissue engineering[J]. Acta biomaterialia, 2011, 7(1): 234-243.

[210] Maleki H, Gharehaghaji A A, Moroni L, et al. Influence of the solvent type on the morphology and mechanical properties of electrospun PLLA yarns[J]. Biofabrication, 2013, 5(3): 035014.

[211] Zhao Y, Liu B, Bi H, et al. The Degradation Properties of MgO Whiskers/PLLA Composite In Vitro[J]. International journal of molecular sciences, 2018, 19(9): 2740.

[212] Bai L, Zhao X, Bao R Y, et al. Effect of temperature, crystallinity and molecular chain orientation on the thermal conductivity of polymers: a case study of PLLA[J]. Journal of materials science, 2018, 53(14): 10543-10553.

[213] Takahashi K, Sawai D, Yokoyama T, et al. Crystal transformation from the α-to the β-form upon tensile drawing of poly (l-lactic acid)[J]. Polymer, 2004, 45(14): 4969-4976.

[214] Shieh Y T, Liu G L, Twu Y K, et al. Effects of carbon nanotubes on dynamic mechanical property, thermal property, and crystal structure of poly (L-lactic acid)[J]. Journal of Polymer Science Part B: Polymer Physics, 2010, 48(2): 145-152.

[215] Pei A, Zhou Q, Berglund L A. Functionalized cellulose nanocrystals as biobased nucleation agents in poly (l-lactide)(PLLA)-Crystallization and mechanical property effects[J]. Composites Science and Technology, 2010, 70(5): 815-821.

[216] Gay S, Arostegui S, Lemaitre J. Preparation and characterization of dense nanohydroxyapatite/PLLA composites[J]. Materials Science and Engineering: C, 2009, 29(1): 172-177.

[217] Lin Z, Wu J, Qiao W, et al. Precisely controlled delivery of magnesium ions thru sponge-like monodisperse PLGA/nano-MgO-alginate core-shell microsphere device to enable in-situ bone regeneration[J]. Biomaterials, 2018, 174: 1-16.

[218] Shuai C, Guo W, Gao C, et al. An nMgO containing scaffold: antibacterial activity, degradation properties and cell responses[J]. International Journal of Bioprinting, 2017, 4(1).

[219] Qi F, Chen N, Wang Q. Preparation of PA11/BaTiO3 nanocomposite powders with improved processability, dielectric and piezoelectric properties for use in selective laser sintering[J]. Materials & Design, 2017, 131: 135-143.

[220] Park S D, Todo M, Arakawa K, et al. Effect of crystallinity and loading-rate on mode I fracture behavior of poly (lactic acid)[J]. Polymer, 2006, 47(4): 1357-1363.

[221] Yang Y, Yu W, Duan H, et al. Realization of reinforcing and toughening poly (phenylene sulfide) with rigid silica nanoparticles[J]. Journal of Polymer Research, 2016, 23(9): 188.

[222] Zhao C, Wu H, Ni J, et al. Development of PLA/Mg composite for orthopedic implant: tunable degradation and enhanced mineralization[J]. Composites Science and Technology, 2017, 147: 8-15.

[223] Yang J, Cao X, Zhao Y, et al. Enhanced pH stability, cell viability and reduced degradation rate of poly (L-lactide)-based composite in vitro: Effect of modified magnesium oxide nanoparticles [J]. Journal of Biomaterials science, Polymer edition, 2017, 28(5): 486-503.

[224] Peng D, Qin W, Wu X, et al. Improvement of the resistance performance of carbon/cyanate ester composites during vacuum electron radiation by reduced graphene oxide modified TiO_2 [J]. RSC Advances, 2015, 5 (94): 77138-77146.

[225] Liu G, Zhou T, Liu W, et al. Enhanced desulfurization performance of PDMS membranes by incorporating silver decorated dopamine nanoparticles[J]. Journal of Materials Chemistry A, 2014, 2(32): 12907-12917.

[226] Cebe P, Hong S D. Crystallization behaviour of poly (ether-ether-ketone) [J]. Polymer, 1986, 27(8): 1183-1192.

[227] Miyata T, Masuko T. Crystallization behaviour of poly (L-lactide) [J]. Polymer, 1998, 39 (22): 5515-5521.

[228] Zhang Z, Wang C, Yang Z, et al. Crystallization behavior and melting characteristics of PP nucleated by a novel supported β-nucleating agent[J]. Polymer, 2008, 49(23): 5137-5145.

[229] Zhao Y, Qiu Z, Yang W. Effect of functionalization of multiwalled nanotubes on the crystallization and hydrolytic degradation of biodegradable poly (L-lactide)[J]. The Journal of Physical Chemistry B, 2008, 112 (51): 16461-16468.

[230] Vasanthan N, Ly H, Ghosh S. Impact of nanoclay on isothermal cold crystallization kinetics and polymorphism of poly (L-lactic acid) nanocomposites [J]. The Journal of Physical Chemistry B, 2011, 115 (31): 9556-9563.

[231] Senior J, Delgado C, Fisher D, et al. Influence of surface hydrophilicity of liposomes on their interaction with plasma protein and clearance from the circulation: studies with poly (ethylene glycol)-coated vesicles[J]. Biochimica et Biophysica Acta (BBA)-Biomembranes, 1991, 1062(1): 77-82.

[232] Guan J, Gao C, Feng L, et al. Surface modification of polyurethane for promotion of cell adhesion and growth 1: Surface photo-grafting with N, N-dimethylaminoethyl methacrylate and cytocompatibility of the modified surface[J]. Journal of Materials Science: Materials in Medicine, 2001, 12(5): 447-452.

[233] Wang X, Song G, Lou T. Fabrication and characterization of nano-composite scaffold of PLLA/silane modified hydroxyapatite[J]. Medical engineering & physics, 2010, 32(4): 391-397.

[234] Shuai C, Li Y, Feng P, et al. Positive feedback effects of Mg on the hydrolysis of poly-l-lactic acid (PLLA): Promoted degradation of PLLA scaffolds[J]. Polymer Testing, 2018, 68: 27-33.

[235] Fletcher N H J. Size effect in heterogeneous nucleation[J]. The Journal of chemical physics, 1958, 29(3):

572-576.

［236］Sing S L, Yeong W Y, Wiria F E, et al. Direct selective laser sintering and melting of ceramics: a review ［J］. Rapid Prototyping Journal, 2017, 23(3): 611-623.

［237］Wang X, Shi J, Feng Z, et al. Visible emission characteristics from different defects of ZnS nanocrystals［J］. Physical Chemistry Chemical Physics, 2011, 13(10): 4715-4723.

［238］Tan J, Wang D, Cao H, et al. Effect of Local Alkaline Microenvironment on the Behaviors of Bacteria and Osteogenic Cells［J］. ACS applied materials & interfaces, 2018, 10(49): 42018-42029.

［239］Yuan W, Li B, Chen D, et al. Formation Mechanism, Corrosion Behavior, and Cytocompatibility of Microarc Oxidation Coating on Absorbable High-Purity Zinc［J］. ACS Biomaterials Science & Engineering, 2019.

［240］Wagener V, Schilling A, Mainka A, et al. Cell adhesion on surface-functionalized magnesium［J］. ACS applied materials & interfaces, 2016, 8(19): 11998-12006.

［241］Kraemer M, Schilling M, Eifler R, et al. Corrosion behavior, biocompatibility and biomechanical stability of a prototype magnesium-based biodegradable intramedullary nailing system ［J］. Materials Science and Engineering: C, 2016, 59: 129-135.

［242］Peng F, Li H, Wang D, et al. Enhanced Corrosion Resistance and Biocompatibility of Magnesium Alloy by Mg-Al-Layered Double Hydroxide［J］. Acs Applied Materials & Interfaces, 2016, 8(51): 35033-35044.

［243］Vahidgolpayegani A, Wen C, Hodgson P, et al. 2 - Production methods and characterization of porous Mg and Mg alloys for biomedical applications［J］. Metallic Foam Bone, 2017, 47(11): 25-82.

［244］Valiev R Z, Estrin Y, Horita Z, et al. Producing bulk ultrafine-grained materials by severe plastic deformation ［J］. Journal of Plasticity Engineering, 2006, 58(4): 33-39.

［245］Atrens A, Johnston S, Shi Z, et al. Understanding Mg corrosion in the body for biodegradable medical implants［J］. Scripta Materialia, 2018, 154: 92-100.

［246］Song G L, Atrens A. Corrosion mechanisms of magnesium alloys［J］. Advanced engineering materials, 1999, 1(1): 11-33.

［247］Bobbert F, Lietaert K, Eftekhari A A, et al. Additively manufactured metallic porous biomaterials based on minimal surfaces: A unique combination of topological, mechanical, and mass transport properties［J］. Acta biomaterialia, 2017, 53: 572-584.

［248］Zhu D, Su Y, Young M L, et al. Biological responses and mechanisms of human bone marrow mesenchymal stem cells to Zn and Mg biomaterials［J］. ACS applied materials & interfaces, 2017, 9(33): 27453-27461.

［249］Bondarenko A, Angrisani N, Meyer-Lindenberg A, et al. Magnesium-based bone implants: Immunohistochemical analysis of peri-implant osteogenesis by evaluation of osteopontin and osteocalcin expression［J］. Journal of biomedical materials research Part A, 2014, 102(5): 1449-1457.

［250］Hu H, Nie X, Ma Y: Corrosion and surface treatment of magnesium alloys, Magnesium Alloys-Properties in Solid and Liquid States: IntechOpen, 2014.

［251］Yang L-j, Wei Y-h, Hou L-f, et al. Corrosion behaviour of die-cast AZ91D magnesium alloy in aqueous sulphate solutions［J］. Corrosion Science, 2010, 52(2): 345-351.

［252］Atrens A, Song G L, Liu M, et al. Review of recent developments in the field of magnesium corrosion［J］. Advanced Engineering Materials, 2015, 17(4): 400-453.

［253］Shi Z, Jia J X, Atrens A. Galvanostatic anodic polarisation curves and galvanic corrosion of high purity Mg in 3.5% NaCl saturated with Mg (OH) 2［J］. Corrosion Science, 2012, 60: 296-308.

［254］Zhao D, Witte F, Lu F, et al. Current status on clinical applications of magnesium-based orthopaedic implants: A review from clinical translational perspective［J］. Biomaterials, 2017, 112: 287-302.

[255] Xu Y, Wu Q, Sun Y, et al. Three-dimensional self-assembly of graphene oxide and DNA into multifunctional hydrogels[J]. ACS nano, 2010, 4(12): 7358-7362.

[256] Stankovich S, Dikin D A, Piner R D, et al. Synthesis of graphene-based nanosheets via chemical reduction of exfoliated graphite oxide[J]. carbon, 2007, 45(7): 1558-1565.

[257] Nair R R, Blake P, Grigorenko A N, et al. Fine structure constant defines visual transparency of graphene [J]. Science, 2008, 320(5881): 1308-1308.

[258] Bian Y, Bian Z-Y, Zhang J-X, et al. Effect of the oxygen-containing functional group of graphene oxide on the aqueous cadmium ions removal[J]. Applied Surface Science, 2015, 329: 269-275.

[259] Wilson N R, Pandey P A, Beanland R, et al. Graphene oxide: structural analysis and application as a highly transparent support for electron microscopy[J]. ACS nano, 2009, 3(9): 2547-2556.

[260] Wei N, Peng X, Xu Z. Understanding water permeation in graphene oxide membranes[J]. ACS applied materials & interfaces, 2014, 6(8): 5877-5883.

[261] Pei S, Cheng H-M. The reduction of graphene oxide[J]. Carbon, 2012, 50(9): 3210-3228.

[262] Li Y, Gao W, Ci L, et al. Catalytic performance of Pt nanoparticles on reduced graphene oxide for methanol electro-oxidation[J]. Carbon, 2010, 48(4): 1124-1130.

[263] Shuai C, Feng P, Wu P, et al. A combined nanostructure constructed by graphene and boron nitride nanotubes reinforces ceramic scaffolds[J]. Chemical Engineering Journal, 2017, 313: 487-497.

[264] Yan S J, Zou X W, Zhang M G. Preparation of La-Mg-Ni Hydrogen Storage Composite Alloys by Mechanical Alloying[C]. Advanced Materials Research, 2013: 2707-2712.

[265] Song J, Gao H, Zhu G, et al. The preparation and characterization of polycaprolactone/graphene oxide biocomposite nanofiber scaffolds and their application for directing cell behaviors[J]. Carbon, 2015, 95: 1039-1050.

[266] Zhao J, Xie X, Zhang C. Effect of the graphene oxide additive on the corrosion resistance of the plasma electrolytic oxidation coating of the AZ31 magnesium alloy[J]. Corrosion Science, 2017, 114: 146-155.

[267] Ikhe A B, Kale A B, Jeong J, et al. Perfluorinated polysiloxane hybridized with graphene oxide for corrosion inhibition of AZ31 magnesium alloy[J]. Corrosion Science, 2016, 109: 238-245.

[268] Rashad M, Pan F, Asif M. Exploring mechanical behavior of Mg-6Zn alloy reinforced with graphene nanoplatelets[J]. Materials Science and Engineering: A, 2016, 649: 263-269.

[269] Tong L, Zhang J, Xu C, et al. Enhanced corrosion and wear resistances by graphene oxide coating on the surface of Mg-Zn-Ca alloy[J]. Carbon, 2016, 109: 340-351.

[270] Turan M E, Sun Y, Akgul Y, et al. The effect of GNPs on wear and corrosion behaviors of pure magnesium [J]. Journal of Alloys and Compounds, 2017, 724: 14-23.

[271] Abidin N I Z, Rolfe B, Owen H, et al. The in vivo and in vitro corrosion of high-purity magnesium and magnesium alloys WZ21 and AZ91[J]. Corrosion Science, 2013, 75: 354-366.

[272] Abidin N I Z, Martin D, Atrens A. Corrosion of high purity Mg, AZ91, ZE41 and Mg2Zn0. 2Mn in Hanks solution at room temperature[J]. Corrosion Science, 2011, 53(3): 862-872.

[273] Zhou W, Shen T, Aung N N. Effect of heat treatment on corrosion behaviour of magnesium alloy AZ91D in simulated body fluid[J]. Corrosion Science, 2010, 52(3): 1035-1041.

[274] Gao J, Guan S, Ren Z, et al. Homogeneous corrosion of high pressure torsion treated Mg-Zn-Ca alloy in simulated body fluid[J]. Materials Letters, 2011, 65(4): 691-693.

[275] Gu X, Zhou W, Zheng Y, et al. Corrosion fatigue behaviors of two biomedical Mg alloys-AZ91D and WE43-in simulated body fluid[J]. Acta Biomaterialia, 2010, 6(12): 4605-4613.

[276] Shi Z, Jia J X, Atrens A. Galvanostatic anodic polarization curves and galvanic corrosion of AZ31B in 0.01 M Na2SO4 saturated with Mg (OH) 2[J]. Advanced Engineering Materials, 2012, 14(5): 324-334.

[277] Mathaudhu S N, Luo A A, Neelameggham N R, et al. An Hydrogen Evolution Method for the Estimation of the Corrosion Rate of Magnesium Alloys[M]. 2014.

[278] Park H S, Ha H W, Ruoff R S, et al. On the improvement of photoelectrochemical performance and finite element analysis of reduced graphene oxide-BiVO 4 composite electrodes[J]. Journal of Electroanalytical Chemistry, 2014, 716(716): 8-15.

[279] Safarpour M, Khataee A, Vatanpour V. Thin film nanocomposite reverse osmosis membrane modified by reduced graphene oxide/TiO$_2$ with improved desalination performance[J]. Journal of Membrane Science, 2015, 489(5): 43-54.

[280] Zeng R, Liu Z, Zhang F, et al. Corrosion resistance of in-situ Mg-Al hydrotalcite conversion film on AZ31 magnesium alloy by one-step formation[J]. Transactions of Nonferrous Metals Society of China, 2015, 25 (6): 1917-1925.

[281] Atrens A, Song G L, Shi Z, et al. Understanding the Corrosion of Mg and Mg Alloys[J]. 2017.

[282] Atrens A D, Gentle I, Atrens A. Possible dissolution pathways participating in the Mg corrosion reaction[J]. Corrosion Science, 2015, 92: 173-181.

[283] Shi Z, Jia J X, Atrens A. Galvanostatic anodic polarisation of WE43[J]. Journal of Magnesium & Alloys, 2014, 2(3): 197-202.

[284] Raucci M G, Giugliano D, Longo A, et al. Comparative facile methods for preparing graphene oxide-hydroxyapatite for bone tissue engineering[J]. Journal of Tissue Engineering & Regenerative Medicine, 2016, 11(8): n/a-n/a.

[285] Shi Y, Li M, Liu Q, et al. Electrophoretic deposition of graphene oxide reinforced chitosan-hydroxyapatite nanocomposite coatings on Ti substrate[J]. Journal of Materials Science: Materials in Medicine, 2016, 27 (3): 48.

[286] Shi Z, Liu M, Atrens A. Measurement of the corrosion rate of magnesium alloys using Tafel extrapolation[J]. Corrosion science, 2010, 52(2): 579-588.

[287] Song G, Atrens A. Understanding magnesium corrosion-a framework for improved alloy performance[J]. Advanced engineering materials, 2003, 5(12): 837-858.

[288] El Essawy N A, Konsowa A H, Elnouby M, et al. A novel one-step synthesis for carbon-based nanomaterials from polyethylene terephthalate (PET) bottles waste[J]. Journal of the Air & Waste Management Association, 2017, 67(3): 358-370.

[289] Chen X, Liu L, Pan F, et al. Microstructure, electromagnetic shielding effectiveness and mechanical properties of Mg-Zn-Cu-Zr alloys[J]. Materials Science and Engineering: B, 2015, 197: 67-74.

[290] Xia X, Chen Q, Zhao Z, et al. Microstructure, texture and mechanical properties of coarse-grained Mg-Gd-Y-Nd-Zr alloy processed by multidirectional forging[J]. Journal of Alloys and Compounds, 2015, 623: 62-68.

[291] Cheng W, Ma S, Bai Y, et al. Corrosion behavior of Mg-6Bi-2Sn alloy in the simulated body fluid solution: The influence of microstructural characteristics[J]. Journal of Alloys and Compounds, 2018, 731: 945-954.

[292] Zhu Y, Yu G, Hu B, et al. Electrochemical behaviors of the magnesium alloy substrates in various pretreatment solutions[J]. Applied Surface Science, 2010, 256(9): 2988-2994.

[293] Sanchez A H M, Luthringer B J C, Feyerabend F, et al. Mg and Mg alloys: how comparable are in vitro and in vivo corrosion rates? A review[J]. Acta biomaterialia, 2015, 13: 16-31.

[294] Long T, Zhang X, Huang Q, et al. Novel Mg-based alloys by selective laser melting for biomedical

applications: microstructure evolution, microhardness and in vitro degradation behaviour[J]. Virtual and Physical Prototyping, 2018, 13(2): 71-81.

[295] Cipriano A F, Sallee A, Guan R G, et al. A comparison study on the degradation and cytocompatibility of Mg-4Zn-x Sr alloys in direct culture[J]. ACS Biomaterials Science & Engineering, 2017, 3(4): 540-550.

[296] Córdoba L C, Montemor M F, Coradin T. Silane/TiO_2 coating to control the corrosion rate of magnesium alloys in simulated body fluid[J]. Corrosion Science, 2016, 104: 152-161.

[297] Zhang Y, Liu X, Jamali S S, et al. The effect of treatment time on the ionic liquid surface film formation: Promising surface coating for Mg alloy AZ31[J]. Surface and Coatings Technology, 2016, 296: 192-202.

[298] Yang P, Gai S, Lin J. Functionalized mesoporous silica materials for controlled drug delivery[J]. Chemical Society Reviews, 2012, 41(9): 3679-3698.

[299] Akbay E, Ölmez T G. Sonochemical synthesis and loading of PbS nanoparticles into mesoporous silica[J]. Materials Letters, 2018, 215: 263-267.

[300] Wang J, Yang M, Lu Y, et al. Surface functionalization engineering driven crystallization behavior of polyethylene glycol confined in mesoporous silica for shape-stabilized phase change materials[J]. Nano Energy, 2016, 19: 78-87.

[301] Xu Y, Gao D, Feng P, et al. A mesoporous silica composite scaffold: Cell behaviors, biomineralization and mechanical properties[J]. Applied Surface Science, 2017, 423: 314-321.

[302] McCarty M F. Reported anti atherosclerotic activity of silicon may reflect increased endothelial synthesis of heparan sulfate proteoglycans[J]. Medical hypotheses, 1997, 49(2): 175-176.

[303] Gu D D, Meiners W, Wissenbach K, et al. Laser additive manufacturing of metallic components: materials, processes and mechanisms[J]. International materials reviews, 2012, 57(3): 133-164.

[304] Shuai C, Yang Y, Wu P, et al. Laser rapid solidification improves corrosion behavior of Mg-Zn-Zr alloy[J]. Journal of Alloys and Compounds, 2017, 691: 961-969.

[305] Xia K, Pan H, Wang T, et al. Effect of Ca/P ratio on the structural and corrosion properties of biomimetic CaP coatings on ZK60 magnesium alloy[J]. Materials Science and Engineering: C, 2017, 72: 676-681.

[306] Sing S L, Wiria F E, Yeong W Y. Selective laser melting of lattice structures: A statistical approach to manufacturability and mechanical behavior[J]. Robotics and Computer-Integrated Manufacturing, 2018, 49: 170-180.

[307] Wei K, Gao M, Wang Z, et al. Effect of energy input on formability, microstructure and mechanical properties of selective laser melted AZ91D magnesium alloy[J]. Materials Science and Engineering: A, 2014, 611: 212-222.

[308] Xiong G, Nie Y, Ji D, et al. Characterization of biomedical hydroxyapatite/magnesium composites prepared by powder metallurgy assisted with microwave sintering[J]. Current Applied Physics, 2016, 16(8): 830-836.

[309] Huang Y, Liu D, Anguilano L, et al. Fabrication and characterization of a biodegradable Mg-2Zn-0.5 Ca/β-TCP composite[J]. Materials Science and Engineering: C, 2015, 54: 120-132.

[310] Wang X, Zhang P, Dong L H, et al. Microstructure and characteristics of interpenetrating β-TCP/Mg-Zn-Mn composite fabricated by suction casting[J]. Materials & Design (1980-2015), 2014, 54: 995-1001.

[311] Gu D, Wang H, Dai D, et al. Densification behavior, microstructure evolution, and wear property of TiC nanoparticle reinforced AlSi10Mg bulk-form nanocomposites prepared by selective laser melting[J]. Journal of Laser Applications, 2015, 27(S1): S17003.

[312] Aghajani K, Tayebi H A. Synthesis of SBA-15/PAni mesoporous composite for adsorption of reactive dye from

aqueous media: RBF and MLP networks predicting models[J]. Fibers and Polymers, 2017, 18(3): 465-475.

[313] Huang K, Cai S, Xu G, et al. Sol-gel derived mesoporous 58S bioactive glass coatings on AZ31 magnesium alloy and in vitro degradation behavior[J]. Surface and Coatings Technology, 2014, 240: 137-144.

[314] Park J H, Schwartz Z, Olivares-Navarrete R, et al. Enhancement of surface wettability via the modification of microtextured titanium implant surfaces with polyelectrolytes[J]. Langmuir, 2011, 27(10): 5976-5985.

[315] López-Noriega A, Arcos D, Vallet-Regí M. Functionalizing mesoporous bioglasses for long-term anti-osteoporotic drug delivery[J]. Chemistry-A European Journal, 2010, 16(35): 10879-10886.

[316] Huang K, Cai S, Xu G, et al. Preparation and characterization of mesoporous 45S5 bioactive glass-ceramic coatings on magnesium alloy for corrosion protection[J]. Journal of Alloys and Compounds, 2013, 580: 290-297.

[317] Wu Z, Tang T, Guo H, et al. In vitro degradability, bioactivity and cell responses to mesoporous magnesium silicate for the induction of bone regeneration[J]. Colloids and Surfaces B: Biointerfaces, 2014, 120: 38-46.

[318] Hench L L. Bioceramics: from concept to clinic[J]. Journal of the american ceramic society, 1991, 74(7): 1487-1510.

[319] Lee S, Yun H S, Kim S H. The comparative effects of mesoporous silica nanoparticles and colloidal silica on inflammation and apoptosis[J]. Biomaterials, 2011, 32(35): 9434-9443.

[320] Gil-Santos A, Marco I, Moelans N, et al. Microstructure and degradation performance of biodegradable Mg-Si-Sr implant alloys[J]. Materials Science and Engineering: C, 2017, 71: 25-

[321] Keyvani A, Zamani M, Fattah-alhosseini A, et al. Microstructure and corrosion resistance of MAO coatings on AZ31 magnesium[J]. Materials Research Express, 2018, 5(8): 086510.

[322] Li C-J, Sun H-F, Cheng S, et al. The corrosion behavior of cold drawn pure magnesium mini-tube for biomedical application[J]. Materials Research Express, 2018, 6(2): 026539.

[323] Annur D, Erryani A, Lestari F P, et al. Microstructure and corrosion study of porous Mg-Zn-Ca alloy in simulated body fluid[J]. Materials Research Express, 2017, 4(3): 034006.

[324] Xu S, Teng X, Zhou G, et al. Effect of solution treatment on mechanical and corrosion resistance properties of Mg-Zn-Nd-xCa alloy[J]. Materials Research Express, 2017, 4(12): 126510.

[325] Uddin M S, Rosman H, Hall C, et al. Enhancing the corrosion resistance of biodegradable Mg-based alloy by machining-induced surface integrity: influence of machining parameters on surface roughness and hardness [J]. International Journal of Advanced Manufacturing Technology, 2016: 1-14.

[326] Xin R, Luo Y, Zuo A, et al. Texture effect on corrosion behavior of AZ31 Mg alloy in simulated physiological environment[J]. Materials Letters, 2012, 72(7): 1-4.

[327] Toghyani S, Khodaei M. Fabrication and characterization of magnesium scaffold using different processing parameters[J]. Materials Research Express, 2018, 5(3): 035407.

[328] Witecka A, Yamamoto A. Influence of SaOS-2 cells on corrosion behavior of cast Mg-2. 0Zn0. 98Mn magnesium alloy[J]. Colloids and Surfaces B: Biointerfaces.

[329] Rosalbino F, . , Negri S, DE, Scavino G, . , et al. Microstructure and in vitro degradation performance of Mg-Zn-Mn alloys for biomedical application[J]. Journal of Biomedical Materials Research Part A, 2013, 101A(3): 704-711.

[330] Gobara M, Shamekh M, Akid R. Improving the corrosion resistance of AZ91D magnesium alloy through reinforcement with titanium carbides and borides[J]. Journal of Magnesium and Alloys, 2015, 3(2): 112-120.

［331］Zheng-rong Q, Qiang Z, Li-li T, et al. Comparison of degradation behavior and the associated bone response of ZK60 and PLLA in vivo［J］. Journal of Biomedical Materials Research Part A, 2014, 102(5): 1255-1263.

［332］Han P, Cheng P, Zhang S, et al. Invitro and invivo studies on the degradation of high-purity Mg (99. 99wt. %) screw with femoral intracondylar fractured rabbit model［J］. Biomaterials, 2015, 64: 57-69.

［333］Raman R K S. The role of microstructure in localized corrosion of magnesium alloys［J］. Metallurgical & Materials Transactions A, 2004, 35(8): 2525-2531.

［334］Virtanen S. Biodegradable Mg and Mg alloys: Corrosion and biocompatibility［J］. Materials Science & Engineering B, 2011, 176(20): 1600-1608.

［335］Johnston S, Shi Z, Dargusch M S, et al. Influence of surface condition on the corrosion of ultra-high-purity Mg alloy wire［J］. Corrosion Science, 2016, 108: 66-75.

［336］Singer F, Schlesak M, Mebert C, et al. Corrosion Properties of Polydopamine Coatings Formed in One-Step Immersion Process on Magnesium［J］. Acs Appl Mater Interfaces, 2015, 7(48): 26758-26766.

［337］Du H, Wei Z, Liu X, et al. Effects of Zn on the microstructure, mechanical property and bio-corrosion property of Mg-3Ca alloys for biomedical application［J］. Materials Chemistry and Physics, 2011, 125(3): 568-575.

［338］Lu F, Ma A, Jiang J, et al. Enhanced mechanical properties and rolling formability of fine-grained Mg-Gd-Zn-Zr alloy produced by equal-channel angular pressing［J］. Journal of Alloys & Compounds, 2015, 643: 28-33.

［339］Wang J F, Song P F, Pan F S, et al. Microstructure and phase composition of as-cast Mg-9Er-6Y-xZn-0. 6Zr alloys［J］. Transactions of Nonferrous Metals Society of China, 2013, 23(4): 889-895.

［340］Liu K, Wang X, Wen K. Effect of isothermal homogenization on microstructure and mechanical properties of the Mg-5Y-4Gd-0. 5Zn-0. 4Zr alloy［J］. Materials & Design (1980-2015), 2013, 52: 1035-1042.

［341］Guangli B I, Fang D, Zhao L, et al. An elevated temperature Mg-Dy-Zn alloy with long period stacking ordered phase by extrusion［J］. Materials Science & Engineering A, 2011, 528(10): 3609-3614.

［342］Xu D, Han E-H, Xu Y. Effect of long-period stacking ordered phase on microstructure, mechanical property and corrosion resistance of Mg alloys: A review［J］. Progress in Natural Science: Materials International, 2016, 26(2): 117-128.

［343］Kishida K, Yokobayashi H, Inui H. A formation criterion for Order-Disorder (OD) phases of the Long-Period Stacking Order (LPSO)-type in Mg-Al-RE (Rare Earth) Ternary Systems［J］. Scientific Reports, 2017, 7(1): 12294.

［344］Umantsev A, Ode M. Formation of long-period stacking fault structures in magnesium alloys［J］. Computational Materials Science, 2016, 124: 173-182.

［345］Li J H, Barrirero J, Sha G, et al. Precipitation hardening of an Mg-5Zn-2Gd-0. 4Zr (wt. %) alloy［J］. Acta Materialia, 2016, 108: 207-218.

［346］Huang S, Wang J, Hou F, et al. Effect of Gd and Y contents on the microstructural evolution of long period stacking ordered phase and the corresponding mechanical properties in Mg-Gd-Y-Zn-Mn alloys［J］. Materials Science and Engineering: A, 2014, 612: 363-370.

［347］Shuai C, Yang Y, Peng S, et al. Nd-induced honeycomb structure of intermetallic phase enhances the corrosion resistance of Mg alloys for bone implants［J］. J Mater Sci Mater Med, 2017, 28(9): 130.

［348］Kim Y M, Chang D Y, Kim H S, et al. Key factor influencing the ignition resistance of magnesium alloys at elevated temperatures［J］. Scripta Materialia, 2011, 65(11): 958-961.

［349］Wang J, Witte F, Xi T, et al. Recommendation for modifying current cytotoxicity testing standards for biodegradable magnesium-based materials[J]. Acta Biomaterialia, 2015, 21: 237-249.

[350] Jia Z, Xiong P, Shi Y, et al. Inhibitor encapsulated, self-healable and cytocompatible chitosan multilayer coating on biodegradable Mg alloy: a pH-responsive design[J]. J. Mater. Chem. B.

[351] Shi L L, Huang Y, Yang L, et al. Mechanical properties and corrosion behavior of Mg-Gd-Ca-Zr alloys for medical applications[J]. Journal of the Mechanical Behavior of Biomedical Materials, 2015, 47: 38-48.

[352] Hu Y, Zou S, Chen W, et al. Mineralization and drug release of hydroxyapatite/poly (l-lactic acid) nanocomposite scaffolds prepared by Pickering emulsion templating[J]. Colloids & Surfaces B Biointerfaces, 2014, 122: 559-565.

[353] Wu Q, Tang Y, Chen H, et al. In vitro and in vivo research of osteoblastic induced rat mesenchymal stem cells cultured onβ-TCP/PLLA porous scaffold[J]. Chinese Journal of Materials Research, 2006, 20(5): 538-543.

[354] Sabir M I, Xu X, Li L. A review on biodegradable polymeric materials for bone tissue engineering applications [J]. Journal of Materials Science, 2009, 44(21): 5713-5724.

[355] Shuai C, Shuai C, Feng P, et al. Silane Modified Diopside for Improved Interfacial Adhesion and Bioactivity of Composite Scaffolds[J]. Molecules, 2017, 22(4): 511.

[356] Pei F, Peng S, Ping W, et al. A space network structure constructed by tetraneedlelike ZnO whiskers supporting boron nitride nanosheets to enhance comprehensive properties of poly(L-lacti acid) scaffolds[J]. Scientific Reports, 2016, 6: 33385.

[357] Revie R W. 30. Microbiological Degradation of Polymeric Materials[M]. John Wiley & Sons, Inc., 2011: págs. 62-63.

[358] Ozdil D, Aydin H M. Polymers for medical and tissue engineering applications[J]. Journal of Chemical Technology & Biotechnology, 2015, 89(12): 1793-1810.

[359] I Iguez-franco F, Auras R, Dolan K, et al. Chemical recycling of poly(lactic acid) by water-ethanol solutions [J]. Polymer Degradation & Stability, 2018.

[360] Shuai C, Wu P, Zhong Y, et al. Polyetheretherketone/poly (glycolic acid) blend scaffolds with biodegradable properties[J]. Journal of Biomaterials Science Polymer Edition, 2016, 27(14): 1434-1446.

[361] Sun H, Qu T, Zhnag X, et al. Designing biomaterials for in situ periodontal tissue regeneration [J]. Biotechnology Progress, 2012, 28(1): 3-20.

[362] Tan L, Yu X, Wan P, et al. Biodegradable Materials for Bone Repairs: A Review[J]. Journal of Materials Science & Technology, 2013, 29(6): 503-513.

[363] Velde K V D, Kiekens P. Biopolymers: overview of several properties and consequences on their applications [J]. Polymer Testing, 2002, 21(4): 433-442.

[364] Zhang K, Wang H, Chen H, et al. Fabrication of silk fibroin blended P(LLA-CL) nanofibrous scaffolds for tissue engineering[J]. Journal of Biomedical Materials Research Part A, 2010, 93(3): 984.

[365] Vieira A, Vieira J, Ferra J, et al. Mechanical study of PLA-PCL fibers during in vitro degradation[J]. Journal of the mechanical behavior of biomedical materials, 2011, 4(3): 451-460.

[366] Hakkarainen M, Albertsson A C, Karlsson S. Weight losses and molecular weight changes correlated with the evolution of hydroxyacids in simulated in vivo degradation of homo- and copolymers of PLA and PGA[J]. Polymer Degradation & Stability, 2013, 52(3): 283-291.

[367] Mulvey R E. Modern ate chemistry: applications of synergic mixed alkali-metal-magnesium or-zinc reagents in synthesis and structure building[J]. Organometallics, 2006, 25(5): 1060-1075.

[368] Mulvey R E. ChemInform Abstract: s-Block Metal Inverse Crowns: Synthetic and Structural Synergism in

Mixed Alkali Metal-Magnesium (or Zinc) Amide Chemistry[J]. Cheminform, 2001, 32(40): 1049-1056.

[369] Cifuentes S C, Gavil N R, Lierlich M, et al. In vitro degradation of biodegradable polylactic acid/magnesium composites: relevance of Mg particle shape[J]. Acta Biomaterialia, 2016, 32(6): 348.

[370] Li H, Wu T, Zheng Y, et al. Fabrication and characterization of Mg/P(LLA-CL)-blended nanofiber scaffold [J]. Journal of Biomaterials Science Polymer Edition, 2014, 25(10): 1013-1027.

[371] Butt M S, Bai J, Wan X, et al. Mg alloy rod reinforced biodegradable poly-lactic acid composite for load bearing bone replacement[J]. Surface & Coatings Technology, 2016, 309.

[372] Hl G, Km H, R S, et al. Guidelines for the use of vitamins, trace elements, calcium, magnesium, and phosphorus in infants and children receiving total parenteral nutrition: report of the Subcommittee on Pediatric Parenteral Nutrient Requirements from the Committee on Clinical Pra[J]. The American journal of clinical nutrition, 1988, 48(5): 1324-1342.

[373] Wong H M, Chu P K, Leung F K L, et al. Engineered polycaprolactone-magnesium hybrid biodegradable porous scaffold for bone tissue engineering[J]. Progress in Natural Science: Materials International, 2014, 24 (5): 561-567.

[374] Brown A, Zaky S, Jr R H, et al. Porous magnesium/PLGA composite scaffolds for enhanced bone regeneration following tooth extraction[J]. Acta Biomaterialia, 2015, 11: 543-553.

[375] Cifuentes S C, Frutos E, Gonz Lez-carrasco J L, et al. Novel PLLA/magnesium composite for orthopedic applications: a proof of concept[J]. Materials Letters, 2012, 74(5): 239-242.

[376] Cifuentes S C, Lieblich M, L Pez F A, et al. Effect of Mg content on the thermal stability and mechanical behaviour of PLLA/Mg composites processed by hot extrusion[J]. Materials Science & Engineering C, 2017, 72: 18.

[377] Kim S M, Kang M H, Kim H E, et al. Innovative micro-textured hydroxyapatite and poly(l-lactic)-acid polymer composite film as a flexible, corrosion resistant, biocompatible, and bioactive coating for Mg implants [J]. Materials Science & Engineering C Materials for Biological Applications, 2017, 81: 97.

[378] Shi Y J, Pei J, Zhang J, et al. Enhanced corrosion resistance and cytocompatibility of biodegradable Mg alloys by introduction of Mg(OH)2 particles into poly (L-lactic acid) coating[J]. Scientific Reports, 2017, 7: 41796.

[379] Du G, Li J, Wang Z B, et al. Effect of Magnesium Addition on Behavior of Collision and Agglomeration between Solid Inclusion Particles on H13 Steel Melts[J]. Steel Research International, 2017, 88(3).

[380] Feng P, Peng S, Wu P, et al. A nano-sandwich construct built with graphene nanosheets and carbon nanotubes enhances mechanical properties of hydroxyapatite-polyetheretherketone scaffolds[J]. International Journal of Nanomedicine, 2016, 11(default): 3487-3500.

[381] Neumann I A, Ribeiro A M. Biodegradable poly (l-lactic acid) (PLLA) and PLLA-3-arm blend membranes: The use of PLLA-3-arm as a plasticizer[J]. Polymer Testing, 2017.

[382] Shuai C, Shuai C, Wu P, et al. Characterization and Bioactivity Evaluation of (Polyetheretherketone/ Polyglycolicacid)-Hydroyapatite Scaffolds for Tissue Regeneration[J]. Materials, 2016, 9(11): 934.

[383] Indulekha K, Thomas D, Supriya N, et al. Inherently flame retardant vinyl bearing hyperbranched polysiloxanes having improved thermal stability-Ceramization and analysis of associated thermal properties[J]. Polymer Degradation & Stability, 2018, 147: 12-24.

[384] Cifuentes S C, Frutos E, Benavente R, et al. Assessment of mechanical behavior of PLA composites reinforced with Mg micro-particles through depth-sensing indentations analysis[J]. J Mech Behav Biomed Mater, 2017, 65: 781-790.

[385] Hollister S J. Porous scaffold design for tissue engineering[J]. Nature Materials, 2005, 4(7): 518.

[386] Jiang S, Wang H, Chu C, et al. Synthesis of antimicrobial Nisin-phosphorylated soybean protein isolate/poly (L-lactic acid)/ZrO$_2$ membranes [J]. International Journal of Biological Macromolecules, 2015, 72: 502-509.

[387] Stahl T. Development of a Biodegradable Polymer-Metal Composite as a Novel Biomaterial[J]. 2016.

[388] Wan P, Yuan C, Tan L L, et al. Fabrication and evaluation of bioresorbable PLLA/magnesium and PLLA/ magnesium fluoride hybrid composites for orthopedic implants[J]. Composites Science & Technology, 2014, 98: 36-43.

[389] Bhang S H, Lim J S, Choi C Y, et al. The behavior of neural stem cells on biodegradable synthetic polymers [J]. Journal of Biomaterials Science Polymer Edition, 2007, 18(2): 223-239.

[390] Chen Y, Song Y, Zhang S, et al. Interaction between a high purity magnesium surface and PCL and PLA coatings during dynamic degradation[J]. Biomedical Materials, 2011, 6(2): 025005.

[391] Nembach E. Particle strengthening of metals and alloys[J]. Materials Science & Technology, 1997, 3(5): 329-337.

[392] Lee C J, Huang J C, Hsieh P J. Mg based nano-composites fabricated by friction stir processing[J]. Scripta Materialia, 2006, 54(7): 1415-1420.

[393] Y. H, Cheng, Y. F, et al. In vitro Study on Biodegradable AZ31 Magnesium Alloy Fibers Reinforced PLGA Composite[J]. Journal of Materials Science & Technology, 2013, 29(6): 545-550.

[394] Zreiqat H, Howlett C R, Zannettino A, et al. Mechanisms of magnesium-stimulated adhesion of osteoblastic cells to commonly used orthopaedic implants[J]. Journal of Biomedical Materials Research, 2002, 62(2): 175-184.

[395] Banin E, Hughes D, O. P. Kuipers, Editorial: Bacterial pathogens, antibiotics and antibiotic resistance, FEMS Microbiol. Rev., 41 (2017).

[396] E. Anes, Acting on Actin During Bacterial Infection, 2017.

[397] B. Nabil, E. A. Ahmida, C. Christine, V. Julien, A. Abdelkrim, Polyfunctional cotton fabrics with catalytic activity and antibacterial capacity, Chem. Eng. J., (2018).

[398] D. L. Boschetto, L. Lerin, R. Cansian, S. B. C. Pergher, M. D. Luccio, Preparation and antimicrobial activity of polyethylene composite films with silver exchanged zeolite-Y, Chem. Eng. J., 204-206 (2012) 210-216.

[399] Yongjun, Qiao, Zhongjun, Zhai, Limei, Chen, Hong, Cytocompatible 3D chitosan/hydroxyapatite composites endowed with antibacterial properties: toward a self-sterilized bone tissue engineering scaffold, Sci Bulletin, 60 (2015) 1193-1202.

[400] H. Chen, G. Lan, L. Ran, Y. Xiao, K. Yu, B. Lu, F. Dai, D. Wu, F. Lu, A novel wound dressing based on a Konjac glucomannan/silver nanoparticle composite sponge effectively kills bacteria and accelerates wound healing, Carbohydr. Polym., 183 (2018) 70.

[401] D. Zhao, Y. Gao, S. Nie, Z. Liu, F. Wang, P. Liu, S. Hu, Self-assembly of honeycomb-like calcium-aluminum-silicate-hydrate (C-A-S-H) on ceramsite sand and its application in photocatalysis, Chem. Eng. J., (2018).

[402] X. Zhou, W. Weng, B. Chen, W. Feng, W. Wang, W. Nie, L. Chen, X. Mo, J. Su, C. He, Mesoporous silica nanoparticles/gelatin porous composite scaffolds with localized and sustained release of vancomycin for treatment of infected bone defects, Journal of Materials Chemistry B, 6 (2018).

[403] P. Cheng, Y. Liu, Z. Yi, X. Wang, M. Li, Q. Liu, K. Liu, D. Wang, In situ prepared nanosized Pt-Ag/

PDA/PVA- co -PE nanofibrous membrane for highly-efficient catalytic reduction of p -nitrophenol, Composites Communications, 9 (2018) 11-16.

[404] A. Hoppe, N. S. Güldal, A. R. Boccaccini, A review of the biological response to ionic dissolution products from bioactive glasses and glass-ceramics, Biomaterials, 32 (2011) 2757-2774.

[405] Kargozar S, Montazerian M, Hamzehlou S, et al. Mesoporous bioactive glasses (MBGs): Promising platforms for antibacterial strategies[J]. Acta Biomater, 2018.

[406] X. Wang, F. Cheng, J. Liu, J. H. Smått, D. Gepperth, M. Lastusaari, C. Xu, L. Hupa, Biocomposites of copper-containing mesoporous bioactive glass and nanofibrillated cellulose: biocompatibility and angiogenic promotion in chronic wound healing application, Acta Biomater., 46 (2016) 286-298.

[407] Y. Liu, S. Yang, S. N. Yin, L. Feng, Y. Zang, H. Xue, In situ construction of fibrous AgNPs/g-C 3 N 4 aerogel toward light-driven CO x -free methanol dehydrogenation at room temperature, Chem. Eng. J., 334 (2017).

[408] B. Pant, P. Pokharel, A. P. Tiwari, P. S. Saud, M. Park, Z. K. Ghouri, S. Choi, S. J. Park, H. Y. Kim, Characterization and antibacterial properties of aminophenol grafted and Ag NPs decorated graphene nanocomposites, Ceram. Int., 41 (2015) 5656-5662.

[409] B. Bhaduri, M. Engel, T. Polubesova, W. Wu, B. Xing, B. Chefetz, Dual functionality of an Ag-Fe$_3$O$_4$-carbon nanotube composite material: Catalytic reduction and antibacterial activity, Journal of Environmental Chemical Engineering, 6 (2018) 4103-4113.

[410] U. Farooq, M. Danish, S. Lu, M. Naqvi, Z. Qiu, Q. Sui, A step forward towards synthesizing a stable and regeneratable nanocomposite for remediation of trichloroethene, Chem. Eng. J., 347 (2018).

[411] S. Du, Y. Luo, Z. Liao, W. Zhang, X. Li, T. Liang, F. Zuo, K. Ding, New insights into the formation mechanism of gold nanoparticles using dopamine as a reducing agent, J. Colloid Interface Sci., 523 (2018) 27-34.

[412] Cong Y, Xia T, Zou M, et al. Mussel-inspired polydopamine coating as a versatile platform for synthesizing polystyrene/Ag nanocomposite particles with enhanced antibacterial activities[J]. J Mater Chem B, 2014, 2 (22):3450.

[413] W. Xia, J. Chang, Well-ordered mesoporous bioactive glasses (MBG): a promising bioactive drug delivery system, J. Control. Release, 110 (2006) 522-530.

[414] Y. Xu, P. Wu, P. Feng, W. Guo, W. Yang, C. Shuai, Interfacial reinforcement in a poly-l-lactic acid/mesoporous bioactive glass scaffold via polydopamine, Colloids Surf. B Biointerfaces, (2018) 45-53.

[415] Faure E, FalentinDaudré, Céline, Jérôme, Christine, et al. Catechols as versatile platforms in polymer chemistry[J]. Prog Polym Sci, 2013, 38(1):236-270.

[416] P. Prieto, V. Nistor, K. Nouneh, M. Oyama, M. Abd-Lefdil, R. Díaz, XPS study of silver, nickel and bimetallic silver-nickel nanoparticles prepared by seed-mediated growth, Appl. Surf. Sci., 258 (2012) 8807-8813.

[417] H. F. Teoh, P. Dzung, W. Q. Lim, J. H. Chua, K. K. Lee, Z. Hu, H. Tan, E. S. Tok, C. H. Sow, Microlandscaping on a graphene oxide film via localized decoration of Ag nanoparticles, Nanoscale, 6 (2014) 3143-3149.

[418] A. Gupta, A. R. Koirala, B. Joshi, S. Khanal, B. Gupta, N. Parajuli, Synthesis of Silver Nanoparticles Using Leaves of Taraxacum officinale and Their Antimicrobial Activities, Advanced Science, 9 (2017) 221-228.

[419] O. J. Garcíaricard, J. C. Silvamartínez, A. J. Hernándezmaldonado, Systematic evaluation of textural

properties, activation temperature and gas uptake of Cu2 (pzdc) 2L [L = dipyridyl-based ligands] porous coordination pillared-layer networks, Dalton Trans. , 41 (2012) 8922-8930.

[420] L. Xia, M. Xu, G. Cheng, L. Yang, Y. Guo, D. Li, D. Fang, Q. Zhang, H. Liu, Facile construction of Ag nanoparticles encapsulated into carbon nanotubes with robust antibacterial activity, Carbon, 130 (2018) 775-781.

[421] L. Zhang, Z. Liu, Y. Wang, R. Xie, X. J. Ju, W. Wang, L. Lin, L. Y. Chu, Facile immobilization of Ag nanoparticles on microchannel walls in microreactors for catalytic applications, Chem. Eng. J. , 309 (2017) 691-699.

[422] M. E. Lynge, d. W. R. Van, A. Postma, B. Städler, Polydopamine--a nature-inspired polymer coating for biomedical science, Nanoscale, 3 (2011) 4916-4928.

[423] H. Xu, X. Liu, G. Su, B. Zhang, D. Wang, Electrostatic repulsion-controlled formation of polydopamine-gold Janus particles, Langmuir the Acs Journal of Surfaces & Colloids, 28 (2012) 13060-13065.

[424] M. Trchová, J. Stejskal, The reduction of silver nitrate to metallic silver inside polyaniline nanotubes and on oligoaniline microspheres, Synth. Met. , 160 (2010) 1479-1486.

[425] S. Zhu, H. Sun, H. Geng, D. Liu, X. Zhang, Q. Cai, X. Yang, Dual functional polylactide-hydroxyapatite nanocomposites for bone regeneration with nano-silver being loaded: Via reductive polydopamine, Rsc Advances, 6 (2016) 91349-91360.

[426] Wu C, Zhang G, Xia T, et al. Bioinspired synthesis of polydopamine/Ag nanocomposite particles with antibacterial activities[J]. Mat Sci Eng-C Mater, 2015, 55:155-165.

[427] Hild N, Tawakoli P N, Halter J G, et al. pH-dependent antibacterial effects on oral microorganisms through pure PLGA implants and composites with nanosized bioactive glass[J]. Acta Biomater. , 2013, 9(11):9118-9125.

[428] Wu C, Ramaswamy Y, Zhu Y, et al. The effect of mesoporous bioactive glass on the physiochemical, biological and drug-release properties of poly (dl-lactide-co-glycolide) films [J]. Biomaterials, 2009, 30 (12):2199-2208.

[429] Boccaccini A R, Maquet V. Bioresorbable and bioactive polymer/Bioglass® composites with tailored pore structure for tissue engineering applications[J]. Compos Sci. Technol. , 2003, 63(16):2417-2429.

[430] D. Mcshan, P. C. Ray, H. Yu, Molecular toxicity mechanism of nanosilver, J. Food Drug Anal. , 22 (2014) 116-127.

[431] J. S. Kim, E. Kuk, K. N. Yu, J. H. Kim, S. J. Park, H. J. Lee, S. H. Kim, Y. K. Park, Y. H. Park, C. Y. Hwang, Antimicrobial effects of silver nanoparticles, Nanomedicine Nanotechnology Biology & Medicine, 3 (2007) 95-101.

[432] X. Zhu, D. Wu, W. Wang, F. Tan, P. K. Wong, X. Wang, X. Qiu, X. Qiao, Highly effective antibacterial activity and synergistic effect of Ag-MgO nanocomposite against Escherichia coli, J. Alloys Compd. , 684 (2016) 282-290.

[433] I. V. Sukhorukova, A. N. Sheveyko, N. V. Shvindina, E. A. Denisenko, S. G. Ignatov, D. Shtansky, Approaches for Controlled Ag + Ion Release: Influence of Surface Topography, Roughness, and Bactericide Content, ACS Appl. Mater. Interfaces, 9 (2017) 4259-4271.

[434] Z. Wang, S. Liu, J. Ma, G. Qu, X. Wang, S. Yu, J. He, J. Liu, T. Xia, G. B. Jiang, Silver nanoparticles induced RNA polymerase-silver binding and RNA transcription inhibition in erythroid progenitor cells, ACS Nano, 7 (2013) 4171-4186.

[435] F. Mirzajani, A. Ghassempour, A. Aliahmadi, M. A. Esmaeili, Antibacterial effect of silver nanoparticles on

Staphylococcus aureus, Biometals, 24 (2011) 135-141.

［436］J. J. Lin, W. C. Lin, R. X. Dong, S. H. Hsu, The cellular responses and antibacterial activities of silver nanoparticles stabilized by different polymers, Nanotechnology, 23 (2012) 065102.

［437］S. Yang, J. Wang, H. Tan, F. Zeng, C. Liu, Mechanically robust PEGDA-MSNs-OH nanocomposite hydrogel with hierarchical meso-macroporous structure for tissue engineering, Soft Matter, 8 (2012) 8981.

［438］B. Sarker, J. Hum, S. N. Nazhat, A. R. Boccaccini, Combining Collagen and Bioactive Glasses for Bone Tissue Engineering: A Review, Advanced Healthcare Materials, 4 (2015) 176-194.

［439］D. Schaubroeck, Y. Vercammen, L. V. Vaeck, E. Vanderleyden, P. Dubruel, J. Vanfleteren, Surface characterization and stability of an epoxy resin surface modified with polyamines grafted on polydopamine, Appl. Surf. Sci. , 303 (2014) 465-472.

［440］Ali S, Farooq I, Iqbal K. A review of the effect of various ions on the properties and the clinical applications of novel bioactive glasses in medicine and dentistry［J］. The Saudi Dental J, 2014, 26(1):1-5.

［441］Murphy C, Kolan K, Li W, et al. 3D bioprinting of stem cells and polymer/bioactive glass composite scaffolds for bone tissue engineering［J］. International Journal of Bioprinting, 2017, 3(1): 53-63.

［442］J. Liu, K. He, W. Wu, T. B. Song, M. G. Kanatzidis, In Situ Synthesis of Highly Dispersed and Ultrafine Metal Nanoparticles from Chalcogels, J. Am. Chem. Soc. , 139 (2017) 2900.

［443］Y. T. Li, S. B. Lin, L. C. Chen, H. H. Chen, Antimicrobial activity and controlled release of nanosilvers in bacterial cellulose composites films incorporated with montmorillonites, Cellulose, 24 (2017) 4871-4883.

［444］C. Gao, F. Pei, S. Peng, C. Shuai, Carbon nanotubes, graphene and boron nitride nanotubes reinforced bioactive ceramics for bone repair, Acta Biomaterialia, 61 (2017) 1.

［445］Y. Liu, Y. Fang, X. Liu, X. Wang, B. Yang, Mussel-inspired modification of carbon fiber via polyethyleneimine/polydopamine co-deposition for the improved interfacial adhesion, Composites Science & Technology, 151 (2017).

［446］Y. Ling, W. Li, B. Wang, W. Gan, C. Zhu, M. A. Brady, C. Wang, Epoxy resin reinforced with nanothin polydopamine-coated carbon nanotubes: a study of the interfacial polymer layer thickness, Rsc Advances, 6 (2016) 31037-31045.

［447］Shuai C, Guo W, Wu P, et al. A graphene oxide-Ag co-dispersing nanosystem: Dual synergistic effects on antibacterial activities and mechanical properties of polymer scaffolds［J］. Chemical Engineering Journal, 2018, 347: 322-333.

［448］El-kady A M, Saad E A, El-hady B M A, et al. Synthesis of silicate glass/poly (L-lactide) composite scaffolds by freeze-extraction technique: characterization and in vitro bioactivity evaluation［J］. Ceramics International, 2010, 36(3): 995-1009.

［449］Eltohamy M, Kundu B, Moon J, et al. Anti-bacterial zinc-doped calcium silicate cements: Bone filler［J］. Ceramics International, 2018, 44(11): 13031-13038.

［450］Jayasree R, Kumar T S, Perumal G, et al. Drug and ion releasing tetracalcium phosphate based dual action cement for regenerative treatment of infected bone defects［J］. Ceramics International, 2018, 44 (8): 9227-9235.

［451］Shuai C, Guo W. Calcium Silicate Improved Bioactivity and Mechanical Properties of Poly(3-hydroxybutyrate-co-3-hydroxyvalerate) Scaffolds［J］. Polymers, 2017, 9(12): 175.

［452］Lendvai L, Apostolov A, Karger-kocsis J. Characterization of layered silicate-reinforced blends of thermoplastic starch (TPS) and poly (butylene adipate-co-terephthalate)［J］. Carbohydrate polymers, 2017, 173: 566-572.

[453] Corcione C E, Gervaso F, Scalera F, et al. Highly loaded hydroxyapatite microsphere/PLA porous scaffolds obtained by fused deposition modelling[J]. Ceramics International, 2018.

[454] Heidari F, Razavi M, Bahrololoom M E, et al. Evaluation of the mechanical properties, in vitro biodegradability and cytocompatibility of natural chitosan/hydroxyapatite/nano-Fe_3O_4 composite[J]. Ceramics International, 2018, 44(1): 275-281.

[455] Cyras V P, Manfredi L B, Ton-that M-T, et al. Physical and mechanical properties of thermoplastic starch/montmorillonite nanocomposite films[J]. Carbohydrate Polymers, 2008, 73(1): 55-63.

[456] Balakrishnan H, Hassan A, Imran M, et al. Aging of Toughened Polylactic Acid Nanocomposites: Water Absorption, Hygrothermal Degradation and Soil Burial Analysis[J]. Journal of Polymers and the Environment, 2011, 19(4): 863-875.

[457] Yahiaoui F, Benhacine F, Ferfera-harrar H, et al. Development of antimicrobial PCL/nanoclay nanocomposite films with enhanced mechanical and water vapor barrier properties for packaging applications[J]. Polymer Bulletin, 2014, 72(2): 235-254.

[458] Olad A, Farshi Azhar F. The synergetic effect of bioactive ceramic and nanoclay on the properties of chitosan-gelatin/nanohydroxyapatite-montmorillonite scaffold for bone tissue engineering[J]. Ceramics International, 2014, 40(7): 10061-10072.

[459] Zhang X, Wang H, Liu Z, et al. Fabrication of durable fluorine-free superhydrophobic polyethersulfone (PES) composite coating enhanced by assembled MMT-SiO_2 nanoparticles[J]. Applied Surface Science, 2017, 396: 1580-1588.

[460] Ling Y P, Ool C-H, Matsumoto A, et al. Properties evaluation and fabrication of green clay reformulated from water sludge[J]. Ceramics International, 2018, 44(2): 1411-1419.

[461] Terziĉ A, Pezo L, Andriĉ L, et al. Optimization of bentonite clay mechano-chemical activation using artificial neural network modeling[J]. Ceramics International, 2017, 43(2): 2549-2562.

[462] Shi J, Lou Z, Yang M, et al. An interlayer expansion model for counterion-intercalated montmorillonite from first-principles calculations[J]. Computational Materials Science, 2015, 96: 134-139.

[463] Teich-mcgoldrick S L, Greathouse J A, Jové-colón C F, et al. Swelling Properties of Montmorillonite and Beidellite Clay Minerals from Molecular Simulation: Comparison of Temperature, Interlayer Cation, and Charge Location Effects[J]. The Journal of Physical Chemistry C, 2015, 119(36): 20880-20891.

[464] Yi H, Jia F, Zhao Y, et al. Surface wettability of montmorillonite (0 0 1) surface as affected by surface charge and exchangeable cations: A molecular dynamic study[J]. Applied Surface Science, 2018, 459: 148-154.

[465] Chen C, Liu H, Chen T, et al. An insight into the removal of Pb(II), Cu(II), Co(II), Cd(II), Zn(II), Ag(I), Hg(I), Cr(VI) by Na(I)-montmorillonite and Ca(II)-montmorillonite[J]. Applied Clay Science, 2015, 118: 239-247.

[466] Uddin M K. A review on the adsorption of heavy metals by clay minerals, with special focus on the past decade[J]. Chemical Engineering Journal, 2017, 308: 438-462.

[467] Choi Y-S, Kim K-H, Kim D-G, et al. Synthesis and characterization of self-cross-linkable and bactericidal methacrylate polymers having renewable cardanol moieties for surface coating applications[J]. RSC Adv., 2014, 4(78): 41195-41203.

[468] Wu H, Xie H, He G, et al. Effects of the pH and anions on the adsorption of tetracycline on iron-montmorillonite[J]. Applied Clay Science, 2016, 119: 161-169.

[469] Zhou C-H, Zhang D, Tong D-S, et al. Paper-like composites of cellulose acetate-organo-montmorillonite for

removal of hazardous anionic dye in water[J]. Chemical Engineering Journal, 2012, 209: 223-234.

[470] Boehm R D, Daniels J, Stafslien S, et al. Polyglycolic acid microneedles modified with inkjet-deposited antifungal coatings[J]. Biointerphases, 2015, 10(1): 011004.

[471] Hopp B, Smausz T, Kecskeméti G, et al. Femtosecond pulsed laser deposition of biological and biocompatible thin layers[J]. Applied Surface Science, 2007, 253(19): 7806-7809.

[472] Camejo-abreu c, Tabernero V, Alba M D, et al. Enhanced activity of clays and its crucial role for the activity in ethylene polymerization[J]. Journal of Molecular Catalysis A Chemical, 2014, 393(18): 96-104.

[473] Chen K, Guo B, Luo J. Quaternized carboxymethyl chitosan/organic montmorillonite nanocomposite as a novel cosmetic ingredient against skin aging[J]. Carbohydrate polymers, 2017, 173: 100-106.

[474] Feng P, Guo X, Gao C, et al. Diopside modified porous polyglycolide scaffolds with improved properties[J]. RSC Advances, 2015, 5(68): 54822-54829.

[475] Fu S Y, Feng X Q, Lauke B, et al. Effects of particle size, particle/matrix interface adhesion and particle loading on mechanical properties of particulate-polymer composites[J]. Composites Part B Engineering, 2008, 39(6): 933-961.

[476] Yang J, Zhao J-J, Han C-R, et al. Keys to enhancing mechanical properties of silica nanoparticle composites hydrogels: The role of network structure and interfacial interactions[J]. Composites Science and Technology, 2014, 95: 1-7.

[477] Bikiaris D N. Nanocomposites of aliphatic polyesters: An overview of the effect of different nanofillers on enzymatic hydrolysis and biodegradation of polyesters[J]. Polymer Degradation and Stability, 2013, 98(9): 1908-1928.

[478] Sailema-palate G P, Vidaurre A, Campillo-fernández A J, et al. A comparative study on Poly (ε-caprolactone) film degradation at extreme pH values[J]. Polymer Degradation and Stability, 2016, 130: 118-125.

[479] Shie M Y, Ding S J, Chang H C. The role of silicon in osteoblast-like cell proliferation and apoptosis[J]. Acta Biomaterialia, 2011, 7(6): 2604-2614.

[480] Magallanesperdomo M, De aza A H, Mateus A Y, et al. In vitro study of the proliferation and growth of human bone marrow cells on apatite-wollastonite-2M glass ceramics[J]. Acta Biomaterialia, 2010, 6(6): 2254-2263.

[481] Zhai W, Lu H, Wu C, et al. Stimulatory effects of the ionic products from Ca-Mg-Si bioceramics on both osteogenesis and angiogenesis in vitro[J]. Acta Biomaterialia, 2013, 9(8): 8004-8014.

[482] Hengne A, Malawadkar A, Biradar N, et al. Surface synergism of an Ag-Ni/ZrO$_2$ nanocomposite for the catalytic transfer hydrogenation of bio-derived platform molecules[J]. Rsc Advances, 2014, 4(19): 9730-9736.

[483] Le Ouay B, Stellacci F. Antibacterial activity of silver nanoparticles: A surface science insight[J]. Nano Today, 2015, 10(3): 339-354.

[484] Marambiojones C, Hoek E M V. A review of the antibacterial effects of silver nanomaterials and potential implications for human health and the environment[J]. Journal of Nanoparticle Research, 2010, 12(5): 1531-1551.

[485] Dang W, Li T, Li B, et al. A bifunctional scaffold with CuFeSe2 nanocrystals for tumor therapy and bone reconstruction[J]. Biomaterials, 2018, 160: 92-106.

[486] Ma H, Jiang C, Zhai D, et al. A bifunctional biomaterial with photothermal effect for tumor therapy and bone regeneration[J]. Advanced Functional Materials, 2016, 26(8): 1197-1208.

[487] Zhang Y, Zhai D, Xu M, et al. 3D-printed bioceramic scaffolds with a Fe_3O_4/graphene oxide nanocomposite interface for hyperthermia therapy of bone tumor cells[J]. Journal of Materials Chemistry B, 2016, 4(17): 2874-2886.

[488] Ding D, Xie Y, Li K, et al. Black plasma-sprayed Ta2O5 coatings with photothermal effect for bone tumor therapy[J]. Ceramics International, 2018, 44(11): 12002-12006.

[489] Lu Y, Li M, Li L, et al. High-activity chitosan/nano hydroxyapatite/zoledronic acid scaffolds for simultaneous tumor inhibition, bone repair and infection eradication[J]. Materials Science and Engineering: C, 2018, 82: 225-233.

[490] Ma H, Li T, Huan Z, et al. 3D printing of high-strength bioscaffolds for the synergistic treatment of bone cancer[J]. NPG Asia Materials, 2018: 1.

[491] Li M, Wang W, Zhu Y, et al. Molecular and cellular mechanisms for zoledronic acid-loaded magnesium-strontium alloys to inhibit giant cell tumors of bone[J]. Acta biomaterialia, 2018, 77: 365-379.

[492] Kawanishi S, Hiraku Y, Pinlaor S, et al. Oxidative and nitrative DNA damage in animals and patients with inflammatory diseases in relation to inflammation-related carcinogenesis[J]. Biological chemistry, 2006, 387 (4): 365-372.

[493] Song J, Li J, Qiao J, et al. PKD prevents H_2O_2-induced apoptosis via NF-κB and p38 MAPK in RIE-1 cells [J]. Biochemical and biophysical research communications, 2009, 378(3): 610-614.

[494] Chen G, Wang F, Trachootham D, et al. Preferential killing of cancer cells with mitochondrial dysfunction by natural compounds[J]. Mitochondrion, 2010, 10(6): 614-625.

[495] Pelicano H, Carney D, Huang P. ROS stress in cancer cells and therapeutic implications[J]. Drug resistance updates, 2004, 7(2): 97-110.

[496] Li Z-Y, Yang Y, Ming M, et al. Mitochondrial ROS generation for regulation of autophagic pathways in cancer[J]. Biochemical and biophysical research communications, 2011, 414(1): 5-8.

[497] Wang H, Zhang Y, Du Y. Ovarian and breast cancer spheres are similar in transcriptomic features and sensitive to fenretinide[J]. BioMed research international, 2013, 2013.

[498] Shen L, Lan Z, Sun X, et al. Proteomic analysis of lanthanum citrate-induced apoptosis in human cervical carcinoma SiHa cells[J]. Biometals, 2010, 23(6): 1179-1189.

[499] Yu L, Xiong J, Guo L, et al. The effects of lanthanum chloride on proliferation and apoptosis of cervical cancer cells: involvement of let-7a and miR-34a microRNAs[J]. Biometals, 2015, 28(5): 879-890.

[500] Zhang H, Wang C, Zhu L, et al. Growth and Characterization of Series Nd: Gd x La 1-x VO 4 (x = 0.80, 0.60, 0.45) Crystals[J]. Journal of materials research, 2002, 17(3): 556-562.

[501] Sze A, Erickson D, Ren L, et al. Zeta-potential measurement using the Smoluchowski equation and the slope of the current-time relationship in electroosmotic flow[J]. Journal of colloid and interface science, 2003, 261 (2): 402-410.

[502] Hu J, Jia X, Li Q, et al. Binding of La3 + to calmodulin and its effects on the interaction between calmodulin and calmodulin binding peptide, polistes mastoparan[J]. Biochemistry, 2004, 43(10): 2688-2698.

[503] Dong S, Zhao Y, Liu H, et al. Duality of effect of La^{3+} on mitochondrial permeability transition pore depending on the concentration[J]. Biometals, 2009, 22(6): 917.

[504] Heffeter P, Jakupec M A, K Rner W, et al. Anticancer activity of the lanthanum compound [tris (1, 10-phenanthroline) lanthanum (III)] trithiocyanate (KP772; FFC24)[J]. Biochemical pharmacology, 2006, 71(4): 426-440.

[505] Hongwei C, Sisun L, Lifang M, et al. Inhibitory effect of lanthanum chloride on migration and invasion of

cervical cancer cells[J]. Journal of Rare Earths, 2013, 31(1): 94-100.

[506] Liu L, Gebresellasie K, Collins B, et al. Degradation rates of pure zinc, magnesium, and magnesium alloys measured by volume loss, mass loss, and hydrogen evolution[J]. Applied Sciences, 2018, 8(9): 1459.

[507] Parande G, Manakari V, Gupta H, et al. Magnesium-β-tricalcium phosphate composites as a potential orthopedic implant: A mechanical/damping/immersion perspective[J]. Metals, 2018, 8(5): 343.

[508] Xiong H, Liang Z, Wang Z, et al. Mechanical Properties and Degradation Behavior of Mg (100-7x) Zn6xYx (x = 0.2, 0.4, 0.6, 0.8) Alloys[J]. Metals, 2018, 8(4): 261.

[509] Cao N Q, Pham D N, Kai N, et al. In vitro corrosion properties of Mg matrix in situ composites fabricated by spark plasma sintering[J]. Metals, 2017, 7(9): 358.

[510] Yang Y, Wu P, Wang Q, et al. The enhancement of Mg corrosion resistance by alloying Mn and laser-melting [J]. Materials, 2016, 9(4): 216.

[511] Sun W, Zhang G, Tan L, et al. The fluoride coated AZ31B magnesium alloy improves corrosion resistance and stimulates bone formation in rabbit model[J]. Materials Science and Engineering: C, 2016, 63: 506-511.

[512] Pu S, Chen M, Chen Y, et al. Zirconium ions integrated in 1-hydroxyethylidene-1, 1-diphosphonic acid (HEDP) as a metalorganic-like complex coating on biodegradable magnesium for corrosion control[J]. Corrosion Science, 2018, 144: 277-287.

[513] Weizbauer A, Seitz J-M, Werle P, et al. Novel magnesium alloy Mg-2La caused no cytotoxic effects on cells in physiological conditions[J]. Materials Science and Engineering: C, 2014, 41: 267-273.

[514] Myrissa A, Agha N A, Lu Y, et al. In vitro and in vivo comparison of binary Mg alloys and pure Mg[J]. Materials Science and Engineering: C, 2016, 61: 865-874.

[515] Zhang Y, Li J-Y, Liaw P K, et al. Effects of heat treatment on the mechanical properties and corrosion behaviour of the Mg-2Zn-0.2 Mn-xNd alloys[J]. Journal of Alloys and Compounds, 2018, 769: 552-565.

[516] Zhang Y, Li J, Lai H, et al. Effect of homogenization on microstructure characteristics, corrosion and biocompatibility of Mg-Zn-Mn-xCa alloys[J]. Materials, 2018, 11(2): 227.

[517] Jiang B, Xiang Q, Atrens A, et al. Influence of crystallographic texture and grain size on the corrosion behaviour of as-extruded Mg alloy AZ31 sheets[J]. Corrosion Science, 2017, 126: 374-380.

[518] Ding Y, Lin J, Wen C, et al. Mechanical properties, in vitro corrosion and biocompatibility of newly developed biodegradable Mg-Zr-Sr-Ho alloys for biomedical applications[J]. Scientific reports, 2016, 6: 31990.

[519] Willbold E, Gu X, Albert D, et al. Effect of the addition of low rare earth elements (lanthanum, neodymium, cerium) on the biodegradation and biocompatibility of magnesium[J]. Acta biomaterialia, 2015, 11: 554-562.

[520] Fitzpatrick L A. Differences in the actions of calcium versus lanthanum to influence parathyroid hormone release[J]. Endocrinology, 1990, 127(2): 711-715.

[521] Weiss G B. Cellular pharmacology of lanthanum[J]. Annual review of pharmacology, 1974, 14(1): 343-354.

[522] Liu H, Yuan L, Yang X, et al. La3 + , Gd3 + and Yb3 + induced changes in mitochondrial structure, membrane permeability, cytochrome c release and intracellular ROS level[J]. Chemico-biological interactions, 2003, 146(1): 27-37.

[523] Orzolek A, Wysocki P, Strzezek J, et al. Superoxide dismutase (SOD) in boar spermatozoa: Purification, biochemical properties and changes in activity during semen storage (16 C) in different extenders[J].

reproductive biology, 2013, 13(1): 34-40.

[524] Perillo B, Di Santi A, Cernera G, et al. Nuclear receptor-induced transcription is driven by spatially and timely restricted waves of ROS: the role of Akt, IKKα, and DNA damage repair enzymes[J]. Nucleus, 2014, 5(5): 482-491.

[525] Clement J A. Studies of Bioactive Natural Products and Mechanism-Based Bioassays [D]. Virginia Tech, 2005.

[526] Dhand C, Ong S T, Dwivedi N, et al. Bio-inspired in situ crosslinking and mineralization of electrospun collagen scaffolds for bone tissue engineering[J]. Biomaterials, 2016, 104: 323-338.

[527] Naveena N. Biomimetic composites and stem cells interaction for bone and cartilage tissue regeneration[J]. Journal of Materials Chemistry, 2012, 22(12): 5239-5253.

[528] Praemer A, Furner S, Rice D P. Musculoskeletal conditions in the United States [J]. Musculoskeletal Conditions in the United States, 1992.

[529] Caterini R, Potenza V, Ippolito E, et al. Treatment of recalcitrant atrophic non-union of the humeral shaft with BMP-7, autologous bone graft and hydroxyapatite pellets[J]. Injury-international Journal of the Care of the Injured, 2016, 47: S71-S77.

[530] Schwartz A M, Schenker M L, Ahn J, et al. Building better bone: The weaving of biologic and engineering strategies for managing bone loss[J]. Journal of Orthopaedic Research, 2017, 35(9): 1855.

[531] Bone R C, Balk R A, Cerra F B, et al. Definitions for Sepsis and Organ Failure and Guidelines for the Use of Innovative Therapies in Sepsis[J]. Chest, 1992, 101(6): 1644-1655.

[532] Hu K, Olsen B R. The roles of vascular endothelial growth factor in bone repair and regeneration[J]. Bone, 2016, 91: 30-38.

[533] Yang F, Wang J, Hou J, et al. Bone regeneration using cell-mediated responsive degradable PEG - based scaffolds incorporating with rhBMP-2[J]. Biomaterials, 2013, 34(5): 1514-1528.

[534] Rumpler M, Woesz A, F, Manjubala I, et al. Three-dimensional growth behavior of osteoblasts on biomimetic hydroxylapatite scaffolds[J]. Journal of Biomedical Materials Research Part A, 2010, 81A(1): 40-50.

[535] Zhang H, Ahmad M, Gronowicz G. Effects of transforming growth factor-beta 1 (TGF-1) on in vitro mineralization of human osteoblasts on implant materials[J]. Biomaterials, 2003, 24(12): 2013-2020.

[536] Zhu Y, Yang Q, Yang M, et al. Protein Corona of Magnetic Hydroxyapatite Scaffold Improves Cell Proliferation via Activation of Mitogen-Activated Protein Kinase Signaling Pathway[J]. Acs Nano, 2017, 11(4): 3690.

[537] Puricelli E, Dutra N B, Ponzoni D. Histological evaluation of the influence of magnetic field application in autogenous bone grafts in rats[J]. Head & Face Medicine, 2009, 5(1): 1-6.

[538] Kim I S, Song J K, Zhang Y L, et al. Biphasic electric current stimulates proliferation and induces VEGF production in osteoblasts[J]. Biochimica Et Biophysica Acta Molecular Cell Research, 2006, 1763(9): 907-916.

[539] Panseri S, Russo A, Sartori M, et al. Modifying bone scaffold architecture in vivo with permanent magnets to facilitate fixation of magnetic scaffolds[J]. Bone, 2013, 56(2): 432-439.

[540] Jiang P, Zhang Y, Zhu C, et al. Fe_3O_4/BSA particles induce osteogenic differentiation of mesenchymal stem cells under static magnetic field[J]. Acta Biomaterialia, 2016, 46: 141-150.

[541] Wang J, An Y, Li F, et al. The effects of pulsed electromagnetic field on the functions of osteoblasts on implant surfaces with different topographies[J]. Acta Biomaterialia, 2014, 10(2): 975-985.

[542] Hu W W, Hsu Y T, Cheng Y C, et al. Electrical stimulation to promote osteogenesis using conductive

polypyrrole films[J]. Mater Sci Eng C Mater Biol Appl, 2014, 37(4): 28-36.

[543] Clark C C, Wang W, Brighton C T. Up-regulation of expression of selected genes in human bone cells with specific capacitively coupled electric fields[J]. Journal of Orthopaedic Research, 2014, 32(7): 894-903.

[544] Li J K, Chang W H, Lin J C, et al. Cytokine release from osteoblasts in response to ultrasound stimulation [J]. Biomaterials, 2003, 24(13): 2379-2385.

[545] Liu C, Abedian R, Meister R, et al. Influence of perfusion and compression on the proliferation and differentiation of bone mesenchymal stromal cells seeded on polyurethane scaffolds[J]. Biomaterials, 2012, 33(4): 1052-1064.

[546] Chang W H, Chen L J, Lin F H. Effect of pulse-burst electromagnetic field stimulation on osteoblast cell activities[J]. Bioelectromagnetics, 2010, 25(6): 457-465.

[547] Rosenberg J N, Turchetta J. Magnetic coil stimulation of the brachial plexus[J]. Archives of Physical Medicine & Rehabilitation, 1993, 74(9): 928.

[548] Balint R, Cassidy N J, Cartmell S H. Electrical stimulation: a novel tool for tissue engineering[J]. Tissue Engineering Part B Reviews, 2013, 19(1): 48-57.

[549] Supronowicz P R, Ajayan P M, Ullmann K R, et al. Novel current-conducting composite substrates for exposing osteoblasts to alternating current stimulation[J]. Journal of Biomedical Materials Research Part A, 2010, 59(3): 499-506.

[550] Zhao Z, Watt C, Karystinou A, et al. Directed migration of human bone marrow mesenchymal stem cells in a physiological direct current electric field[J]. European Cells & Materials, 2011, 22: 344.

[551] Mogil R J, Kaste S C, Jr F R, et al. Effect of Low-Magnitude, High-Frequency Mechanical Stimulation on BMD Among Young Childhood Cancer Survivors: A Randomized Clinical Trial[J]. Jama Oncology, 2016, 2 (7): 908.

[552] Baskett P J. Advances in cardiopulmonary resuscitation[M]. Springer-Verlag, 1977: 200.

[553] Bars D L, Gozariu M, Cadden S W. Animal Models of Nociception[J]. Pharmacological Reviews, 2001, 53 (4): 597-652.

[554] Athanasiou K A, Zhu C, Lanctot D R, et al. Fundamentals of biomechanics in tissue engineering of bone[J]. Tissue Engineering, 2000, 6(4): 361-381.

[555] Zhang J, Ding C, Ren L, et al. The effects of static magnetic fields on bone[J]. Progress in Biophysics & Molecular Biology, 2014, 114(3): 146.

[556] Wieland D C, Krywka C, Mick E, et al. Investigation of the inverse piezoelectric effect of trabecular bone on a micrometer length scale using synchrotron radiation[J]. Acta Biomaterialia, 2015, 25: 339.

[557] Papachroni K K, Karatzas D N, Papavassiliou K A, et al. Mechanotransduction in osteoblast regulation and bone disease[J]. Trends in Molecular Medicine, 2009, 15(5): 208.

[558] Kotani H, Kawaguchi H, Shimoaka T, et al. Strong static magnetic field stimulates bone formation to a definite orientation in vitro and in vivo[J]. Journal of Bone & Mineral Research, 2002, 17(10): 1814-1821.

[559] Markov M S, Hazlewood C F. Electromagnetic field dosimetry for clinical application[J]. Environmentalist, 2009, 29(2): 161-168.

[560] Luben R A, Cain C D, Chen C Y, et al. Effects of Electromagnetic Stimuli on Bone and Bone Cells in vitro: Inhibition of Responses to Parathyroid Hormone by Low-Energy Low-Frequency Fields[J]. Proceedings of the National Academy of Sciences of the United States of America, 1982, 79(13): 4180-4184.

[561] Adams C S, Mansfiele K, Perlot R L, et al. Matrix regulation of skeletal cell apoptosis. Role of calcium and phosphate ions[J]. Journal of Biological Chemistry, 2001, 276(23): 20316-20322.

[562] W Jcik-piotrowica K, Kaszuba-zwoi Ska J, Rokita E, et al. Cell viability modulation through changes of Ca (2 +)-dependent signalling pathways[J]. Progress in Biophysics & Molecular Biology, 2016, 121(1): 45-53.

[563] Zhang X, Liu X, Pan L, et al. Magnetic fields at extremely low-frequency (50 Hz, 0.8 mT) can induce the uptake of intracellular calcium levels in osteoblasts [J]. Biochemical & Biophysical Research Communications, 2010, 396(3): 662-666.

[564] Pounder N M, Harrison A J. Low intensity pulsed ultrasound for fracture healing: a review of the clinical evidence and the associated biological mechanism of action[J]. Ultrasonics, 2008, 48(4): 330-338.

[565] Otter M W, Mcleod K J, Rubin C T. Effects of electromagnetic fields in experimental fracture repair[J]. Clinical Orthopaedics & Related Research, 1998, 355S(355 Suppl): 90-104.

[566] Brighton C T, Wang W, Selees R, et al. Signal transduction in electrically stimulated bone cells[J]. Journal of Bone & Joint Surgery American Volume, 2001, 83-A(10): 1514.

[567] Kim I S, Song J K, Song Y M, et al. Novel effect of biphasic electric current on in vitro osteogenesis and cytokine production in human mesenchymal stromal cells[J]. Tissue Eng Part A, 2009, 15(9): 2411-2422.

[568] Xu J, Wang W, Clark C C, et al. Signal transduction in electrically stimulated articular chondrocytes involves translocation of extracellular calcium through voltage-gated channels 1[J]. Osteoarthritis & Cartilage, 2009, 17(3): 397-405.

[569] Zhuang H, Wang W, Seldes R M, et al. Electrical stimulation induces the level of TGF-beta1 mRNA in osteoblastic cells by a mechanism involving calcium/calmodulin pathway[J]. Biochem Biophys Res Commun, 1997, 237(2): 225-229.

[570] Hroniktupaj M, Rice W L, Croningolomb M, et al. Osteoblastic differentiation and stress response of human mesenchymal stem cells exposed to alternating current electric fields[J]. Biomedical Engineering Online, 2011, 10(1): 9.

[571] Baylink D J, Finkelman R D, Mohan S. Growth factors to stimulate bone formation[J]. Journal of Bone & Mineral Research, 1993, 8(S2): S565-S572.

[572] Pelissier P, Masquelet A C, Bareille R, et al. Induced membranes secrete growth factors including vascular and osteoinductive factors and could stimulate bone regeneration[J]. Journal of Orthopaedic Research, 2010, 22(1): 73-79.

[573] Fitzsimmons R J, Strong D D, Mohan S, et al. Low-amplitude, low-frequency electric field-stimulated bone cell proliferation may in part be mediated by increased IGF-II release[J]. Journal of Cellular Physiology, 1992, 150(1): 84.

[574] Ijiri K, Matsunaga S, Fukudt T, et al. Indomethacin inhibition of ossification induced by direct current stimulation[J]. Journal of Orthopaedic Research, 1995, 13(1): 123-131.

[575] Ignatius A, Blessing H, Liedert A, et al. Tissue engineering of bone: effects of mechanical strain on osteoblastic cells in type I collagen matrices[J]. Biomaterials, 2005, 26(3): 311.

[576] Knippenberg M, Helder M N, Doulabi B Z, et al. Adipose tissue-derived mesenchymal stem cells acquire bone cell-like responsiveness to fluid shear stress on osteogenic stimulation[J]. Tissue Engineering Part A, 2005, 11(12): 1780-1788.

[577] Morita Y, Watanabe S, Ju Y, et al. Determination of optimal cyclic uniaxial stretches for stem cell-to-tenocyte differentiation under a wide range of mechanical stretch conditions by evaluating gene expression and protein synthesis levels[J]. Acta of Bioengineering & Biomechanics, 2013, 15(3): 71.

[578] Tsuzuki T, Okabe K, Kajiya H, et al. Osmotic membrane stretch increases cytosolic Ca(2 +) and inhibits

bone resorption activity in rat osteoclasts[J]. Japanese Journal of Physiology, 2000, 50(1): 67-76.

[579] Lianyun X U. Investigation of pressure loading rates on streaming potentials in bone[J]. Chinese Science: Technical Science, 2011, 54(6): 1376-1381.

[580] Hsu S H, Chang J C. The static magnetic field accelerates the osteogenic differentiation and mineralization of dental pulp cells[J]. Cytotechnology, 2010, 62(2): 143-155.

[581] Yamamoto Y, Ohsaki Y, Goto T, et al. Effects of static magnetic fields on bone formation in rat osteoblast cultures[J]. Journal of Dental Research, 2003, 82(12): 962.

[582] Aliabouzar M, Zhang L G, Sarkar K. Lipid Coated Microbubbles and Low Intensity Pulsed Ultrasound Enhance Chondrogenesis of Human Mesenchymal Stem Cells in 3D Printed Scaffolds[J]. Scientific Reports, 2016, 6: 37728.

[583] Jian Z, Chong D, Peng S. Alterations of Mineral Elements in Osteoblast During Differentiation Under Hypo, Moderate and High Static Magnetic Fields[J]. Biological Trace Element Research, 2014, 162(1-3): 153.

[584] Di S, Tian Z, Qian A, et al. Large gradient high magnetic field affects FLG29.1 cells differentiation to form osteoclast-like cells[J]. International Journal of Radiation Biology, 2012, 88(11): 806.

[585] Huang J, Liu W, Liang Y, et al. Preparation and biocompatibility of diphasic magnetic nanocomposite scaffold[J]. Materials Science & Engineering C, 2018, 87: 70.

[586] Yun H M, Ahn S J, Park K R, et al. Magnetic nanocomposite scaffolds combined with static magnetic field in the stimulation of osteoblastic differentiation and bone formation[J]. Biomaterials, 2016, 85: 88-98.

[587] Feng S W, Lo Y J, Chang W J, et al. Static magnetic field exposure promotes differentiation of osteoblastic cells grown on the surface of a poly-L-lactide substrate[J]. Medical & Biological Engineering & Computing, 2010, 48(8): 793-798.

[588] Yan J L, Zhou J, Ma H P, et al. Pulsed electromagnetic fields promote osteoblast mineralization and maturation needing the existence of primary cilia[J]. Molecular & Cellular Endocrinology, 2015, 404: 132-140.

[589] Zhou J, Xue-yan L I, Chen K M, et al. Effect of Sinusoidal Electricity Magnetic Field at Different Intensity on the Differentiation and Collagen-I, BMP-2 mRNA Expression of Osteoblasts in Vitro[J]. Chinese Journal of Medical Physics, 2010.

[590] Kamolmatyakul S, Jinorose U, Prinyaroj P, et al. Responses of human normal osteoblast cells and osteoblast-like cell line, MG-63 cells, to pulse electromagnetic field (PEMF)[J]. Songklanakarin Journal of Science & Technology, 2008, 30(1): 25-29.

[591] Diniz P, Shomura K, Soejima K, et al. Effects of pulsed electromagnetic field (PEMF) stimulation on bone tissue like formation are dependent on the maturation stages of the osteoblasts[J]. Bioelectromagnetics, 2002, 23(5): 398-405.

[592] Wang P, Liu J, Yang Y, et al. Differential intensity-dependent effects of pulsed electromagnetic fields on RANKL-induced osteoclast formation, apoptosis, and bone resorbing ability in RAW264.7 cells[J]. Bioelectromagnetics, 2017.

[593] Chang K, Hongshong C W, YU Y H, et al. Pulsed electromagnetic field stimulation of bone marrow cells derived from ovariectomized rats affects osteoclast formation and local factor production[J]. Bioelectromagnetics, 2004, 25(2): 134-141.

[594] Banks T A, Luckman P S, Frith J E, et al. Effects of electric fields on human mesenchymal stem cell behaviour and morphology using a novel multichannel device[J]. Integrative Biology Quantitative Biosciences from Nano to Macro, 2015, 7(6): 693.

[595] Creecy C M, O'neill C F, Arulanandam B P, et al. Mesenchymal stem cell osteodifferentiation in response to alternating electric current[J]. Tissue Engineering Part A, 2013, 19(3-4): 467-474.

[596] Wang X, Gao Y, Shi H, et al. Influence of the intensity and loading time of direct current electric field on the directional migration of rat bone marrow mesenchymal stem cells[J]. Medical Frontiers, 2016, 10(3): 286.

[597] Grunert P C, Jonitz-heincke A, Su Y, et al. Establishment of a novel in vitro test setup for electric and magnetic stimulation of human osteoblasts[J]. Cell Biochemistry & Biophysics, 2014, 70(2): 805-817.

[598] Jin G H, Kim G H. The effect of sinusoidal AC electric stimulation of 3D PCL/CNT and PCL/β-TCP based bio-composites on cellular activities for bone tissue regeneration[J]. Journal of Materials Chemistry B, 2013, 1(10): 1439-1452.

[599] Rubin C, Bolander M, Ryaby J P, et al. The use of low-intensity ultrasound to accelerate the healing of fractures[J]. Journal of Bone & Joint Surgery American Volume, 2001, 83-A(2): 259.

[600] Sant'anna E F, Leven R M, Virdi A S, et al. Effect of low intensity pulsed ultrasound and BMP-2 on rat bone marrow stromal cell gene expression [J]. Journal of Orthopaedic Research Official Publication of the Orthopaedic Research Society, 2005, 23(3): 646.

[601] Yang R S, Lin W L, Chen Y Z, et al. Regulation by ultrasound treatment on the integrin expression and differentiation of osteoblasts[J]. Bone, 2005, 36(2): 276-283.

[602] Sun J S, Hong R C, Chang W H, et al. In vitro effects of low-intensity ultrasound stimulation on the bone cells[J]. Journal of Biomedical Materials Research Part B Applied Biomaterials, 2015, 57(3): 449-456.

[603] Korstjens C M, Nolte P A, Burger E H, et al. Stimulation of bone cell differentiation by low-intensity ultrasound--a histomorphometric in vitro study[J]. Journal of Orthopaedic Research, 2004, 22(3): 495-500.

[604] Xuan Z, Castro N J, Wei Z, et al. Improved Human Bone Marrow Mesenchymal Stem Cell Osteogenesis in 3D Bioprinted Tissue Scaffolds with Low Intensity Pulsed Ultrasound Stimulation[J]. Sci Rep, 2016, 6: 32876.

[605] Aliabouzar M, Lee S J, Zhou X, et al. Effects of Scaffold Microstructure and Low Intensity Pulsed Ultrasound on Chondrogenic Differentiation of Human Mesenchymal Stem Cells [J]. Biotechnology & Bioengineering, 2018, 115(2).

[606] Tang L L, Wang Y L, Pan J, et al. The effect of step-wise increased stretching on rat calvarial osteoblast collagen production[J]. Journal of Biomechanics, 2004, 37(1): 157-161.

[607] Jagodzinski M, Drescher M, Zeichen J, et al. Effects of cyclic longitudinal mechanical strain and dexamethasone on osteogenic differentiation of human bone marrow stromal cells [J]. European Cells & Materials, 2004, 7: 35.

[608] Kearney E M, Farrell E, Prendergast P J, et al. Tensile strain as a regulator of mesenchymal stem cell osteogenesis[J]. Annals of Biomedical Engineering, 2010, 38(5): 1767-1779.

[609] Sanchez C, Pesesse L, Gabay O, et al. Regulation of subchondral bone osteoblast metabolism by cyclic compression[J]. Arthritis & Rheumatology, 2012, 64(4): 1193.

[610] Li J, Rose E, Frances D, et al. Effect of oscillating fluid flow stimulation on osteocyte mRNA expression[J]. Journal of Biomechanics, 2012, 45(2): 247-251.

[611] Liu X, Zhang X, Lee I. A quantitative study on morphological responses of osteoblastic cells to fluid shear stress[J]. Journal of Biochemistry and Biophysics, 2010, 42(3): 195-201.

[612] Li P, Ma Y C, Shen H L, et al. Cytoskeletal reorganization mediates fluid shear stress-induced ERK5 activation in osteoblastic cells[J]. Cell Biology International, 2012, 36(3): 229-236.

[613] Stiehler M, B nger C, Baatrup A, et al. Effect of dynamic 3-D culture on proliferation, distribution, and osteogenic differentiation of human mesenchymal stem cell[J]. Journal of Biomedical Materials Research Part

A, 2009, 89A(1): 96-107.

[614] Chen G, Rui X, Chang Z, et al. Responses of MSCs to 3D Scaffold Matrix Mechanical Properties under Oscillatory Perfusion Culture[J]. Acs Applied Materials & Interfaces, 2017, 9(2).

[615] Shah F A, Snis A, Matic A, et al. 3D printed Ti6Al4V implant surface promotes bone maturation and retains a higher density of less aged osteocytes at the bone-implant interface[J]. Acta Biomaterialia, 2016, 30: 357-367.

[616] Lee J W, Kang K S, Lee S H, et al. Bone regeneration using a microstereolithography-produced customized poly (propylene fumarate)/diethyl fumarate photopolymer 3D scaffold incorporating BMP-2 loaded PLGA microspheres[J]. Biomaterials, 2011, 32(3): 744-752.

[617] Peng F, Yy X, Wei M. In vitro cell performance on hydroxyapatite particles/poly(-lactic acid) nanofibrous scaffolds with an excellent particle along nanofiber orientation [J]. Acta Biomaterialia, 2011, 7(6): 2585-2592.

[618] Perez R A, El-fiqi A, Park J H, et al. Therapeutic bioactive microcarriers: co-delivery of growth factors and stem cells for bone tissue engineering[J]. Acta Biomaterialia, 2014, 10(1): 520-530.

[619] Seyednejad H, Gawlitta D, Kuiper R V, et al. Invivo biocompatibility and biodegradation of 3D-printed porous scaffolds based on a hydroxyl-functionalized poly(ε-caprolactone)[J]. Biomaterials, 2012, 33(17): 4309-4318.

[620] Yang W F, Long L, Wang R, et al. Surface-Modified Hydroxyapatite Nanoparticle-Reinforced Polylactides for Three-Dimensional Printed Bone Tissue Engineering Scaffolds [J]. Journal of Biomedical Nanotechnology, 2018.

[621] Wang H, Zhao S, Zhou J, et al. Biocompatibility and osteogenic capacity of borosilicate bioactive glass scaffolds loaded with Fe_3O_4 magnetic nanoparticles[J]. Journal of Materials Chemistry B, 2015, 3(21): 4377-4387.

[622] He L, Zhao P, Han Q, et al. Surface modification of poly- l -lactic acid fibrous scaffolds by a molecular-designed multi-walled carbon nanotube multilayer for enhancing cell interactions[J]. Carbon, 2013, 56(56): 224-234.

[623] Wu C, Xia L, Han P, et al. Graphene-oxide-modified β-tricalcium phosphate bioceramics stimulate in vitro and in vivo osteogenesis[J]. Carbon, 2015, 93: 116-129.

[624] Zhang J, Zhao S, Zhu M, et al. 3D-Printed Magnetic Fe_3O_4/MBG/PCL Composite Scaffolds with Multifunctionality of Bone Regeneration, Local Anticancer Drug Delivery and Hyperthermia[J]. Journal of Materials Chemistry B, 2014, 2(43): 7583-7595.

[625] Arjmand M, Ardeshirylajimi A, Maghsoudi H, et al. Osteogenic differentiation Potential of Mesenchymal Stem Cells cultured on Nanofibrous Scaffold Improved in the Presence of Pulsed Electromagnetic Field[J]. Journal of Cellular Physiology, 2017.

[626] Sun S, Titushkin I, Cho M. Regulation of mesenchymal stem cell adhesion and orientation in 3D collagen scaffold by electrical stimulus[J]. Bioelectrochemistry, 2006, 69(2): 133-141.

[627] Midura R J, Ibiwoye M O, Powell K A, et al. Pulsed electromagnetic field treatments enhance the healing of fibular osteotomies[J]. Journal of Orthopaedic Research, 2005, 23(5): 1035-1046.

[628] Friedenberg Z B, Harlow M C, Brighton C T. Healing of nonunion of the medial malleolus by means of direct current: a case report[J]. Journal of Trauma & Acute Care Surgery, 1971, 11(10): 883-885.

[629] Paterson D C, Lewis G N, Cass C A. Treatment of delayed union and nonunion with an implanted direct current stimulator[J]. Clin Orthop Relat Res, 1980, &NA;(148): 117-128.

[630] Nolte P A, Van D K A, Patka P, et al. Low-intensity pulsed ultrasound in the treatment of nonunions[J]. Journal of Trauma, 2001, 51(4): 693.

[631] Yan Q C, Tomita N, Ikada Y. Effects of static magnetic field on bone formation of rat femurs[J]. Medical Engineering & Physics, 1998, 20(6): 397-402.

[632] Xu S, Tomita N, Ohata R, et al. Static magnetic field effects on bone formation of rats with an ischemic bone model[J]. Biomed Mater Eng, 2001, 11(3): 257-263.

[633] Xu S, Okano H, Tomita N, et al. Recovery Effects of a 180 mT Static Magnetic Field on Bone Mineral Density of Osteoporotic Lumbar Vertebrae in Ovariectomized Rats[J]. Evidence-based complementary and alternative medicine: eCAM, 2011, 2011(4136): 1-8.

[634] Shen W W, Zhao J H. Pulsed electromagnetic fields stimulation affects BMD and local factor production of rats with disuse osteoporosis[J]. Bioelectromagnetics, 2010, 31(2): 113-119.

[635] Taniguchi N, Kanai S, Kawamoto M, et al. Study on Application of Static Magnetic Field for Adjuvant Arthritis Rats[J]. Evidence-based Complementary and Alternative Medicine, 2004, 1(2): 187.

[636] Taniguchi N, Kanai S. Efficacy of static magnetic field for locomotor activity of experimental osteopenia[J]. Evidence-based complementary and alternative medicine: eCAM, 2007, 4(1): 99.

[637] Puricelli E, Ulbrich L M, Ponzoni D, et al. Histological analysis of the effects of a static magnetic field on bone healing process in rat femurs[J]. Head & Face Medicine, 2006, 2(1): 1-9.

[638] Leesungbok R, Ahn S J, Lee S W, et al. The Effects of a Static Magnetic Field on Bone Formation Around a Sandblasted, Large-Grit, Acid-Etched-Treated Titanium Implant[J]. Journal of Oral Implantology, 2013, 39(S1): 248-255.

[639] Inoue N, Ohnishi I, Chen D, et al. Effect of pulsed electromagnetic fields (PEMF) on late-phase osteotomy gap healing in a canine tibial model[J]. Journal of Orthopaedic Research, 2002, 20(5): 1106-1114.

[640] El-hakim I E, Azim A M, El-hassan M F, et al. Preliminary investigation into the effects of electrical stimulation on mandibular distraction osteogenesis in goats[J]. Int J Oral Maxillofac Surg, 2004, 33(1): 42-47.

[641] Fredericks D C, Smucker J, Petersen E B, et al. Effects of direct current electrical stimulation on gene expression of osteopromotive factors in a posterolateral spinal fusion model[J]. Spine, 2007, 32(2): 174-181.

[642] Park S H, Silva M. Neuromuscular electrical stimulation enhances fracture healing: results of an animal model [J]. Journal of Orthopaedic Research, 2004, 22(2): 382.

[643] Chen S C, Lai C H, Chan W P, et al. Increases in bone mineral density after functional electrical stimulation cycling exercises in spinal cord injured patients[J]. Disability & Rehabilitation, 2005, 27(22): 1337-1341.

[644] Azuma Y, Ito M, Harada Y, et al. Low-Intensity Pulsed Ultrasound Accelerates Rat Femoral Fracture Healing by Acting on the Various Cellular Reactions in the Fracture Callus[J]. Journal of Bone & Mineral Research, 2001, 16(4): 671-680.

[645] Takikawa S, Matsui N, Kokubu T, et al. Low-intensity pulsed ultrasound initiates bone healing in rat nonunion fracture model[J]. Journal of Ultrasound in Medicine Official Journal of the American Institute of Ultrasound in Medicine, 2001, 20(3): 197-205.

[646] Fritton J C, Myers E R, Wright T M, et al. Loading induces site-specific increases in mineral content assessed by microcomputed tomography of the mouse tibia[J]. Bone, 2005, 36(6): 1030-1038.

[647] Lambers F M, Schulte F A, Kuhn G, et al. Mouse tail vertebrae adapt to cyclic mechanical loading by increasing bone formation rate and decreasing bone resorption rate as shown by time-lapsed in vivo imaging of

dynamic bone morphometry[J]. Bone, 2011, 49(6): 1340-1350.

[648] Peptan A I, Lopez A, Kopher R A, et al. Responses of intramembranous bone and sutures upon in vivo cyclic tensile and compressive loading[J]. Bone, 2008, 42(2): 432-438.

[649] Jing D, Shen G, Huang J, et al. Circadian rhythm affects the preventive role of pulsed electromagnetic fields on ovariectomy-induced osteoporosis in rats[J]. Bone, 2010, 46(2): 487.

[650] Sanchez C, Gabay O, Salvat C, et al. Mechanical loading highly increases IL-6 production and decreases OPG expression by osteoblasts[J]. Osteoarthritis Cartilage, 2009, 17(4): 473-481.

[651] Aydin N, Bezer M. The effect of an intramedullary implant with a static magnetic field on the healing of the osteotomised rabbit femur[J]. International Orthopaedics, 2011, 35(1): 135-141.

[652] Saifzadeh S, Hobbenaghi R, Jalali F S S, et al. Effect of a static magnetic field on bone healing in the dog: radiographic and histopathological studies[J]. Iranian Journal of Veterinary Research, 2007, 8(1): 8-15.

[653] Zhang H, Gan L, Zhu X, et al. Moderate-intensity 4mT static magnetic fields prevent bone architectural deterioration and strength reduction by stimulating bone formation in streptozotocin-treated diabetic rats[J]. Bone, 2018, 107: 36.

[654] Zhang J, Meng X, Ding C, et al. Regulation of osteoclast differentiation by static magnetic fields[J]. Journal of Bioelectricity, 2016, 36(1): 8-19.

[655] Cai Q, Shi Y, Shan D, et al. Osteogenic differentiation of MC3T3-E1 cells on poly(L-lactide)/Fe$_3$O$_4$ nanofibers with static magnetic field exposure[J]. Mater Sci Eng C Mater Biol Appl, 2015, 55: 166-173.

[656] Boda S K, Thrivikraman G, BASU B. Magnetic field assisted stem cell differentiation - role of substrate magnetization in osteogenesis[J]. Journal of Materials Chemistry B, 2015, 3(16): 3150-3168.

[657] Singh R K, Patel K D, Lee J H, et al. Potential of magnetic nanofiber scaffolds with mechanical and biological properties applicable for bone regeneration[J]. Plos One, 2014, 9(4): e91584.

[658] Lei T, Liang Z, Li F, et al. Pulsed electromagnetic fields(PEMF) attenuate changes in vertebral bone mass, architecture and strength in ovariectomized mice[J]. Bone, 2017, 108: 10.

[659] Adams E. Apparatus and method for invasive electrical stimulation of bone fractures: US, 1986.

[660] Yonemori K, Matsunaga S, Ishidou Y, et al. Early effects of electrical stimulation on osteogenesis[J]. Bone, 1996, 19(2): 173.

[661] Szewczenko J. Influence of bone union electrostimulation on corrosion of bone stabilizer in rabbits[J]. Archives of Materials Science & Engineering, 2007, 28(5).

[662] Jr B T, Black J, Brighton C T, et al. Electrical osteogenesis by low direct current[J]. Journal of Orthopaedic Research Official Publication of the Orthopaedic Research Society, 1983, 1(2): 120.

[663] Brighton C T, Hozack W J, Brager M D, et al. Fracture healing in the rabbit fibula when subjected to various capacitively coupled electrical fields[J]. Journal of Orthopaedic Research Official Publication of the Orthopaedic Research Society, 1985, 3(3): 331-340.

[664] Brighton C T, Pollack S R. Treatment of recalcitrant non-union with a capacitively coupled electrical field. A preliminary report[J]. Journal of Bone & Joint Surgery American Volume, 1985, 67(4): 577-585.

[665] Fitzsimmons R J, Strong D D, Mohan S, et al. Low-amplitude, low-frequency electric field-stimulated bone cell proliferation may in part be mediated by increased IGF-II release[J]. Journal of Cellular Physiology, 1992, 150(1): 84-89.

[666] Romano C L, Romano D, Logoluso N. Low-intensity pulsed ultrasound for the treatment of bone delayed union or nonunion: a review[J]. Ultrasound in Medicine & Biology, 2009, 35(4): 529-536.

[667] Naruse K, Mikuni-takagaki Y, Azuma Y, et al. Anabolic Response of Mouse Bone-Marrow-Derived Stromal

Cell Clone ST2 Cells to Low-Intensity Pulsed Ultrasound ☆ [J]. Biochemical & Biophysical Research Communications, 2000, 268(1): 216-220.

[668] Iwashina T, Mochida J, Miyazaki T, et al. Low-intensity pulsed ultrasound stimulates cell proliferation and proteoglycan production in rabbit intervertebral disc cells cultured in alginate[J]. Biomaterials, 2006, 27 (3): 354-361.

[669] Fermor B, Weinberg J B, Pisetsky D S, et al. The effects of static and intermittent compression on nitric oxide production in articular cartilage explants[J]. Journal of Orthopaedic Research Official Publication of the Orthopaedic Research Society, 2001, 19(4): 729.

[670] Zhong Z, Zeng X L, Ni J H, et al. Comparison of the biological response of osteoblasts after tension and compression[J]. European Journal of Orthodontics, 2013, 35(1): 59-65.

[671] Jiang J, Zhao L G, Teng Y J, et al. ERK5 signalling pathway is essential for fluid shear stress-induced COX-2 gene expression in MC3T3-E1 osteoblast [J]. Molecular & Cellular Biochemistry, 2015, 406 (1-2): 237-243.

[672] Tan S D, Vries T J D, Kuijpers-jagtman A M, et al. Osteocytes subjected to fluid flow inhibit osteoclast formation and bone resorption[J]. Bone, 2007, 41(5): 745.

[673] You L, Temiyasathit S, Lee P, et al. Osteocytes as mechanosensors in the inhibition of bone resorption due to mechanical loading[J]. Bone, 2008, 42(1): 172-179.

[674] Kim C H, You L, Yellowley C E, et al. Oscillatory fluid flow-induced shear stress decreases osteoclastogenesis through RANKL and OPG signaling[J]. Bone, 2006, 39(5): 1043.

[675] Cheung W Y, Liu C, Tonelli-zasarsky R M, et al. Osteocyte apoptosis is mechanically regulated and induces angiogenesis in vitro[J]. Journal of Orthopaedic Research, 2015, 29(4): 523-530.

[676] Wang F, Yang Y, Ling Y, Liu J, Cai X, Zhou X, Tang X, Liang B, Chen Y, Chen H, Injectable and thermally contractible hydroxypropyl methyl cellulose/Fe_3O_4 for magnetic hyperthermia ablation of tumors, Biomaterials, 128 (2017) 84.

[677] Yallapu M. M, Othman S. F, Curtis E. T, Gupta B. K, Jaggi M, Chauhan S. C, Multi-functional Magnetic Nanoparticles for Magnetic Resonance Imaging and Cancer Therapy, Biomaterials, 32 (2011) 1890-1905.

[678] Li S, Shao C, Gu W, Wang R, Zhang J, Lai J, Li H, Ye L, Targeted imaging of brain gliomas using multifunctional Fe_3O_4/MnO nanoparticles, Rsc Advances, 5 (2015) 33639-33645.

[679] Perez R, Patel K, Kim H. W, Novel magnetic nanocomposite injectables: calcium phosphate cements impregnated with ultrafine magnetic nanoparticles for bone regeneration, Rsc Advances, 5 (2015) 13411-13419.

[680] De Santis R, D'Amora U, Russo T, Ronca A, Gloria A, Ambrosio L, 3D fibre deposition and stereolithography techniques for the design of multifunctional nanocomposite magnetic scaffolds, Journal of Materials Science: Materials in Medicine, 26 (2015) 250.

[681] Banobre-López M, Pineiro-Redondo Y, Sandri M, Tampieri A, De Santis R, Dediu V. A, Rivas J, Hyperthermia induced in magnetic scaffolds for bone tissue engineering, IEEE Transactions on Magnetics, 50 (2014) 1-7.

[682] Bock N, Riminucci A, Dionigi C, Russo, Tampieri A, Landi E, Goranov V. A, Marcacci M, Dediu V, A novel route in bone tissue engineering: magnetic biomimetic scaffolds, Acta Biomaterialia, 6 (2010) 786-796.

[683] De Santis R, Gloria A, Russo T, d'Amora U, Zeppetelli S, Dionigi C, Sytcheva A, Herrmannsdörfer T, Dediu V, Ambrosio L, A basic approach toward the development of nanocomposite magnetic scaffolds for

advanced bone tissue engineering, J. Appl. Polym. Sci., 122 (2011) 3599-3605.

[684] Shrestha B. K, Shrestha S, Tiwari A. P, Kim J. I, Ko S. W, Kim H. J, Chan H. P, Kim C. S, Bio-inspired hybrid scaffold of zinc oxide-functionalized multi-wall carbon nanotubes reinforced polyurethane nanofibers for bone tissue engineering, Materials & Design, (2017).

[685] Zhang F, Song Q, Huang X, Li F, Wang K, Tang Y, Hou C, Shen H, A Novel High Mechanical Property PLGA Composite Matrix Loaded with Nanodiamond-Phospholipid Compound for Bone Tissue Engineering, Acs Appl Mater Interfaces, 8 (2015) 1087-1097.

[686] Choi D, Wang D, Bae I. T, Xiao J, Nie Z, Wang W, Viswanathan V. V, Lee Y. J, Zhang J. G, Graff G. L, LiMnPO4 nanoplate grown via solid-state reaction in molten hydrocarbon for Li-ion battery cathode, Nano Lett., 10 (2010) 2799.

[687] Liu X, Ma D, Tang H, Tan L, Xie Q, Zhang Y, Ma M, Yao S, Polyamidoamine dendrimer and oleic acid-functionalized graphene as biocompatible and efficient gene delivery vectors, Acs Applied Materials & Interfaces, 6 (2014) 8173.

[688] A. L. W. †, N. J. T. And, †, Stephen O'Brien, Spectroscopic Characterization of the Surface of Iron Oxide Nanocrystals, Chem. Mater., 17 (2005) 325-328.

[689] Cabaço M. I, Besnard M, Danten Y, Coutinho J. A. P, Solubility of CO_2 in 1-butyl-3-methyl-imidazolium-trifluoro acetate ionic liquid studied by Raman spectroscopy and DFT investigations, J. Phys. Chem. B, 115 (2011) 3538.

[690] Jadhav N. V, Prasad A. I, Kumar A, Mishra R, Dhara S, Babu K, Prajapat C, Misra N, Ningthoujam R, Pandey B, Synthesis of oleic acid functionalized Fe_3O_4 magnetic nanoparticles and studying their interaction with tumor cells for potential hyperthermia applications, Colloids and Surfaces B: Biointerfaces, 108 (2013) 158-168.

[691] Shahabadi N, Falsafi M, Mansouri K, Improving antiproliferative effect of the anticancer drug cytarabine on human promyelocytic leukemia cells by coating on Fe_3O_4 @ SiO_2 nanoparticles, Colloids & Surfaces B Biointerfaces, 141 (2016) 213-222.

[692] Chandrappa K. G, Venkatesha T. V, Electrochemical bulk synthesis of Fe_3O_4 and α-Fe_2O_3 nanoparticles and its Zn Co α Fe_2O_3 composite thin films for corrosion protection, Materials & Corrosion, 65 (2014) 509-521.

[693] Vasile E, Serafim A, Dragusin D. M, Petrea C, Iovu H, Stancu I. C, Apatite formation on active nanostructured coating based on functionalized gold nanoparticles, J. Nanopart. Res., 14 (2012) 1-14.

[694] Rana S, Ram S, Seal S, Roy S. K, Surface structure and topology in surface stabilized Co-nanoparticles with a thin Al_2O_3 amorphous layer, Appl. Surf. Sci., 236 (2004) 141-154.

[695] Biswas S, And V. K. S, Ram S, Fecht H. J, Nanorods of Silver-Coated Magnetic CrO_2 Particles from a Polymer Template in Hot Water, Journal of Physical Chemistry C, 111 (2007) 7593-7598.

[696] Shete P. B, Patil R. M, Tiwale B. M, Pawar S. H, Water dispersible oleic acid-coated Fe_3O_4 nanoparticles for biomedical applications, Journal of Magnetism & Magnetic Materials, 377 (2015) 406-410.

[697] Kim U. -J, Park J, Kim H. J, Wada M, Kaplan D. L, Three-dimensional aqueous-derived biomaterial scaffolds from silk fibroin, Biomaterials, 26 (2005) 2775-2785.

[698] Murphy C. M, Haugh M. G, O'Brien F. J, The effect of mean pore size on cell attachment, proliferation and migration in collagen-glycosaminoglycan scaffolds for bone tissue engineering, Biomaterials, 31 (2010) 461-466.

[699] Mandal B. B, Kundu S. C, Cell proliferation and migration in silk fibroin 3D scaffolds, Biomaterials, 30 (2009) 2956-2965.

[700] Kim H. J, Kim U. -J, Vunjak-Novakovic G, Min B. -H, Kaplan D. L, Influence of macroporous protein scaffolds on bone tissue engineering from bone marrow stem cells, Biomaterials, 26 (2005) 4442-4452.

[701] Li D, Wang J, Chen F, Jing H, Fe$_3$O$_4$@ SiO$_2$ supported aza-crown ether complex cation ionic liquids: preparation and applications in organic reactions, RSC Advances, 7 (2017) 4237-4242.

[702] Lu Y, Yin Y, And B. T. M, Xia Y, Modifying the Surface Properties of Superparamagnetic Iron Oxide Nanoparticles through A Sol-Gel Approach, Nano Lett. , 2 (2002) 183-186.

[703] Ramazani A, Khoobi M, Sadri F, Tarasi R, Shafiee A, Aghahosseini H, Sang W. J, Efficient and selective oxidation of alcohols in water employing palladium supported nanomagnetic Fe$_3$O$_4$@ hyperbranched polyethylenimine (Fe$_3$O$_4$@ HPEI. Pd) as a new organic-inorganic hybrid nanocatalyst, Appl. Organomet. Chem. , 32 (2017).

[704] Jiang F, Zhang Y, Wang Z, Wang W, Xu Z, Wang Z, Combination of magnetic and enhanced mechanical properties for copolymer-grafted magnetite composite thermoplastic elastomers, Acs Appl Mater Interfaces, 7 (2015) 10563-10575.

[705] Hong R. Y, Pan T. T, Han Y. P, Zhang S. Z, Li H. Z, Ding J, Graft polymerization synthesis and application of magnetic Fe$_3$O$_4$/polyacrylic acid composite nanoparticles, J. Appl. Polym. Sci. , 106 (2010) 1439-1447.

[706] Hou C, Song S, Zhou X, Wei J, Li T, Electromagnetic and mechanical properties of Fe$_3$O$_4$-coated amorphous carbon nanotube/polyvinyl chloride composites, Compos. Interfaces, 23 (2016) 1-7.

[707] Yin G, Zhao D, Ren Y, Zhang L, Zhou Z, Li Q, A convenient process to fabricate gelatin modified porous PLLA materials with high hydrophilicity and strength, Biomaterials Science, 4 (2015) 310.

[708] Liu Z, Jia L, Yan Z, Bai L, Plasma-treated electrospun nanofibers as a template for the electrostatic assembly of silver nanoparticles, (2018).

[709] Tan W. L, Bakar M. A, The effects of magnetite particles and lithium triflate on the thermal behavior and degradation of epoxidized natural rubber (ENR-50), American-Eurasian Journal of Sustainable Agriculture, 8 (2014) 111-122.

[710] Tang S, Hu K, Sun J, Li Y, Guo Z, Liu M, Liu Q, Zhang F, Gu N, High quality multicellular tumor spheroid induction platform based on anisotropic magnetic hydrogel, ACS applied materials & interfaces, 9 (2017) 10446-10452.

[711] Hao S, Zhang Y, Meng J, Liu J, Wen T, Gu N, Xu H, Integration of a Superparamagnetic Scaffold and Magnetic Field To Enhance the Wound-Healing Phenotype of Fibroblasts, ACS applied materials & interfaces, 10 (2018) 22913-22923.

[712] Liu X, Zhang J, Tang S, Sun J, Lou Z, Yang Y, Wang P, Li Y, Gu N, Growth enhancing effect of LBL-assembled magnetic nanoparticles on primary bone marrow cells, Science China Materials, 59 (2016) 901-910.

[713] Guo Z, Hu K, Sun J, Zhang T, Zhang Q, Song L, Zhang X, Gu N, Fabrication of hydrogel with cell adhesive micropatterns for mimicking the oriented tumor-associated extracellular matrix, ACS applied materials & interfaces, 6 (2014) 10963-10968.

[714] Hu K, Zhou N, Li Y, Ma S, Guo Z, Cao M, Zhang Q, Sun J, Zhang T, Gu N, Sliced magnetic polyacrylamide hydrogel with cell-adhesive microarray interface: a novel multicellular spheroid culturing platform, ACS applied materials & interfaces, 8 (2016) 15113-15119.

[715] Long T, Guo Y. P, Tang S, Guo Y. J, Zhu Z. A, Emulsion fabrication of magnetic mesoporous carbonated hydroxyapatite microspheres for treatment of bone infection, Rsc Advances, 4 (2014) 11816-11825.

[716] Yuan H, Wang Y, Zhou S. M, Lou S, Fabrication of superparamagnetic Fe$_3$O$_4$ hollow microspheres with a

high saturation magnetization, Chem. Eng. J., 175 (2011) 555-560.

[717] Chen W, Long T, Guo Y. J, Zhu Z. A, Guo Y. P, Magnetic hydroxyapatite coatings with oriented nanorod arrays: hydrothermal synthesis, structure and biocompatibility, Journal of Materials Chemistry B, 2 (2014) 1653-1660.

[718] Sapirlekhovitser Y, Rotenberg M. Y, Jopp J, Friedman G, Polyak B, Cohen S, Magnetically actuated tissue engineered scaffold: insights into mechanism of physical stimulation, Nanoscale, 8 (2016) 3386-3399.

[719] Zeng X. B, Hu H, Xie L. Q, Lan F, Jiang W, Wu Y, Gu Z. W, Magnetic responsive hydroxyapatite composite scaffolds construction for bone defect reparation, International Journal of Nanomedicine, 7 (2012) 3365.

[720] Wong D. S, Li J, Yan X, Wang B, Li R, Zhang L, Bian L, Magnetically Tuning Tether Mobility of Integrin Ligand Regulates Adhesion, Spreading, and Differentiation of Stem Cells, Nano Lett., 17 (2017) 1685.

[721] Tang B, Zhuang J, Wang L, Zhang B, Lin S, Jia F, Dong L, Wang Q, Cheng K, Weng W, Harnessing Cell Dynamic Responses on Magnetoelectric Nanocomposite Films to Promote Osteogenic Differentiation, ACS applied materials & interfaces, 10 (2018) 7841-7851.

[722] Shuai C, Yang W, Peng S, Gao C, Guo W, Lai Y, Feng P, Physical stimulations and their osteogenesis-inducing mechanisms, International Journal of Bioprinting, 4 (2018).

[723] Guo Y. -P, Long T, Tang S, Guo Y. -J, Zhu Z. -A, Hydrothermal fabrication of magnetic mesoporous carbonated hydroxyapatite microspheres: biocompatibility, osteoinductivity, drug delivery property and bactericidal property, Journal of Materials Chemistry B, 2(2014) 2899-2909.